T0359102

Meningioma

Editors

RANDY L. JENSEN
GABRIEL ZADA

NEUROSURGERY
CLINICS OF NORTH AMERICA

www.neurosurgery.theclinics.com

Consulting Editors
RUSSELL R. LONSER
DANIEL K. RESNICK

July 2023 • Volume 34 • Number 3

ELSEVIER

1600 John F. Kennedy Boulevard • Suite 1800 • Philadelphia, Pennsylvania, 19103-2899

http://www.theclinics.com

NEUROSURGERY CLINICS OF NORTH AMERICA Volume 34, Number 3
July 2023 ISSN 1042-3680, ISBN-13: 978-0-323-93849-5

Editor: Stacy Eastman
Developmental Editor: Akshay Samson

Neurosurgery Clinics of North America (ISSN 1042-3680) is published quarterly by Elsevier Inc., 360 Park Avenue South, New York, NY 10010-1710. Months of issue are January, April, July, and October. Business and Editorial Offices: 1600 John F. Kennedy Blvd., Suite 1800, Philadelphia, PA 19103-2899. Customer Service Office: 11830 Westline Industrial Drive, St. Louis, MO 63146. Periodicals postage paid at New York, NY, and additional mailing offices. Subscription prices are $451.00 per year (US individuals), $821.00 per year (US institutions), $484.00 per year (Canadian individuals), $1,019.00 per year (Canadian institutions), $562.00 per year (international individuals), $1,019.00 per year (international institutions), $100.00 per year (US students), $255.00 per year (international students), and $100.00 per year (Canadian students). International air speed delivery is included in all *Clinics* subscription prices. All prices are subject to change without notice. **POSTMASTER:** Send address changes to *Neurosurgery Clinics of North America*, Elsevier Periodicals Customer Service, 11830 Westline Industrial Drive, St. Louis, MO 63146. **Customer Service: 1-800-654-2452 (US and Canada). From outside the US and Canada, call: 1-314-453-7041. Fax: 1-314-453-5170. E-mail: JournalsCustomerService-usa@elsevier.com (for print support) and journalsonlinesupport-usa@elsevier.com (for online support).**

Reprints. For copies of 100 or more, of articles in this publication, please contact the Commercial Reprints Department, Elsevier Inc., 360 Park Avenue South, New York, NY 10010-1710. Tel. 212-633-3874; Fax: 212-633-3820; E-mail: reprints@elsevier.com.

Neurosurgery Clinics of North America is covered in *MEDLINE/PubMed (Index Medicus), EMBASE/Excerpta Medica, and Current Contents/Clinical Medicine (CC/CM).*

Contributors

CONSULTING EDITORS

RUSSELL R. LONSER, MD
Professor and Chair, Department of
Neurological Surgery, The Ohio State
University Wexner Medical Center, Columbus,
Ohio, USA

DANIEL K. RESNICK, MD, MS
Professor and Vice Chairman, Program
Director, Department of Neurosurgery,
University of Wisconsin-Madison School of
Medicine and Public Health, Madison,
Wisconsin, USA

EDITORS

RANDY L. JENSEN, MD, PhD, MHPE
Professor of Neurosurgery, Radiation
Oncology and Oncological Sciences, Director
of Neurological Cancers Center, Huntsman
Cancer Institute, Department of Neurosurgery,
Clinical Neurosciences Center, University of
Utah, Salt Lake City, Utah, USA

GABRIEL ZADA, MD, MS
Professor of Neurosurgery, Otolaryngology,
and Medicine, Co-Director, USC Pituitary
Center, Co-Director, USC Radiosurgery
Center, Neuro-Oncology and Endoscopic
Pituitary/Skull Base Program, Department of
Neurological Surgery, Keck School of Medicine
of USC, Los Angeles, California, USA

AUTHORS

DAVID AGYAPONG, BS
School of Medicine, Robert Wood Johnson
Medical School, New Brunswick, New Jersey,
USA

MOHAMMED A. AZAB, MBBS
Boise State University, Boise, Idaho, USA

MICHAEL A. BAMIMORE, DO
Department of Neurological Surgery, Mayo
Clinic, Jacksonville, Florida, USA; Department
of Neurological Surgery, Cooper University
Hospital, Camden, New Jersey, USA

ILARIA BOVE, MD
Research Fellow, Department of Neurological
Surgery, University of Southern California,
Keck School of Medicine of USC, Los Angeles,
California, USA; Division of Neurosurgery,
Department of Neurological Sciences,
Università degli Studi di Napoli Federico II,
Naples, Italy

PRISCILLA K. BRASTIANOS, MD
Center for Cancer Research, Massachusetts
General Hospital Cancer Center, Harvard
Medical School, Boston, Massachusetts, USA

KAROL P. BUDOHOSKI, MD, PhD
Department of Neurosurgery, Clinical
Neurosciences Center, University of Utah, Salt
Lake City, Utah, USA

KAISORN L. CHAICHANA, MD
Department of Neurological Surgery, Mayo
Clinic, Jacksonville, Florida, USA

STEPHANIE CHEOK, MD
Department of Neurological Surgery, University
of Southern California, Keck School of
Medicine of USC, Los Angeles, California, USA

KYRIL COLE, MPH
School of Medicine, University of Utah, Salt
Lake City, Utah, USA

WILLIAM T. COULDWELL, MD, PhD
Department of Neurosurgery, Clinical
Neurosciences Center, University of Utah, Salt
Lake City, Utah, USA

CHRIS CUTLER, BS
Chicago Medical School, Rosalind Franklin
University of Medicine and Science, North
Chicago, Illinois, USA

ASHISH DAHAL, AB
Center for Cancer Research, Massachusetts
General Hospital Cancer Center, Harvard
Medical School, Boston, Massachusetts,
USA

CHRISTIAN DAVIDSON, MD
Department of Pathology, University of Utah,
Sandy, Utah, USA

CHLOE DUMOT, MD, PhD
Department of Neurological Surgery, University
of Virginia Health System, Charlottesville,
Virginia, USA

IAN F. DUNN, MD
Department of Neurosurgery, University of
Oklahoma Health Sciences Center, Oklahoma
City, Oklahoma, USA

EMMA EARL, BS
School of Medicine, University of Utah, Salt
Lake City, Utah, USA

MATTHEW FINDLAY, BS
School of Medicine, University of Utah, Salt
Lake City, Utah, USA

ELENA GRECO, MD
Department of Radiology, Mayo Clinic,
Jacksonville, Florida, USA

CHADWIN HANNA, BS
Department of Neurosurgery, University of
Florida, Gainesville, Florida, USA

DOMINIQUE HIGGINS, MD, PhD
Department of Neurosurgery, Assistant
Professor, University of North Carolina,
USA

RAYMOND Y. HUANG, MD, PhD
Associate Professor, Department of Radiology,
Brigham and Women's Hospital, Harvard
Medical School, Boston, Massachusetts,
USA

NAZANIN IJAD, BSc
Center for Cancer Research, Massachusetts
General Hospital Cancer Center, Harvard
Medical School, Boston, Massachusetts,
USA

MICHAEL E. IVAN, MD, MBS
Department of Neurosurgery, University of
Miami, University of Miami Brain Tumor
Initiative, Miami, Florida, USA

RANDY L. JENSEN, MD, PhD, MHPE
Professor of Neurosurgery, Radiation
Oncology and Oncological Sciences, Director
of Neurological Cancers Center, Huntsman
Cancer Institute, Department of Neurosurgery,
Clinical Neurosciences Center, University of
Utah, Salt Lake City, Utah, USA

ADRIAN E. JIMENEZ, BS
Department of Neurosurgery, Johns Hopkins
School of Medicine, Baltimore, Maryland,
USA

TAREQ A. JURATLI, MD
Department of Neurosurgery, Carl Gustav
Carus University Hospital, TU Dresden,
Germany; Department of Neurosurgery,
Translational Neuro-Oncology Laboratory,
Massachusetts General Hospital Cancer
Center, Harvard Medical School, Boston,
Massachusetts, USA

MICHAEL KARSY, MD, PhD, MSC
Department of Neurosurgery, Clinical
Neurosciences Center, University of Utah, Salt
Lake City, Utah, USA

MAJID KHAN, BS
Reno School of Medicine, University of
Nevada, Reno, Nevada, USA

ALBERT E. KIM, MD
Center for Cancer Research, Massachusetts
General Hospital Cancer Center, Harvard
Medical School, Boston, Massachusetts,
USA

KIHONG KIM, MD
Department of Neurosurgery, Los Angeles,
California, USA

RICARDO J. KOMOTAR, MD
Department of Neurosurgery, University of
Miami, University of Miami Brain Tumor
Initiative, Miami, Florida, USA

GRACE LEE, MD
Harvard Medical School, Department of
Radiation Oncology, Massachusetts General
Hospital, Boston, Massachusetts, USA

MICHELLE LIN, MD
Department of Neurological Surgery, Keck
School of Medicine of USC, University of
Southern California, Los Angeles, California,
USA

ERIK K. LOKEN, MD, PhD
Instructor, Department of Radiology, Brigham
and Women's Hospital, Harvard Medical
School, Boston, Massachusetts, USA

BRANDON LUCKE-WOLD, MD, PhD
Department of Neurosurgery, University of
Florida, Gainesville, Florida, USA

WILLIAM J. MACK, MD
Department of Neurological Surgery, Keck
School of Medicine of USC, University of
Southern California, Los Angeles, California,
USA

NATALIE MAHGEREFTEH, HSD
Department of Neurosurgery, Los Angeles,
California, USA

YELENA MALKHASYAN, BS
Department of Neurosurgery, Los Angeles,
California, USA

GEORGIOS MANTZIARIS, MD
Department of Neurological Surgery, University
of Virginia Health System, Charlottesville,
Virginia, USA

LINA MARENCO-HILLEMBRAND, MD
Department of Neurological Surgery, Mayo
Clinic, Jacksonville, Florida, USA

JOE MENDEZ, MD
Department of Neurosurgery, Huntsman
Cancer Institute, University of Utah, Salt Lake
City, Utah, USA

ERIK H. MIDDLEBROOKS, MD
Departments of Neurological Surgery and
Radiology, Mayo Clinic, Jacksonville, Florida,
USA

KHASHAYAR MOZAFFARI, BS
Department of Neurosurgery, Los Angeles,
California, USA

DEBRAJ MUKHERJEE, MD, MPH
Department of Neurosurgery, Johns Hopkins
School of Medicine, Baltimore, Maryland, USA

VINCENT NGUYEN, MD
Department of Neurological Surgery, Keck
School of Medicine of USC, University of
Southern California, Los Angeles, California,
USA

ALI H. PALEJWALA, MD
Department of Neurosurgery, University of
Oklahoma Health Sciences Center, Oklahoma
City, Oklahoma, USA

PANAYIOTIS E. PELARGOS, MD
Department of Neurosurgery, University of
Oklahoma Health Sciences Center, Oklahoma
City, Oklahoma, USA

STYLIANOS PIKIS, MD
Department of Neurological Surgery, University
of Virginia Health System, Charlottesville,
Virginia, USA

VIJAY M. RAVINDRA, MD, MSPH
Department of Neurosurgery, Clinical
Neurosciences Center, University of Utah, Salt
Lake City, Utah, USA; Department of
Neurosurgery, University of California, San
Diego, La Jolla, California, USA; Department of
Neurosurgery, Naval Medical Center San
Diego, San Diego, California, USA

KRISHNAN RAVINDRAN, MD
Department of Neurological Surgery, Mayo
Clinic, Jacksonville, Florida, USA

CAMERON A. RAWANDUZY, MD
Department of Neurosurgery, Clinical
Neurosciences Center, University of Utah, Salt
Lake City, Utah, USA

ROBERT C. RENNERT, MD
Department of Neurosurgery, Clinical
Neurosciences Center, University of Utah, Salt
Lake City, Utah, USA

JACOB J. RUZEVICK, MD
Department of Neurological Surgery, University
of Southern California, Keck School of
Medicine of USC, Los Angeles, California, USA

MEIC H. SCHMIDT, MD, MBA
Department of Neurosurgery, University of
New Mexico, Albuquerque, New Mexico, USA

ASHISH H. SHAH, MD
Assistant Professor, Department of
Neurosurgery, University of Miami, Director
of Clinical Trials and Translational
Research, University of Miami Brain Tumor
Initiative, Miami, Florida, USA

JASON SHEEHAN, MD, PhD
Department of Neurological Surgery, University
of Virginia Health System, Charlottesville,
Virginia, USA

HELEN A. SHIH, MD
Harvard Medical School, Department of
Radiation Oncology, Massachusetts General
Hospital, Boston, Massachusetts,
USA

SHERWIN A. TAVAKOL, MD, MPH
Department of Neurosurgery, University of
Oklahoma Health Sciences Center, Oklahoma
City, Oklahoma, USA

ZOE TETON, MD
Department of Neurosurgery, Los Angeles,
California, USA

HIROAKI WAKIMOTO, MD, PhD
Center for Cancer Research, Massachusetts
General Hospital Cancer Center, Harvard
Medical School, Boston, Massachusetts,
USA

**ALEXANDER WINKLER-SCHWARTZ, MD,
PhD**
Department of Neurosurgery, Clinical
Neurosciences Center, University of Utah, Salt
Lake City, Utah, USA

ZHIYUAN XU, MD
Department of Neurological Surgery, University
of Virginia Health System, Charlottesville,
Virginia, USA

ISAAC YANG, MD
Professor, Departments of Neurosurgery,
Radiation Oncology, and Head and Neck
Surgery, Jonsson Comprehensive Cancer
Center, Los Angeles Biomedical Research
Institute, Harbor-UCLA Medical Center, David
Geffen School of Medicine, Los Angeles, Los
Angeles, California, USA

GABRIEL ZADA, MD, MS
Professor of Neurosurgery, Otolaryngology,
and Medicine, Co-Director, USC Pituitary
Center, Co-Director, USC Radiosurgery
Center, Neuro-Oncology and Endoscopic
Pituitary/Skull Base Program, Department of
Neurological Surgery, Keck School of Medicine
of USC, Los Angeles, California, USA

XIAOCHUN ZHAO, MD
Department of Neurosurgery, University of
Oklahoma Health Sciences Center, Oklahoma
City, Oklahoma, USA

Contents

Meningiomas are the most common intracranial tumor. This article reviews various aspects of the pathology of these tumors, from their frozen section appearance to the various subtypes a pathologist may come across at the microscope. Special emphasis is placed on the importance of CNS World Health Organization grading by light microscopic means to predict biological behavior of these tumors. Furthermore, relevant literature concerning the potential impact that DNA methylation profiling of these tumors and the possibility that this molecular testing modality might be the next step in refinement of our analysis of meningioma is presented.

Meningiomas represent the most common type of benign tumor of the extra-axial compartment. Although most meningiomas are benign World Health Organization (WHO) grade 1 lesions, the increasingly prevalent of WHO grade 2 lesion and occasional grade 3 lesions show worsened recurrence rates and morbidity. Multiple medical treatments have been evaluated but show limited efficacy. We review the status of medical management in meningiomas, highlighting successes and failures of various treatment options. We also explore newer studies evaluating the use of immunotherapy in management.

Noninvasive imaging methods are used to accurately diagnose meningiomas and track their growth and location. These techniques, including computed tomography, MRI, and nuclear medicine, are also being used to gather more information about the biology of the tumors and potentially predict their grade and impact on prognosis. In this article, we will discuss the current and developing uses of these imaging techniques including additional analysis using radiomics in the diagnosis and treatment of meningiomas, including treatment planning and prediction of tumor behavior.

The rise in availability of neuroimaging has led to an increase in incidentally discovered meningiomas. These tumors are typically asymptomatic and tend to display slow growth. Treatment options include observation with serial monitoring, radiation, and surgery. Although optimal management is unclear, clinicians recommend a conservative approach, which preserves quality of life and limits unnecessary intervention. Several risk factors have been investigated for their potential utility in the development of prognostic models for risk assessment. Herein, the authors review the current literature on incidental meningiomas, focusing their discussion on potential predictive factors for tumor growth and appropriate management practices.

Although benign in histology, the hypervascularity and skull base location of meningiomas can make them surgically challenging lesions. Preoperative endovascular embolization with superselective microcatheterization of vascular pedicles may be efficacious in decreasing intraoperative transfusion requirements with equivocal postoperative functional benefit. The potential benefits of preoperative embolization should be weighed against the risks of ischemic complications. Appropriate patient selection is critical. All patients should be monitored closely postembolization, and a course of steroids can be considered to minimize neurologic symptoms.

Meningiomas are the most common intracranial extra-axial primary tumor. Although most are low grade and slow growing, resection can be technically challenging, particularly when located at the skull base. Appropriate craniotomy and approach selection are of paramount importance to minimize brain retraction, optimize exposure, and achieve complete resection. This article summarizes various craniotomies and their approaches to meningiomas, and illustrates some nuances in performing these techniques with cadaveric dissection and operative videos.

Traditionally, resection of anterior skull base meningiomas has been achieved by transcranial approaches; however, morbidity related (ie, brain retraction, sagittal sinus damage, optic nerve manipulation, and cosmetic healing) represent a limit of the approach. Minimally invasive techniques including supraorbital and endonasal endoscopic approaches (EEA) have gained consensus as surgical corridors provide direct access to the tumor via a midline approach in carefully selected patients. The supraorbital approach requires some retraction of the rectus gyrus, but it offers minimal risk of postoperative CSF leak or sinonasal morbidity compared to EEA.

Intraventricular meningiomas (IVM) are intracranial tumors that originate from collections of arachnoid cells within the choroid plexus. The incidence of meningiomas is estimated to be about 97.5 per 100,000 individuals in the United States with IVMs constituting 0.7% to 3%. Positive outcomes have been observed with surgical treatment of intraventricular meningiomas. This review explores elements of surgical care and management of patients with IVM, highlighting nuances in surgical approaches, their indications, and considerations.

Meningiomas are the most common intracranial brain tumor. Spheno-orbital meningiomas are a rare subtype that originate at the sphenoid wing and characteristically extend to the orbit and surrounding neurovascular structures via bony hyperostosis and soft tissue invasion. This review summarizes early characterizations of spheno-orbital meningiomas, presently understood tumor characteristics, and current management strategies.

Meningiomas of the spinal canal are the most common intradural spinal canal tumors encountered in adults and account for 8% of all meningiomas. Patient presentation can vary considerably. Once diagnosed, these lesions are primarily treated surgically, but depending on location and pathological features, chemotherapy and radiosurgery may be required. Emerging modalities may represent adjuvant therapies. In this article, we review the current management of meningiomas of the spinal column.

Meningiomas are the most prevalent primary tumor of central nervous system origin, and although most of these neoplasms are benign, a small proportion exemplifies an aggressive profile characterized by high recurrence rates, pleomorphic histology, and overall resistance to standard treatment. Standard initial therapy for malignant meningiomas includes maximal safe surgical resection followed by focal radiation. The role for chemotherapy during recurrence of these aggressive meningiomas is less clear. Prognosis is poor, and recurrence of malignant meningiomas is high. This article provides an overview of atypical and anaplastic "malignant" meningiomas, their treatment, and ongoing research looking for more effective treatments.

Meningiomas, the most prevalent primary intracranial tumor, arise from the arachnoid cap cells in the meninges, the membranes that surround the brain and the spinal cord. The field has long sought effective predictors of meningioma recurrence and malignant transformation, as well as therapeutic targets to guide intensified treatment such as early radiation or systemic therapy. Novel and more targeted approaches are currently being tested in numerous clinical trials for patients who have progressed after surgery and/or radiation. In this review, the authors discuss relevant molecular drivers that have therapeutic implications and examine recent clinical trial data evaluating targeted therapies and immunotherapies.

Meningiomas are thought to originate from the meningothelial cells of the arachnoid mater and are the most common primary brain tumor in adults. Histologically confirmed meningiomas occur with an incidence of 9.12/100,000 population and account for 39% of all primary brain tumors and 54.5% of all non-malignant brain tumors. Risk factors for meningioma include age 65 years and older, female gender, African-American race, history of exposure to head and neck ionizing radiation, and certain genetic disorders such as neurofibromatosis II. Intracranial meningiomas are the most commonly benign, WHO Grade I neoplasms. Atypical and anaplastic are considered malignant lesions.

High-grade meningiomas (atypical and anaplastic/malignant) are at increased risk of recurrence following primary treatment with maximum safe surgical resection. Evidence based on several retrospective and prospective observational studies suggests an important role of radiation therapy (RT) in both adjuvant and salvage settings. At present, adjuvant RT is recommended for incompletely resected atypical meningiomas and anaplastic meningiomas irrespective of resection extent with disease control benefit. In completely resected atypical meningiomas, the role of adjuvant RT remains debatable but should be considered given the aggressive and resistant nature of recurrent disease. Randomized trials are currently underway and may guide optimal postoperative management.

Preclinical meningioma models offer a setting to test molecular mechanisms of tumor development and targeted treatment options but historically have been challenging to generate. Few spontaneous tumor models in rodents have been established, but cell culture and in vivo rodent models have emerged along with artificial intelligence, radiomics, and neural networks to differentiate the clinical heterogeneity of meningiomas. We reviewed 127 studies using PRISMA guideline methodology, including laboratory and animal studies, that addressed preclinical modeling. Our evaluation identified that meningioma preclinical models provide valuable molecular insight into disease progression and effective chemotherapeutic and radiation approaches for specific tumor types.

High-value health care has become a widely researched topic within neurosurgery. The concept of "high-value" care involves optimizing resource expenditures relative to patient outcomes, and therefore, high-value care research within neurosurgery has involved identifying prognostic factors for outcomes such as hospital length of stay, discharge disposition, monetary charges/costs incurred during hospitalization, and hospital readmission. The following article will discuss the motivation of high-value health-care research for optimizing the surgical treatment of intracranial meningiomas, highlight recent research investigating high-value care outcomes in patients with intracranial meningioma, and explore future avenues for high-value care research in this patient population.

NEUROSURGERY CLINICS OF NORTH AMERICA

Preface
Meningiomas: An Update on Diagnostic and Therapeutic Approaches

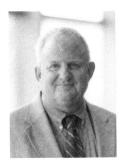
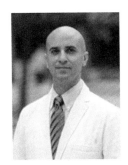

Randy L. Jensen, MD, PhD, MHPE   Gabriel Zada, MD, MS
Editors

Meningiomas are among the most common intracranial tumors. Despite their relatively benign nature, multimodal treatment is often required to treat them because of their invasive nature, varying location, and lack of medical or chemotherapy availability. Advances in imaging, diagnostics, and therapeutics have improved the contemporary care of patients with meningiomas over the past decade. In this issue, we examine the contemporary updates in genomics, epigenomics, pathologic diagnosis, imaging, medical management, and surgical approaches used to treat meningiomas. Special considerations are made for meningiomas in the spine and skull base, with articles to describe the unique features of management of these tumors. Preoperative embolization of meningioma is an ongoing debate and is discussed in this issue. Decision making regarding incidentally found meningiomas is also explored. In addition to standard therapies, such as surgery, radiosurgery, and radiotherapy, we also include a discussion of novel treatment options, including immunotherapy and targeted therapy. Management of atypical, malignant, and treatment-refractory meningiomas is explored, and controversies are outlined. The role of radiotherapy in higher-grade meningiomas is a commonplace question for practicing neurosurgeons and is discussed in detail. Emerging advanced neuroimaging techniques, including preoperative characteristics that may predict consistency of meningiomas, are also reviewed. This collection is rounded out with a review of meningioma models and an in-depth examination of measures of meningioma patient outcome and value-based care. Taken as a whole, these articles provide cutting-edge information to improve the care of patients with meningiomas.

Randy L. Jensen, MD, PhD, MHPE
Huntsman Cancer Institute
University of Utah
5th Floor CNC
175 North Medical Drive
Salt Lake City, UT 84132, USA

Gabriel Zada, MD, MS
USC Pituitary Center
USC Radiosurgery Center
Keck School of Medicine of USC
1520 San Pablo Street #3800
Los Angeles, CA 90033, USA

E-mail addresses:
Randy.jensen@hsc.utah.edu (R.L. Jensen)
gzada@usc.edu (G. Zada)

Neurosurg Clin N Am 34 (2023) xiii
https://doi.org/10.1016/j.nec.2023.04.001
1042-3680/23/© 2023 Published by Elsevier Inc.

Preface

Meningiomas: An Update on Diagnostic and Therapeutic Approaches

Randy L. Jensen, MD, PhD, MHPE   Gabriel Zada, MD, MS
Editors

Histopathologic and Molecular Evaluation of Meningioma

Christian Davidson, MD

KEYWORDS

• Meningioma • Pathology • CNS WHO grading • Methylation

KEY POINTS

- The histopathology of meningiomas is varied.
- CNS World Health Organization grading is used to predict biological behavior and serves as a critical data point in clinical decision-making.
- DNA methylation profiling offers an advanced and potentially more accurate method to predict meningioma clinical behavior.

COMMON HISTOLOGIC FEATURES AND FROZEN SECTION

Meningiomas typically possess spindled-to-epithelioid cells, with the most common histologic features being whorls, nuclear pseudoinclusions, and psammomatous calcifications (see ref[1] and **Fig. 1**). Although not all meningiomas will possess all three, the presence of any one of them in the context of a dural-based mass should tip off the pathologist to a meningothelial neoplasm.

Intraoperative pathology consultation (colloquially known as frozen section) is the neuropathologist's version of acute care. Our neurosurgical colleagues require an answer as quickly as possible, with minimal ability to consult an expert and no opportunity to perform immunohistochemistry (IHC) or molecular testing to refine the diagnosis. Frozen section diagnosis is needed to guide surgical decision-making and is therefore of utmost importance in the treatment of patients with brain tumors. Fortunately, the cardinal histologic features of meningiomas are readily appreciated on both smear preparation and frozen section and should not pose a difficult challenge to a pathologist familiar with these features.

On smearing a meningioma, the nuclei have usual oval, banal, minimally atypical nuclei with smooth nuclear contours and smooth chromatin. Nuclear pseudoinclusions may be seen on smear preparation, but what is most helpful is the nature of meningioma cytoplasm on smear (see **Fig. 1**A). The cytoplasm is faintly eosinophilic and delicate, lending the appearance of tissue paper or "billowing curtains." Whorls and calcifications can also be appreciated (see **Fig. 1**B and C). Taken together with the nuclear features (and the history of a dural-based mass), a diagnosis of meningioma can typically be rendered on smear alone.

Smearing a tumor obviously ruins most evaluation of architecture (whorls excepted). This is where frozen section is most useful. The hallmark histologic features (again, whorls, nuclear pseudoinclusions, and psammomatous calcifications) are often obvious and usually confirm the smear-based diagnostic suspicions.

Although most meningiomas are central nervous system (CNS) World Health Organization (WHO) Grade 1 and therefore portend a favorable prognosis, atypical, or malignant features (see below for details) can be seen on frozen section. One might think that this could put the pathologist is a difficult position, but the reality is that the neurosurgical approach will likely not be altered by the presence of CNS WHO Grade 2 or 3 features. It is therefore best at the time of frozen to mention the

Department of Pathology, University of Utah, Sandy, UT, USA
E-mail address: cjd1041@gmail.com

Neurosurg Clin N Am 34 (2023) 311–318
https://doi.org/10.1016/j.nec.2023.02.001
1042-3680/23/© 2023 Elsevier Inc. All rights reserved.

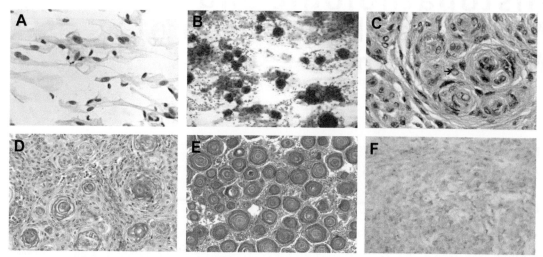

Fig. 1. Cardinal features of meningioma. (*A*) Wispy "billowing curtain" cytoplasm on smearing a meningioma. (*B*) Smeared meningioma showing numerous whorls. (*C*) Whorls and nuclear pseudoinclusions (*arrow*) in a frozen section. (*D*) Whorls in a transitional meningioma. (*E*) Numerous psammomatous calcifications. (*F*) Confirmatory EMA immunohistochemical stain.

high-grade features without labeling the tumor with a CNS WHO Grade. Remember, the pathologist's role during a frozen section of a dural-based tumor (and indeed all neurosurgical resections) is to give information to assist the neurosurgeon's clinical decision-making. Entities such as lymphoma or infection should not be missed, as mandatory testing mandated by these histopathologic suspicions (flow cytometry and cultures, respectively) are standard of care for these patients.

WORLD HEALTH ORGANIZATION CNS TUMOR GRADING CRITERIA
CNS World Health Organization Grade 1 Meningioma

Most meningiomas fall into a CNS WHO Grade 1 classification. If completely resected, these tumors generally show an indolent biologic behavior, with many patients never seeing recurrence.[1]

Meningothelial Meningioma

Meningothelial meningiomas (**Fig. 2**A) are typically composed of epithelioid cells with conspicuous nuclear pseudoinclusions. The cells often form a syncytium, but this is in reality a "pseudosyncytium." Although cell borders are difficult to appreciate on light microscopy, electron microscopy reveals delicate cell processes. Whorls and psammoma bodies are uncommon. These tumors commonly arise at the skull base.

Fibrous Meningioma

Fibrous meningiomas (**Fig. 2**B) show a spindle-cell morphology, with a fascicular growth pattern in a collagen-rich matrix. The cerebral convexities are a common location for this subtype.

Transitional Meningioma

This subtype typically shows a mix of features of both meningothelial meningioma and fibrous meningioma. Whorls and psammoma bodies are readily appreciated in this subtype (see **Fig. 1**D).

Psammomatous Meningioma

Psammomatous meningiomas (**Fig. 2**C) classically arise from the dura of either the sphenoid wing or the spinal column (especially the thoracic spine). This subtype shows numerous psammomatous calcifications, sometimes predominating the tumor to an extant where they obscure the neoplastic meningioma cells.

Angiomatous Meningioma

The angiomatous subtype (**Fig. 2**D) shows numerous blood vessels (typically hyalinized) with intervening space taken up by neoplastic meningothelial cells. Nuclear atypia can be conspicuous, but this is not considered a sign of malignancy. Instead, if it referred to as "degenerative nuclear atypia."

Secretory Meningioma

The hallmark of this subtype is the presence of gland-like formation (**Fig. 2**E), with round, eosinophilic periodic acid-schiff (PAS)-positive and carcinoembryonic antigen (CEA)-immunopositive secretions (**Fig. 2**F). Along with angiomatous and microcystic meningiomas, the adjacent brain

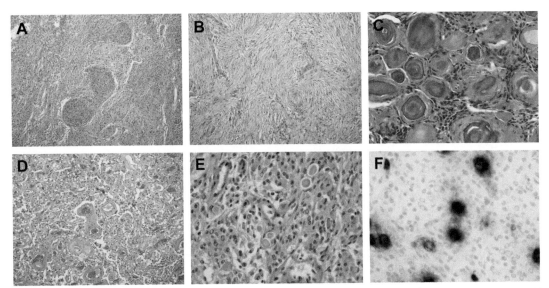

Fig. 2. CNS WHO Grade 1 Subtypes. (*A*). Meningothelial meningioma with pseudosyncytial growth pattern. (*B*). Fibrous meningioma with spindle cell morphology and collagenous matrix. (*C*). Psammomatous meningioma with psammomatous calcifications predominating the histologic picture. (*D*). Angiomatous meningioma with numerous hyalinized blood vessels and intervening neoplastic meningothelial cells. (*E*). Secretory meningioma show eosinophilic secretions. Note the many nuclear pseudoinclusions. (*F*). CEA immunohistochemistry highlighting the secretions of a secretory meningioma.

may show edema out of proportion to the size of the tumor.

Microcystic Meningioma

The microcystic appearance of this subtype is due to the thin, long processes made by oft-vacuolated tumor cells, lending a lacey, cobweb morphology to the tumor. Nuclear atypia and pleomorphism can be prominent, but like the angiomatous subtype (and indeed all WHO Grade 1 subtypes), this is not thought to be a sign of malignancy.

Metaplastic Meningioma

Occasional meningiomas with an angiomatous or microcystic morphology may show differentiation along mesenchymal lineages, with osseous, cartilaginous, and lipomatous tissue. There does not appear to be any clinical significance to this differentiation, as the clinical behavior of these tumors conforms to that of a CNS WHO Grade 1.

Lymphoplasmacyte-Rich Meningioma

This rare subtype shows a marked chronic inflammatory infiltrate, oftentimes obscuring the neoplastic meningioma cells.

CNS WORLD HEALTH ORGANIZATION GRADE 2 MENINGIOMA

Meningiomas assigned a CNS WHO Grade of 2 have a greater likelihood of recurrence.[1] The

CNS WHO Grade is therefore vitally important to recognize, as patients with residual and possibly even gross total resection of CNS WHO Grade 2 meningioma require adjuvant radiation therapy to the tumor bed to prevent progression or recurrence.

There are four broadly grouped ways a neuropathologist can assign a CNS WHO Grade of 2 to a meningothelial tumor. They are:

1. *Increased Mitotic Activity:* A mitotic count of 4 but less than 20 mitoses per 10 high-power fields (HPFs) is diagnostic for atypical meningioma, CNS WHO Grade 2.
2. *Brain Invasion:* Meningiomas that invade the brain parenchyma are deemed atypical meningioma, CNS WHO Grade 2 (unless they have CNS WHO Grade 3 features; see below). Oftentimes, brain invasion is readily apparent on H&E (**Fig. 3**A). However, occasionally, Glial fibrillary acidic protein (GFAP) IHC can be used to demonstrate an invading lobule of meningioma completely surrounded by GFAP-positive brain. Great care should be taken to ensure that the tumor is truly invading the brain parenchyma itself. Some meningiomas follow leptomeningeal blood vessels into the cortex via the Virchow–Robin spaces. Because the Virchow–Robin space is in a continuum of the subarachnoid space, this does not represent true brain invasion.
3. *Morphologic Features:* Excepting a tumor with CNS WHO Grade 3 features (see below), if a

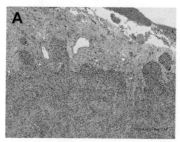 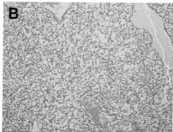 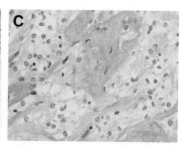

Fig. 3. CNS WHO Grade 2 Subtypes. (*A*) Brain invasion classifies this tumor as an atypical meningioma, CNS WHO Grade 2. (*B*) Chordoid meningioma showing thin trabeculae of tumor cells in the myxoid/mucinous matrix. (*C*). Clear cell meningioma showing tumor cells with clear cytoplasm. Note the sclerotic bands of intervening connective tissue.

meningothelial tumor has 3 (or 4 or 5) of the 5 following histopathologic features, it can reliably be graded as an atypical meningioma, CNS WHO Grade 2.

- Hypercellular foci
- Small cell change
- Necrosis
- Patternless architecture
- Prominent nucleoli

4. *Two CNS WHO Grade 2 Morphologic Subtypes:*
   - *Chordoid Meningioma:* This tumor vaguely resembles chordoma (**Fig. 3**B), with epithelioid cells arranged in loose cords, trabeculae, and small lobules, typically separated by a mucinous matrix. It is common to see meningothelial, fibrous, or transitional subtypes intermixed with the chordoid areas. The pathologist must assess the preponderance of chordoid areas, judging the chordoid areas to make up a preponderance of the histologic patterns.
   - *Clear Cell Meningioma:* This subtype is composed of cells with a clear, glycogen-rich cytoplasm (**Fig. 3**C). The architecture is generally patternless, with psammoma bodies and whorls being indistinct, if present at all. These tumors can have abundant connective tissue, with some tumors showing widespread sclerosis with minimal tumor cells. The cells show minimal nuclear atypia and rare mitotic activity, but this belies their propensity to recur. Clear cell meningioma shows a predilection for the cerebellopontine angle and the lumbosacral spine.

CNS WORLD HEALTH ORGANIZATION GRADE 3 MENINGIOMA

Meningiomas that fulfill the criteria for WHO Grade 3 are frankly malignant tumors with frequent recurrence and a poor prognosis.[1]

Anaplastic (Malignant) Meningioma

These tumors have overtly malignant histopathologic features. These include a mitotic count greater than or equal to 20 mitoses per 10 HPF.[2] In addition, their morphology can appear like that of a carcinoma, sarcoma, or even a melanoma. IHC can sometimes be necessary to establish meningothelial origin, as can deoxyribonucleic acid (DNA) methylation profiling (see below). Alternatively, molecular testing can be employed to assess grade, with both telomerase reverse transcriptase (TERT) promoter mutation[3,4] and homozygous deletion of CDKN2A and/or CDKN2B[4] in and of themselves being diagnostic of a CNS WHO Grade 3 meningioma.

Rhabdoid Meningioma

These aggressive tumors show an ill-defined cytoplasmic inclusion, globular, or fibrillar in texture and typically more eosinophilic that the surrounding cytoplasm.[5] The tumor cells are generally dyscohesive (**Fig. 4**A), and necrosis is often prominent. The nucleoli are often conspicuous, and mitotic figures are numerous. Lower grade morphologies can be admixed with the rhabdoid areas, and much like chordoid meningioma, the rhabdoid cells must comprise a predominance of the tumor to justify this diagnosis. There is no known clinical significance to small foci of rhabdoid cells in otherwise CNS WHO Grade 1 or 2 meningiomas.

Papillary Meningioma

The cardinal feature of this rare subtype of meningioma is a perivascular orientation of meningioma cells, lending a pseudopapillary appearance to the tumor cells (**Fig. 4**B). Rhabdoid cells can often make up the perivascular tumor cells. One must be careful in cases with extensive necrosis, which can result in viable tumor cells "cuffing" blood vessels. This mimic of papillary architecture is not indicative of CNS WHO Grade 3 biolologic behavior.

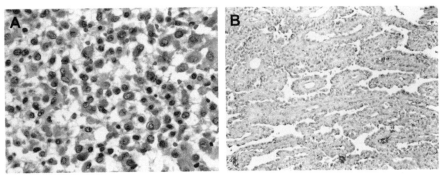

Fig. 4. WHO CNS Grade 3 Subtypes. (*A*) Rhabdoid meningioma with eccentric nuclei, eosinophilic cytoplasmic globules, and a dyscohesive growth pattern. (*B*) Papillary meningioma with neoplastic meningothelial cells lining a delicate fibrovascular core.

DIAGNOSTIC AND PROGNOSTIC IMMUNOHISTOCHEMISTRY

The classic and most well-known immunohistochemical stain to demonstrate meningothelial origin of these tumors is epithelial membrane antigen (EMA) (see **Fig. 1**F). High-grade meningiomas can sometimes show total loss of or markedly decreased EMA staining. Fibrous meningiomas often have minimal EMA staining.[1] Somatostatin receptor 2A (SSTR2A) is another reliable marker of meningiomas but can also be expressed in neuroendocrine tumors. Progesterone receptor is also sometimes employed for diagnostic purposes, but has become less commonly used in recent years.

There are two prognostic IHC stains that have been described. Ki67 (MIB1) labeling over 4% has been associated with a clinical behavior akin to WHO Grade 2, whereas a Ki67 index of 20% or more suggests a clinical behavior akin to WHO Grade 3. A similar breakdown of tumor into mitotic index using phospho-histone H3 has also been reported.[6] A newer IHC marker is a methylation-specific antibody that assesses presence/absence of trimethylation of lysine 27 in the histone-3 protein (H3 K27me3). Katz and colleagues[7] showed that the complete loss of H3 K27me3 in meningiomas was predictive of a more rapid progression. In addition, the loss of H3 K27me3 was associated with a DNA methylation pattern seen in more aggressive meningiomas (see below for discussion of methylation profiling).

HISTOPATHOLOGIC DIFFERENTIAL DIAGNOSES

Multiple tumors can have a similar morphology to various subtypes of meningiomas and require discussion.

Fibrous Meningiomas: With their spindle cells and abundant collagen, fibrous meningiomas can resemble solitary fibrous tumors. This said, EMA and STAT6 IHC can readily distinguish between these two diagnoses. Fibrous meningiomas can also resemble schwannomas, especially given the spindle cells, frequent loss of EMA staining, and often strong S100 staining. Collagen is not typically seen in schwannomas, so this can be a helpful feature. In addition, SSTR2A staining should readily stain meningiomas but spare schwannomas.

Angiomatous Meningioma: These tumors can resemble a vascular malformation, but the presence of interspersed neoplastic meningothelial cells should minimize diagnostic concern for a vascular malformation and instead drive the pathologist to a meningioma diagnosis.

Secretory Meningioma: These can vaguely resemble carcinoma, but immunohistochemical stains (EMA and CEA) should readily demonstrate the meningothelial nature (EMA) and secretory globules (CEA) of this neoplasm.

Lymphoplasmacyte-Rich Meningioma: This neoplasm can resemble nonneoplastic inflammatory conditions. If rich in plasma cells, lymphoplasmacyte-rich meningioma can resemble hypertrophic pachymeningitis, as seen with immunoglobulin G subclass 4 (IgG4)-related disease of the dura and in concert with rheumatoid arthritis or other inflammatory/autoimmune conditions.

Chordoid Meningioma: The obvious microscopic mimic of chordoid meningioma is its namesake, chordoma. The tumor location is generally different between the two: clivus or sacrum for chordoma and supratentorial dural-based mass for chordoid meningioma. IHC is helpful, as chordoma will express brachyury, whereas meningiomas do not. Note that both can express EMA.

CNS WHO Grade 3 Meningiomas: Given the high-grade features present in this grade, tumors such as sarcomas, carcinomas, and melanomas can be brought into the differential. Relevant IHC can readily distinguish between these entities.

DNA METHYLATION PROFILING IN MENINGIOMA
Concept

One of the most promising molecular methods for analysis of nervous system tumors is methylation profiling (methylomics; see ref[8] for excellent review). In the analysis of resected nervous system tumors, methylation profiling can be used in two clinical contexts: (1) molecular classification of a histologically difficult case and/or (2) the elucidation of prognostic factors which may aid in treatment decisions.[8] As meningothelial lineage of meningiomas is generally not histologically challenging to demonstrate, this section covers the possible prognostic implications of methylation profiling of meningiomas.

DNA Methylation

Methylation of DNA generally occurs at Cytosine-phosphate-Guanine (CpG) islands, discrete loci on the genome on which a methyl group is covalently bonded to the C5 position of the cytosine ring by a DNA methyltransferase. Many (but not all) CpG islands are within or near gene promoters. CpG methylation typically blocks the ability of the transcription machinery to sit down on the promoter to create the messenger ribonucleic acid (mRNA) necessary for gene expression. As gene expression is the predominate driver of cellular identity and behavior, the ability to assess methylation patterns in a given tumor could be diagnostically useful. A useful (albeit single-gene) example is the routine assessment of O(6)-methylguanine-DNA methyltransferase (MGMT) promoter methylation in the neuropathologic workup of diffuse gliomas. The MGMT gene encodes the DNA repair enzyme O(6)-methylguanine-DNA methyltransferase (pMGMT). Beside its normal cellular role in DNA repair, pMGMT also removes the lethal DNA adduct formed by the commonly used anti-glioma chemotherapeutic, temozolomide. Removal of the DNA-temozolomide complex from the tumor's DNA reduces the efficacy of the drug. Given that methylated gene promoters inhibit transcription, it should come as no surprise that hypermethylation of the MGMT gene promoter is a positive prognostic factor in the treatment of gliomas. In this scenario, pMGMT is not produced, allowing temozolomide to remain on DNA and result in antitumor toxicity.[9]

With the advent of technology that can examine whole genome methylation profiles (eg, the Illumina 850K methylomics array[10]), the ability has arisen to molecularly define meningiomas. The potentially profound impact of methylation profiling on clinical care arises from one fact: the WHO grading of meningiomas (see above) has pitfalls. Although the WHO-provided guidelines for grading meningiomas are generally predictive of clinical behavior, there are CNS WHO Grade 1 meningiomas that behave in a more aggressive manner. This might not come as a surprise, for instance, given the subjective nature of the assessment of the five "atypical" histologic features.[1,11] We therefore should strive for a more accurate system that can provide our patients with even more well-defined prognostic information. For example, there are occasional histologic CNS WHO Grade 1 meningiomas that behave in a more "atypical" manner. Would it not be helpful to have a system in place ahead of time to inform us of this likely behavior and to treat the patient accordingly? On the flip side, if there are histologic CNS WHO Grade 2 meningiomas that might behave in a more indolent manner, would it not be advantageous to the patient to NOT overtreat this tumor (ie, with radiation)? There is ample evidence that methylation profiling might provide us with a more refined classification system, one which would result in more appropriate clinical decision-making for patients whose tumors have a discrepancy between histologic grade and actual biological behavior.

Clinical Utility

Two reports[12,13] published in 2017 first shed significant light on the power of methylation profiling as a useful diagnostic and prognostic tool in the clinical management of meningioma. Olar and colleagues[12] showed that unsupervised clustering of the methylation profiles of 140 meningiomas classified meningiomas into two subgroups; these groups showed highly divergent recurrence-free survival (RFS) curves. The "molecular methylation unfavorable (MM-UNFAV)" group (the group with a dramatic decrease in RFS) showed copy number variations previously shown to be associated with increase rate of recurrence. The demonstration that methylation profiling could reveal already known copy number variation (CNVs) was solid validation of methylomics in the risk-stratifying of meningiomas.

Sahm and colleagues[13] performed methylation profiling on 497 meningiomas, across all WHO histologic grades, and demonstrated six subgroups with distinct clinical courses: three considered benign, two considered intermediate, and one considered malignant. The six groups spanned the various histologic subtypes, with some WHO Grade 2 meningiomas clustering with benign subgroups, as well as some WHO Grade 1 tumors clustering with the intermediate groups (and, frighteningly, one WHO Grade 1 meningioma clustering with the malignant subgroup). Most striking was their prediction error curves, in which the Brier score (a weighted average of the observed survival status and that predicted by a model, in this case, histology or methylation). When the Brier scores were graphed over time, Sahm and colleagues demonstrated that the error rate for methylation classification of meningiomas was lower than the error rate for CNS WHO histologic grading. This further proves the power (and clinical utility) of methylation profiling in the care of patients with meningioma.

Two more papers published by Nassiri and colleagues[14] and Choudhury and colleagues[15] firmly established methylation profiling as the very near future of meningioma patient care. These papers integrated methylation findings with genetic, transcriptomic, proteomic, and single-cell approaches to discover different molecular subgroups of meningioma. Choudhury and colleagues[15] examined 565 meningiomas and established three subgroups, and although these groups correlated with progression-free survival, Choudhary made note that "DNA methylation grouping does not obviate the importance of meningioma grading".[15] This said, their comprehensive proteogenomic analysis revealed possible therapeutic vulnerabilities, something histologic grading is not capable of doing. Nassiri and colleagues methylomically classified a total of 201 meningiomas into four subgroups.[14] In contrast to Choudhury, Nassiri showed that their molecular groups more accurately predicted clinical outcomes than CNS WHO Grading schemes. The differing impact of methylation profiling on the need for histologic grading must be rectified. So too must be the different number and identity of subgroups these different papers have discovered. A unified, standardized, and broadly accepted methylation scheme must be put forth to establish a certain level of consistency and reduce confusion. It would be beneficial to our neuro-oncology colleagues and their patients if the methylation-based classification of a meningioma depends not on the geographic location of the methylation analysis, but by the actual biology of the tumor itself.

SUMMARY

Meningioma histopathology, while varied, is well-defined. The CNS WHO grading of meningiomas

is also trustworthy and clearly delineated, but some grading criteria can be subjective, which leads to interobserver variability and a possible compromise in patient care. Multiple molecular modalities exist to further refine our classification of meningioma biological behavior. Methylation is the most comprehensively studied molecular tool and is therefore the modality best poised to add to the comprehensive pathologic analysis of this important nervous system tumor.

CLINICS CARE POINTS

- Accurate grading of meningiomas is essential to guide proper treatment decisions.
- Histopathologic analysis is clinically useful to predict the biological behavior of a tumor.
- Genetic or methylomic testing has refined our understanding of the behavior of meningiomas.
- These molecular testing modalities will enhance our ability to predict the clinical course of a given tumor, improving clinical decision-making and therefore, patient care.

DISCLOSURE

Nothing to disclose.

ACKNOWLEDGMENTS

The author would like to thank Drs Qinwen Mao (Professor, Univeristy of Utah) and Cheryl Palmer (Professor Emeritus, Univeristy of Utah) for slides and/or pictures of WHO Grade 2 and 3 meningiomas.

REFERENCES

1. WHO Classification of Tumours Editorial Board. Central nervous system tumours. Lyon (France): International Agency for Research on Cancer; 2021. (WHO classification of tumours series, 5th edition; vol. 6). Available at: https://publications.iarc.fr/601.
2. Perry A, Scheithauer BW, Stafford SL, et al. "Malignancy" in meningiomas: a clinicopathologic study of 116 patients, with grading implications. Cancer 1999;85(9):2046–56.
3. Goutagny S, Nault JC, Mallet M, et al. High incidence of activating TERT promoter mutations in meningiomas undergoing malignant progression. Brain Pathol 2014;24(2):184–9.
4. Simon M, Park TW, Köster G, et al. Alterations of INK4a(p16-p14ARF)/INK4b(p15) expression and

telomerase activation in meningioma progression. J Neuro Oncol 2001;55(3):149–58.

5. Perry A, Scheithauer BW, Stafford SL, et al. Rhabdoid" meningioma: an aggressive variant. Am J Surg Pathol 1998;22(12):1482–90.

6. Olar A, Wani KM, Sulman EP, et al. Mitotic index is an independent predictor of recurrence-free survival in meningioma. Brain Pathol 2015;25(3):266–75.

7. Katz LM, Hielscher T, Liechty B, et al. Loss of histone H3K27me3 identifies a subset of meningiomas with increased risk of recurrence. Acta Neuropathol 2018;135(6):955–63.

8. Galbraith K, Snuderl M. DNA methylation as a diagnostic tool. Acta Neuropathol Commun 2022;10(1): 71.

9. Hegi ME, Diserens AC, Gorlia T, et al. MGMT gene silencing and benefit from temozolomide in glioblastoma. N Engl J Med 2005;352(10):997–1003.

10. Comprehensive coverage for genome-wide DNA methylation studies. In: Illumina Inc. Available at: http//illumine.com/techniques/microarrays/

methylation-arrays.html. Accessed December 4, 2022.

11. Goldbrunner R, Minniti G, Preusser M, et al. EANO guidelines for the diagnosis and treatment of meningiomas. Lancet Oncol 2016;17(9):e383–91.

12. Olar A, Wani KM, Wilson CD, et al. Global epigenetic profiling identifies methylation subgroups associated with recurrence-free survival in meningioma. Acta Neuropathol 2017;133(3):431–44.

13. Sahm F, Schrimpf D, Stichel D, et al. DNA methylation-based classification and grading system for meningioma: a multicentre, retrospective analysis. Lancet Oncol 2017;18(5):682–94.

14. Nassiri F, Liu J, Patil V, et al. A clinically applicable integrative molecular classification of meningiomas. Nature 2021;597(7874):119–25.

15. Choudhury A, Magill ST, Eaton CD, et al. Meningioma DNA methylation groups identify biological drivers and therapeutic vulnerabilities. Nat Genet 2022;54(5):649–59.

Medical Management of Meningiomas

Mohammed A. Azab, MBBS[a], Kyril Cole, MPH[b], Emma Earl, BS[b], Chris Cutler, BS[c],
Joe Mendez, MD[d], Michael Karsy, MD, PhD, MSc[e,*]

KEYWORDS

• Medical management • Meningioma • Radiosurgery • Chemotherapy • Immunotherapy

KEY POINTS

- Alpha-interferon, somatostatin receptor agonists, and vascular endothelial growth factor inhibitors are National Comprehensive Cancer Network–approved medical treatments for meningiomas but show limited clinical impact.
- Previous trialed and failed classes of medical therapy for meningiomas include tyrosine kinase inhibitors (targeting PDGFR, EGFR), hydroxyurea, and chemotherapy.
- Recent genomic studies have identified new driver mutations (TRAF7, SMO, POLR2A, KLF4, AKT1, PI3KCA, NF2, and FAK) with potential impact on treatment.
- Immunomodulation offers a promising avenue for therapeutic treatment in meningioma.

INTRODUCTION

Meningioma is a very common intracranial and spinal tumor that originates from the leptomeningeal arachnoid cap cells.[1] Risk factors include older age, genetic mutations and family disorders, ionizing radiation, and head trauma.[2] Major histopathological classification changes of meningioma occurred in the 2007, 2016, and 2021 World Health Organization (WHO) classifications, with more recent studies better identifying the molecular drivers of this tumor. Fifteen histologic meningioma variants exist, with the majority being WHO grade 1 (80%).[3] The WHO 2016 classification considered brain invasion or the presence of more than 4 mitotic figures or specific subtypes as diagnostic of atypical WHO grade 2 meningioma, resulting in increased incidence of this tumor grade (15%–20%). Grade 3 anaplastic meningioma (1%–3%) has 3 variants and remains rare but has an extremely poor prognosis.[4] The WHO 2021 classification modified WHO 2 tumors to show the presence of 10 or more mitotic figures. The shift in meningioma classification has influenced the incidence of more aggressive tumor types often resulting in potentially wider use of adjuvant radiotherapy. Moreover, further advances in systemic therapies are needed due to limitations in surgery and radiotherapy alone.

In this review, we examine the various medical therapies that have been evaluated in meningiomas (**Table 1**). Many of these agents have had limited success, with results hindered by small study sizes and the variable inclusion criteria. Despite these limitations, previous trials have helped in the ongoing design of the next generation of clinical trials and combination therapies to improve meningioma treatment. We also discuss ongoing clinical trials involving other systemic molecular therapies and immunotherapy agents for the treatment of meningioma (**Table 2**).

[a] Biomolecular Sciences Graduate Program, Boise State University, 1910 University Drive, Boise, ID 83725, USA; [b] School of Medicine, University of Utah, 30 North 1900 East, Salt Lake City, UT 84132, USA; [c] Chicago Medical School, Rosalind Franklin University of Medicine and Science, 3333 N Green Bay Rd., North Chicago, IL 60064, USA; [d] Department of Neurosurgery, Huntsman Cancer Institute, University of Utah, 2000 Circle of Hope Dr., Salt Lake City, UT 84112, USA; [e] Department of Neurosurgery, Clinical Neurosciences Center, University of Utah, 175 North Medical Drive East, Salt Lake City, UT 84132, USA
* Corresponding author. Assistant Professor of Neurosurgery.
E-mail address: neuropub@hsc.utah.edu

Neurosurg Clin N Am 34 (2023) 319–333
https://doi.org/10.1016/j.nec.2023.02.002
1042-3680/23/© 2023 Elsevier Inc. All rights reserved.

Table 1
Summary of studies evaluating medical treatments of meningiomas

Reference	Agent	Mechanism	N	Median PFS	PFS-6
Kim et al,[39] 2012	Hydroxyurea	Ribonucleotide reductase inhibitor	-	-	-
Schrell et al,[26] 1997	Hydroxyurea	Ribonucleotide reductase inhibitor	4	-	-
Newton et al,[27] 2000	Hydroxyurea	Ribonucleotide reductase inhibitor	17	80 wk	-
Mason et al,[28] 2002	Hydroxyurea	Ribonucleotide reductase inhibitor	20	-	-
Rosenthal et al,[29] 2002	Hydroxyurea	Ribonucleotide reductase inhibitor	15	-	-
Loven et al,[30] 2004	Hydroxyurea	Ribonucleotide reductase inhibitor	12	13 mo	-
Hahn et al,[31] 2005	Hydroxyurea with radiotherapy	Ribonucleotide reductase inhibitor	21	-	-
Weston et al,[32] 2006	Hydroxyurea	Ribonucleotide reductase inhibitor	6	-	-
Chamberlain & Johnston,[33] 2011	Hydroxyurea	Ribonucleotide reductase inhibitor	60	4 mo	10%
Chamberlain,[34] 2012	Hydroxyurea	Ribonucleotide reductase inhibitor	35	2 mo	3%
Chamberlain et al,[50] 2004	Temozolomide	Alkylating agent	16	6 mo	0%
Chamberlain et al,[129] 2006	Irinotecan	Topoisomerase 1 inhibitor	16	4.5 mo	6%
Chamberlain,[49] 1996	Cyclophosphamide + adriamycin (doxorubicin) + vincristine (CAV)	Cytotoxic chemotherapy	14	4.6 y	-
Kaba et al,[130] 1997	Interferon-α	Immunomodulator	6	-	-
Muhr et al,[131] 2001	Interferon-α	Immunomodulator	12	-	-
Chamberlain & Glantz,[10] 2008	Interferon-α	Immunomodulator	35	7 mo	54%
Lamberts et al,[1992][46]	Mifepristone (RU486)	Antiprogesterone	12	-	-
Grunberg et al,[43] 1991	Mifepristone (RU486)	Antiprogesterone	14	-	-
Grunberg et al,[44] 2006	Mifepristone (RU486)	Antiprogesterone	28	-	-

Study	Drug	Mechanism	N	Duration	Response
Touat et al, ^ 2014	Mifepristone (RU466)	Antiprogesterone	3	-	-
de Keizer & Smit,[47] 2004	Mifepristone (RU486)	Antiprogesterone	2	-	-
Grunberg & Weiss,[41] 1990	Megestrol acetate	Progesterone receptor agonist	9	-	-
Jaaskelainen et al,[42] 1986	Medroxy-progesterone acetate	Synthetic progesterone	5	-	-
Markwalder et al,[132] 1985	Tamoxifen	Antiestrogen	6	-	-
Goodwin et al,[133] 1993	Tamoxifen	Antiestrogen	21	15.1 mo	-
Runzi et al,[54] 1989	Octreotide	Somatostatin analog	1	-	-
Garcia-Luna et al,[55] 1993	Octreotide	Somatostatin analog	3	-	-
Jaffrain-Rea et al,[56] 1998	Octreotide	Somatostatin analog	1	-	-
Johnson et al,[57] 2011	Octreotide	Somatostatin analog	11	17 wk	-
Chamberlain et al,[7] 2007	Sandostatin LAR	Somatostatin analog	16	5 mo	44%
Norden et al,[59] 2015	Pasireotide LAR	Somatostatin analog	26	20 wk	29%
Simo et al,[58] 2014	Octreotide	Somatostatin analog	9	4.23 mo	44%
Wen et al,[24] 2009	Imatinib	PDGFR TKI	23	2 mo	29.40%
Raizer et al,[23] 2010	Erlotinib	EGFR TKI	1	-	-
Norden et al,[25] 2010	Erlotinib or gefitinib	EGFR TKI	25	10 wk	28%
Reardon et al,[35] 2012	Imatinib and hydroxyurea	PDGFR TKI 1 + ribonucleotide reductase inhibitor	21	7 mo	61.90%
Raizer et al,[23] 2010	Vatalanib (PTL-787)	VEGFR 1 + PDGFR TKI	21	-	37.50%
Raizer et al,[21] 2014	Vatalanib (PTL-787)	VEGFR 1 + PDGFR TKI	25	6.5 mo	37.50%
Kaley et al,[9] 2015	Sunitinib	VEGFR 1 + PDGFR TKI	36	5.2 mo	42%
Puchner et al,[15] 2010	Bevacizumab	Anti-VEGFR antibody	1	-	-
Goutagny et al,[16] 2011	Bevacizumab	Anti-VEGFR antibody	1	-	-
Wilson & Heth,[17] 2012	Bevacizumab + paclitaxel	Anti-VEGFR antibody	1	15 mo	-
Lou et al,[18] 2012	Bevacizumab	Anti-VEGFR antibody	14	17.9 mo	85.70%
Nayak et al,[19] 2012	Bevacizumab	Anti-VEGFR antibody	15	26 wk	43.80%
Nunes et al,[134] 2013	Bevacizumab	Anti-VEGFR antibody	15	15 mo	-
Michael et al,[66] 2017	AZD5363	AKT inhibitor	1	17 mo	-
Shih et al,[135] 2016	Everolimus + bevacizumab	Everolimus (mTOR kinase inhibitor)	17	22 mo	-
Cardona et al,[136] 2019	Everolimus + octreotide	Everolimus (mTOR kinase inhibitor)	31	12.1 mo	58.20%
Brastianos et al,[137] 2022	Pembrolizumab	PD-1 inhibitor	25	7.6 mo	90%

Table 2
Clinical trials of systemic therapy for meningioma

Therapeutic Agent	Therapeutic Target	Tumor Grade	Clinical Trial	Status	Phase	Start date
Nivolumab	Immune check inhibitor	Atypical/malignant	NCT03173950	Recruiting	2	2-Jun-17
Pembrolizumab + SRS	PD-1 inhibitor	Grade 1, 2, 3 and recurrent	NCT04659811	Recruiting	2	9-Dec-20
Nivolumab + ipilimumab + EBRT	PD-1 inhibitor + CTLA-4 inhibitor	Recurrent grade 2 and 3	NCT02648997	Recruiting	2	7-Jan-16
Avelumab + proton therapy + surgery	PD-L1	Recurrent radiation-refractory	NCT03267836	Active (not recruiting)	1 and 2	30-Aug-17
Nivolumab + SRS ± ipilimumab	PD-1 ± CTLA-4	Grade 2, 3 and recurrent	NCT03604978	Recruiting	1 and 2	30-Jul-18
Vismodegib	Inhibits the transmembrane protein Smoothened homolog (SMO)	Recurrent meningioma and NF2 gene mutation	NCT02523014	Recruiting	2	14-Aug-15
Capivasertib	AKT inhibitor					
Abemaciclib	CDK pathway inhibitor					
Ribociclib	CDK4/6-inhibitor	Recurrent grade 2 and 3	NCT02933736	Recruiting	Early 1	14-Oct-16
AZD2014, vistusertib	Dual m-TORC1/2 inhibitor	Recurrent	NCT03071874	Active (not recruiting)	2	7-Mar-17

Abbreviations: EBRT, external beam radiation therapy; SRS, stereotactic radiosurgery.

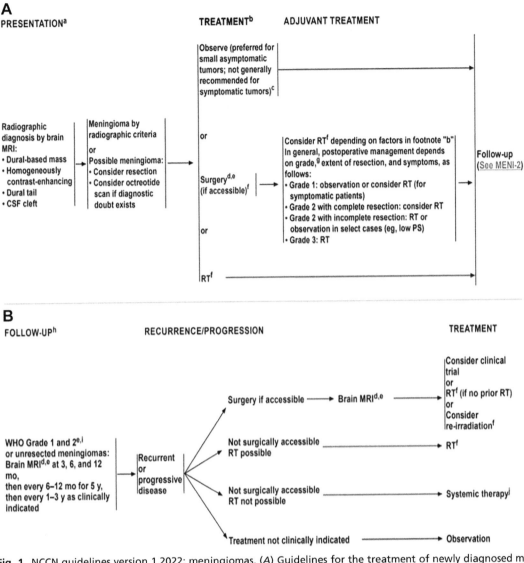

Fig. 1. NCCN guidelines version 1.2022: meningiomas. (*A*) Guidelines for the treatment of newly diagnosed meningioma. For small, asymptomatic lesions, observation is generally recommended after clinical and radiographic evaluation. For larger asymptomatic lesions, resection is typically recommended, particularly when they are in more accessible areas or there are potential neurologic consequences to a conservative approach. Depending on tumor grade, subsequent radiotherapy (RT) may also be recommended. Tumors that are symptomatic are referred for resection when feasible. These patients are monitored closely after surgery and may undergo RT depending on tumor grade and level of resection. (*B*) Guidelines for the treatment of recurrent meningioma. After treatment, patients are followed at 3, 6, and 12 months with contrast-enhanced MRI. After 1 year, the MRIs are repeated every 6 to 12 months for 5 years and then every 1 to 3 years. The management of recurrence depends on individual factors, personalized to the patient. For instance, surgical treatment followed by RT may be used if the recurrence is accessible, whereas RT or chemotherapy, or observation, may be recommended if the lesion is surgically inaccessible. [a]Multidisciplinary input for treatment planning if feasible. [b]Treatment selection should be based on assessment of a variety of interrelated factors, including patient features (eg, age, performance score, comorbidities, treatment preferences), tumor features (eg, size, grade, growth rate, location [proximity to critical structures], potential for causing neurologic consequences if untreated, presence and severity of symptoms), and treatment-related factors (eg, potential for neurologic consequences from surgery/RT, likelihood of complete resection and/or complete irradiation with SRS, treatability of tumor if it progresses, available surgical or radiation oncology expertise and resources). The decision to administer RT after surgery also depends on the extent of resection achieved. Multidisciplinary input for treatment planning is recommended. [c]For asymptomatic meningiomas, observation is preferred for small tumors, with a suggested cutoff of ≤3 cm. Active treatment with surgery

Current Medical Treatments

Current National Comprehensive Cancer Network (NCCN) guidelines (**Fig. 1**) are limited in supporting medical options for primary and recurrent meningioma. Whereas maximal safe gross total resection alone or followed by radiotherapy has yielded 5-year progression-free survival (PFS) rates of 74% to 100% for Grade 2[5,6] and 15% to 57% for grade 3 meningiomas,[6] less benefit is typically reported for these lesions with medical management. For recurrent meningiomas that cannot be treated by surgery or radiation therapy, the current NCCN guidelines recommend only 3 classes of chemotherapeutic agents with partial benefit in clinical trials.[7,8] These agents include alpha-interferon, somatostatin receptor agonists, and vascular endothelial growth factor (VEGF) inhibitors.[7,9,10] Earlier trialed and failed classes of medical therapy for meningiomas include tyrosine kinase inhibitors (targeting PDGFR, EGFR), hormone receptors, hydroxyurea, and chemotherapy. The lack of widely available randomized controlled trials has limited our understanding of systemic therapy in meningioma.[8]

Angiogenic Pathway Inhibitors

VEGF positivity on immunostaining is reported in 79% of meningiomas and correlated with microvascular density and tumor grade.[11–13] The VEGF-targeting agent bevacizumab has been evaluated in several studies and shown median PFS of 26 weeks to 17.9 months and a 6-month PFS (PFS-6) of 37.5% to 85.7%.[8,14–19] However, in these studies, tumor grade, concomitant treatments, and mutational profiles have been heterogeneous. Other angiogenic inhibitors have been trialed as well. A phase 2 trial of vatalanib (PTK787), targeting VEGFR2 and PDGFR2 in 12 patients with WHO grade 2 meningioma, showed radiographic response in 1 patient and stable disease in 9 patients with an overall PFS-6 of 46%.[20]

Another study of 25 patients showed a PFS-6 of 64.3% in WHO grade 2 meningioma and 37.5% in grade 3 meningioma.[21] Sunitinib, targeting VEGFR and PDGFR, showed efficacy in 36 patients with grade 2 and 3 meningioma[9]; however, 4 patients developed intratumoral hemorrhage. One recent study showed VEGFR2 expression correlated with PFS in WHO grade 2 and 3 meningioma and overall survival (OS),[22] suggesting that VEGF may serve as a biomarker of meningioma but may not be a sole target in therapy.

Tyrosine Kinase Receptor Inhibitors

Imatinib (targeting PDGFR)[23] and erlotinib[24,25] and gefitinib[25] (targeting EGFR) have been evaluated in meningioma but have shown limited efficacy. PFS-6 has ranged from 28% to 44% and median PFS has ranged from 8 weeks to 5 months. One study evaluating imatinib in grade 1 and 2 meningioma showed a PFS of 2 months and PFS-6 of 29.4%.[23] Pooled analysis of 2 studies on EGFR inhibitors in 25 patients treated with gefitinib or erlotinib showed a PFS-6 of 29% and OS-12 of 65% for grade 2 to 3 meningiomas.

Hydroxyurea

Hydroxyurea has been widely studied in meningioma. It acts as a ribonucleotide reductase inhibitor of cell cycle progression. It has shown a median PFS of 10 to 80 weeks and PFS-6 of 3% to 10%.[26–35] Hydroxyurea has been used also as concomitant therapy in multiple trials, some including radiotherapy[31] and others involving calcium channel blockers.[36–38] One study of 60 patients with grade 1 meningioma and radiographic progression showed stable disease in 35% and progressive disease in 65% with a median PFS of 4 months.[33] Another study of 13 patients with grade 1 and 2 meningioma showed stable disease in 10 patients and median PFS of 72.4 months.[39] Our group demonstrated in a prospective trial

---

and/or RT is recommended in cases with one or more tumor- and/or treatment-related risk factors, such as proximity to the optic nerve. [d]Postoperative brain MRI within 48 hours after surgery. [e]See Principles of Brain and Spine Tumor Imaging (BRAIN-A). [f]See Principles of Brain Tumor Radiation Therapy (BRAIN-C). [g]WHO Grade 1 = Benign meningioma; WHO Grade 2 = Atypical meningioma; WHO Grade 3 = Malignant (anaplastic) meningioma. [h]Consider less frequent follow-up after 5 to 10 years. [i]More frequent imaging may be required for WHO Grade 3 meningiomas, and for meningiomas of any grade that are treated for recurrence or with systemic therapy. [j]See Principles of Brain and Spinal Cord Tumor Systemic Therapy (BRAIN-D). For asymptomatic meningiomas, observation is preferred for small tumors, with a suggested cutoff of ≤3 cm. Active treatment with surgery and/or RT is recommended in cases with one or more tumor-related and/or treatment-related risk factors, such as proximity to the optic nerve. Principles of brain tumor radiation therapy: WHO grade 1 meningiomas may be treated by fractionated conformal radiotherapy with doses of 45 Gy to 54 Gy. For WHO grade 2, meningiomas undergoing radiation, treatment should be directed to gross tumor (if present), surgical bed, and a margin (1–2 cm) to a dose of 54 Gy to 60 Gy in 1.8 Gy to 2.0 Gy fractions. Consider limiting margin expansion into the brain parenchyma if there is no evidence of brain invasion.

that there was limited benefit in 7 patients using combined hydroxyurea and verapamil with grade 2 and 3 meningioma,[40] with a median PFS of 8 months and PFS-6 of 85%. These results were disappointing in light of preclinical models showing strong efficacy for this drug combination.

Hormone Receptor Targeting Agents

Because of the greater incidence of meningioma in women compared with men (2:1), hormone-mediated tumor development has been posited mechanism that might offer a potent target.[2] A series of 9 patients mostly with grade 1 tumors showed stable radiographic disease with meges-trol use but was limited by short follow-up.[41] Medroxyprogesterone acetate[42] and mifepris-tone[43–47] have been studied in multiple trials without much success, and several recent system-atic reviews found limited evidence for benefit.[43,48]

Chemotherapy

Multiple studies have evaluated systemic chemo-therapy for meningioma use. One study evaluated combined cyclophosphamide, adriamycin (doxo-rubicin), and vincristine (CAV therapy) after surgery in 14 patients with grade 3 meningioma.[49,50] The results showed a median PFS of 4.6 years and PFS-6 of 6%. Another study of 16 patients with re-fractory meningioma treated with the alkylating agent temozolomide showed a median PFS of 5 months.[50] The topoisomerase inhibitor irinote-can[51] and DNA-binding agent trabectedin[52] also showed limited benefit. One possible explanation for the limited effect of chemotherapy in meningi-oma was provided by an in vitro study of multiple chemotherapeutic agents (ie, carmustine, lomus-tine, cisplatin, daunorubicin, dacarbazine, pacli-taxel, temozolomide, topotecan, vincristine, and etoposide) showing limited cell inhibition at clini-cally achievable dosing strategies.[53]

Somatostatin Analogs

Several somatostatin analogs, including octreo-tide, long-acting release (LAR) octreotide (Sandos-tatin LAR), and pasireotide, have been assessed in meningioma.[7,54–59] Somatostatin inhibits multiple neuroendocrine hormones and may target so-matostatin receptors on meningiomas. One study of 16 patients with recurrent meningioma treated with Sandostatin LAR showed a median PFS of 5 months, PFS-6 of 44%, and median OS of 7.5 months.[7] About one-third of patients achieved local control. Another study of 34 patients with pasireotide LAR in recurrent meningiomas showed a PFS-6 of 17% and median PFS of 15 weeks.[59]

Octreotide has also been explored as either a sin-gle[58] or a combined[60] treatment.

GENOMIC STUDIES IN MENINGIOMA

Identification of meningioma molecular profiles can help in stratifying prognosis and devising rational targeted therapy.[61] Several high-impact studies have elucidated new driver mutations of meningioma subtypes (TRAF7, SMO, POLR2A, KLF4, AKT1, PI3KCA, NF2, FAK) with impacts on targeted therapy (**Figs. 2 and 3**).[62–68] Other studies have helped improve stratification of tumor grades by mutational profiles[69–72] and predicted potential druggable targets based on genomic profiling.[73] Genomic analysis of meningioma offers to provide better targeted treatment options; how-ever, these methods are not widely available at all institutions and predicted treatments have not al-ways been validated.

MENINGIOMA MUTATIONS

Improved molecular classification of meningioma may help to expand the role of medical therapy and better explain the limited success of many earlier clinical trials. A subset of low-grade menin-giomas progress or recur uncharacteristically but for unclear reasons.[74] Risk scores may show promise in identifying unique meningioma sub-types, including high-risk WHO grade 1 tumors and low-risk WHO grade 3 tumors.[74] Nassiri and colleagues[75] developed a classification system with 4 consensus molecular phenotype groups (immunogenic, benign NF2 wild-type, hypermeta-bolic, and proliferative) that more accurately pre-dicted outcomes when compared with current grading systems. Their study uncovered group-specific protein targets and revealed that the "immunogenic" phenotype was associated with better clinical outcomes.[75] Schmidt and col-leagues[76] identified 8 differentially expressed genes (eg, PTTG1 and LEPR) associated with poor prognosis.

Classically, NF2 has been implicated in meningi-oma pathogenesis; however, newer studies have improved prediction of more aggressive meningi-omas. NF2 mutations are present in 40% to 60% of sporadic meningiomas, giving rise to NF2 mutant and non-NF2 mutant molecular cate-gories.[77] NF2 mutations are primarily loss of het-erozygosity of chr22q and NF2 mutations in other alleles, in addition to mitotic recombinations, sin-gle deletions, and multiexon deletions.[78] Various studies have associated meningioma recurrence with alterations in CKS2, UBE2C, and TFPI2, and DREAM complex, PI3K-AKT, extracellular matrix

A

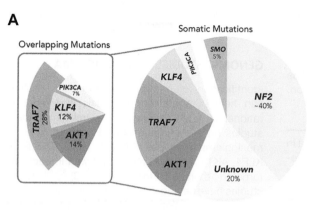

B

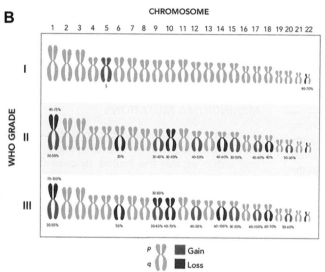

Fig. 2. Major driver mutations in meningioma. (*A*) Recurrent NF2, AKT1, SMO, TRAF7, KLF4, and PIK3CA mutations are collectively present in 80% of grade I meningiomas. Mutations in AKT1, KLF4, and PIK3CA overlap with TRAF7, but not with each other, and largely occur in a mutually exclusive pattern with NF2 and SMO. Oncogenic driver mutations remain unclear for ∼20% of meningiomas. (*B*) Recurrent chromosomal copy number alterations in meningioma. Chromosomal arm-level gains (*red*) and losses (*blue*) are observed with increasing frequency in higher grade meningiomas, compared with grade I meningiomas. §Polysomy 5 is observed in angiomatous subtype of grade I meningiomas. (*From* Bi WL, Zhang M, Wu WW, Mei Y, Dunn IF (2016) Meningioma genomics: diagnostic, prognostic, and therapeutic applications. *Front Surg.* 3:40. https://doi.org/10.3389/fsurg.2016.00040.)

signaling, and cytokine-chemokine signaling mutations.[79,80] Several additional changes in grade 3 meningiomas (H3k27me3, TERT promoter, and CDKN2A/B) predict worsened prognosis.[61] TERT promoter mutations have been associated with grade 1 progressive recurrence.[81] Non-NF2 mutant categories comprise PD1-1/PDL-1, TRAF7, KLF4, AKT1, SMO, and PI3K mutations and have been associated with progression and recurrence.[69,81–86] Additionally, chr1p/14q codeletions and transcription factor mutations have been associated with meningioma recurrence,[87–91] whereas loss of chr1p and chr6q have been associated with progression.[92]

Radiation-induced meningiomas have been associated with NF2 gene rearrangements, loss of chr1p and chr22q, decreased focal gene mutations, and failures within homologous recombination repair machinery.[93,94] Studies regarding meningeal embryologic origins have revealed paraxial mesoderm biomarkers (AKT, KLF4, SMO,

and POLR2A) and neural crest biomarkers (NF2) and the embryonic timeline within prostaglandin D synthase-positive meningioma precursor cells.[95,96] Other studies have identified radiomic signatures within meningiomas that maintain a higher somatic mutational burden, DNA methylation, FOXM1 expression, and TERT promoter mutation.[97,98] Finally, several studies have identified epigenetic factors correlated with meningioma recurrence and progression.[64,99–106]

MENINGIOMA IMMUNOMODULATION

Immunologically, meningiomas are largely composed of tumor-associated macrophages (TAMs), as well as T cells and mast cells.[107,108] Notably, Proctor and colleagues[108] illustrated that M2 TAMs are associated with recurrence. Grund and colleagues[109] found a subset of brain-invasive meningiomas had TAMs or other microglia at the brain–tumor interface, suggesting the

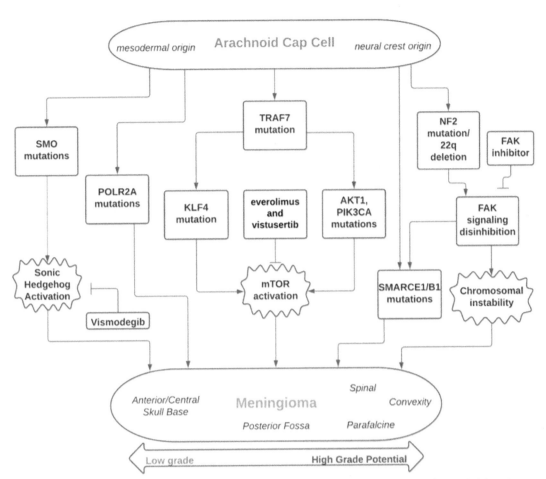

Fig. 3. Genetic drivers of meningioma and potential targetable mutations. (*From* Pawloski JA, Fadel HA, Huang Y-W, Lee IY. Genomic biomarkers of meningioma: a focused review. Int J Molec Sci. 2021; 22(19):10222. https://doi.org/10.3390/ijms221910222.)

driving role of macrophages. High-grade meningiomas maintain increased peripheral myeloid-derived suppressor cells (MDSCs) and PD-L1+ monocytes.[110] In contrast, low-grade meningiomas maintain more "MDSC-like" monocytes with MDSC markers but no T-cell suppressive activity, with an overall increase in functional MDSCs.[111] These findings suggest a crucial role of MDSCs in meningioma induction.

PD-1 and PD-L1 expression on CD4+ and CD8+ cells are directly proportional to tumor grade.[110,112–114] PD-L1 is has been shown to predict worse outcomes and is associated with progression and recurrence.[115,116] Increased regulatory T-cell density is also associated with recurrence, and elevated levels of cytotoxic tumor-infiltrating lymphocytes are associated with prolonged PFS.[113,117] Additionally, meningioma location may affect T-cell infiltration. For example, Zador and colleagues found more oncolytic gamma-delta T-cells in skull base grade 1 meningiomas than in convexity meningiomas.[118] In contrast, Kosugi and colleagues[119] found lower immune cell infiltration in cavernous sinus meningiomas than in convexity meningiomas.

Mast cells have been identified in most high-grade meningiomas, primarily located in perivascular areas, and are associated with peritumoral edema and aggressiveness of meningiomas.[120] Notably, secretory tumors exhibit increased levels of mast cells and edema than nonsecretory tumors.[121] Convexity grade 1 meningiomas maintain more activated mast cells when compared with skull base meningiomas.[118] Additionally, dendritic cells are indicative of worse prognosis, and dendritic cell density is inversely proportional to B-cell density within these tumors.[122] The loss of B-cell presence likely leads to worse outcomes.[74]

Meningioma mutations generate neoantigens that are identified by antigen-presenting cells (APCs) and transferred to major histocompatibility complex molecules. The soluble neoantigen/APC complex travels via meningeal lymph vessels—also home to T-cells, B-cells, and dendritic cells—to deep cervical lymph nodes.[123,124] The contribution of the glymphatic system, draining into deep cervical lymph nodes via periarterial channels, is unclear.[125] Meningeal lymph vessels are much wider than periarterial channels, suggesting an easier path for the soluble neoantigen/APC complex.[126] Meningiomas may also increase permeability to proteins within cerebral vasculature, suggesting a loss of protection by immunoregulatory mechanisms and increased susceptibility to immune clearance.[74]

EMERGING APPROACHES/CLINICAL TRIALS

Immune check proteins (CTLA-4, PD-1, PD-L1) have been the primary target among treatment options for meningiomas. Gelerstein and colleagues[127] described one patient who received nivolumab and saw subsequent decrease in meningioma size. Nidamanuri and colleagues[112] described a retrospective cohort of 3 patients with meningiomas maintaining PD-1 or PD-L1 expressions who received pembrolizumab or nivolumab; they had median PFS of 2 years and median OS of 3 years. In a phase 2 study, Bi and colleagues[128] found nivolumab was well tolerated among patients with high-grade meningiomas that recurred after surgery and radiation. Patients maintained low levels of tumor mutational burden and tumor-infiltrating lymphocytes, and some patients appeared to benefit.[128] Overall, however, nivolumab failed to improve 6-month PFS.[128]

There have been multiple clinical trials evaluating the effectiveness of immunotherapies. These include evaluation of the effect of pembrolizumab on recurrent or residual high-grade meningiomas (NCT03279692) as well as pembrolizumab and stereotactic radiosurgery on grades 1 to 3 and recurrent meningiomas (NCT04659811). Nivolumab with or without ipilimumab and external beam radiation therapy is also being studied to treat recurrent high-grade meningiomas (NCT02648997). Another multi-institution trial is using nivolumab and stereotactic radiosurgery with or without ipilimumab to treat high-grade meningiomas (NCT03604978). Additional agents being examined include avelumab, which is being tested with proton therapy, and surgery to treat recurrent radiation/refractory meningiomas (NCT03267836), and cabozantinib, whose success in treating progressive or recurrent meningiomas is being sought (NCT05425004). Additional clinical trials have aimed to target specific mutations in meningiomas. The Alliance A071401 phase 2 trial (NCT02523014) aims to use SMO, AKT, or NF2 inhibitors for meningiomas harboring these specific mutations.

SUMMARY

Overall, medical treatment and molecular targeting in meningioma has undergone dramatic change because we have improved our understanding of molecular subtypes and biomarkers. These factors may result in improved selection of patients for clinical trials. In addition, newer immunomodulating treatments offer promise for the treatment of meningioma, especially in combination with traditional therapies.

DISCLOSURE

The authors do not report any significant conflicts of interest regarding this article.

DECLARATION OF INTERESTS

No conflicts of interest.

REFERENCES

1. Marosi C, Hassler M, Roessler K, et al. Meningioma. Crit Rev Oncol Hematol 2008;67(2):153–71.
2. Choy W, Kim W, Nagasawa D, et al. The molecular genetics and tumor pathogenesis of meningiomas and the future directions of meningioma treatments. Neurosurg Focus 2011;30(5):E6.
3. Louis DN, Perry A, Reifenberger G, et al. The 2016 World Health Organization Classification of Tumors of the Central Nervous System: a summary. Acta Neuropathol 2016;131(6):803–20.
4. Gritsch S, Batchelor TT, Gonzalez Castro LN. Diagnostic, therapeutic, and prognostic implications of the 2021 World Health Organization classification of tumors of the central nervous system. Cancer 2022;128(1):47–58.
5. Hasan S, Young M, Albert T, et al. The role of adjuvant radiotherapy after gross total resection of atypical meningiomas. World Neurosurg 2015; 83(5):808–15.
6. Sun SQ, Hawasli AH, Huang J, et al. An evidence-based treatment algorithm for the management of WHO Grade II and III meningiomas. Neurosurg Focus 2015;38(3):E3.
7. Chamberlain MC, Glantz MJ, Fadul CE. Recurrent meningioma: salvage therapy with long-acting somatostatin analogue. Neurology 2007;69(10): 969–73.

8. Kaley T, Barani I, Chamberlain M, et al. Historical benchmarks for medical therapy trials in surgery- and radiation-refractory meningioma: a RANO review. Neuro Oncol 2014;16(6):829–40.

9. Kaley TJ, Wen P, Schiff D, et al. Phase II trial of sunitinib for recurrent and progressive atypical and anaplastic meningioma. Neuro Oncol 2015;17(1):116–21.

10. Chamberlain MC, Glantz MJ. Interferon-alpha for recurrent World Health Organization grade 1 intracranial meningiomas. Cancer 2008;113(8):2146–51.

11. Samoto K, Ikezaki K, Ono M, et al. Expression of vascular endothelial growth factor and its possible relation with neovascularization in human brain tumors. Cancer Res 1995;55(5):1189–93.

12. Dharmalingam P, Roopesh Kumar VR, Verma SK. Vascular endothelial growth factor expression and angiogenesis in various grades and subtypes of meningioma. Indian J Pathol Microbiol 2013;56(4):349–54.

13. Lamszus K, Lengler U, Schmidt NO, et al. Vascular endothelial growth factor, hepatocyte growth factor/scatter factor, basic fibroblast growth factor, and placenta growth factor in human meningiomas and their relation to angiogenesis and malignancy. Neurosurgery 2000;46(4):938–47 [discussion: 947-948].

14. Matuschek C, Bölke E, Nawatny J, et al. Bevacizumab as a treatment option for radiation-induced cerebral necrosis. Strahlenther Onkol 2011;187(2):135–9.

15. Puchner MJA, Hans VH, Harati A, et al. Bevacizumab-induced regression of anaplastic meningioma. Ann Oncol 2010;21(12):2445–6.

16. Goutagny S, Raymond E, Sterkers O, et al. Radiographic regression of cranial meningioma in a NF2 patient treated by bevacizumab. Ann Oncol 2011;22(4):990–1.

17. Wilson TJ, Heth JA. Regression of a meningioma during paclitaxel and bevacizumab therapy for breast cancer. J Clin Neurosci 2012;19(3):468–9.

18. Lou E, Sumrall AL, Turner S, et al. Bevacizumab therapy for adults with recurrent/progressive meningioma: a retrospective series. J Neuro Oncol 2012;109(1):63–70.

19. Nayak L, Iwamoto FM, Rudnick JD, et al. Atypical and anaplastic meningiomas treated with bevacizumab. J Neuro Oncol 2012;109(1):187–93.

20. DeBoer R., Grimm S.A., Chandler J., et al., A phase II trial of PTK-787 (PTK/ZK) in recurrent or progressive meningiomas. J Neuro Oncol, 2008;26(15_suppl):2060.

21. Raizer JJ, Grimm SA, Rademaker A, et al. A phase II trial of PTK787/ZK 222584 in recurrent or progressive radiation and surgery refractory meningiomas. J Neuro Oncol 2014;117(1):93–101.

22. Bernatz S, Monden D, Gessler F, et al. Influence of VEGF-A, VEGFR-1-3, and neuropilin 1-2 on progression-free: and overall survival in WHO grade II and III meningioma patients. J Mol Histol 2021;52(2):233–43.

23. Raizer JJ, Abrey LE, Lassman AB, et al. A phase I trial of erlotinib in patients with nonprogressive glioblastoma multiforme postradiation therapy, and recurrent malignant gliomas and meningiomas. Neuro Oncol 2010;12(1):87–94.

24. Wen PY, Yung WK, Lamborn KR, et al. Phase II study of imatinib mesylate for recurrent meningiomas (North American Brain Tumor Consortium study 01-08). Neuro Oncol 2009;11(6):853–60.

25. Norden AD, Raizer JJ, Abrey LE, et al. Phase II trials of erlotinib or gefitinib in patients with recurrent meningioma. J Neuro Oncol 2010;96(2):211–7.

26. Schrell UM, Rittig MG, Anders M, et al. Hydroxyurea for treatment of unresectable and recurrent meningiomas. II. Decrease in the size of meningiomas in patients treated with hydroxyurea. J Neurosurg 1997;86(5):840–4.

27. Newton HB, Slivka MA, Stevens C. Hydroxyurea chemotherapy for unresectable or residual meningioma. J Neuro Oncol 2000;49(2):165–70.

28. Mason WP, Gentili F, Macdonald DR, et al. Stabilization of disease progression by hydroxyurea in patients with recurrent or unresectable meningioma. J Neurosurg 2002;97(2):341–6.

29. Rosenthal MA, Ashley DL, Cher L. Treatment of high risk or recurrent meningiomas with hydroxyurea. J Clin Neurosci 2002;9(2):156–8.

30. Loven D, Hardoff R, Sever ZB, et al. Non-resectable slow-growing meningiomas treated by hydroxyurea. J Neuro Oncol 2004;67(1–2):221–6.

31. Hahn BM, Schrell UM, Sauer R, et al. Prolonged oral hydroxyurea and concurrent 3d-conformal radiation in patients with progressive or recurrent meningioma: results of a pilot study. J Neuro Oncol 2005;74(2):157–65.

32. Weston GJ, Martin AJ, Mufti GJ, et al. Hydroxyurea treatment of meningiomas: a pilot study. Skull Base 2006;16(3):157–60.

33. Chamberlain MC, Johnston SK. Hydroxyurea for recurrent surgery and radiation refractory meningioma: a retrospective case series. J Neuro Oncol 2011;104(3):765–71.

34. Chamberlain MC. Hydroxyurea for recurrent surgery and radiation refractory high-grade meningioma. J Neuro Oncol 2012;107(2):315–21.

35. Reardon DA, Norden AD, Desjardins A, et al. Phase II study of Gleevec® plus hydroxyurea (HU) in adults with progressive or recurrent meningioma. J Neuro Oncol 2012;106(2):409–15.

36. Ragel BT, Gillespie DL, Kushnir V, et al. Calcium channel antagonists augment hydroxyurea- and ru486-induced inhibition of meningioma growth in vivo and in vitro. Neurosurgery 2006;59(5):1109–20 [discussion: 1120-1121].

37. Ragel BT, Couldwell WT, Wurster RD, et al. Chronic suppressive therapy with calcium channel antagonists for refractory meningiomas. Neurosurg Focus 2007;23(4):E10.

38. Jensen RL, Petr M, Wurster RD. Calcium channel antagonist effect on in vitro meningioma signal transduction pathways after growth factor stimulation. Neurosurgery 2000;46(3):692–702 [discussion: 702-703].

39. Kim MS, Yu DW, Jung YJ, et al. Long-term follow-up result of hydroxyurea chemotherapy for recurrent meningiomas. J Korean Neurosurg Soc 2012; 52(6):517–22.

40. Karsy M, Hoang N, Barth T, et al. Combined Hydroxyurea and Verapamil in the Clinical Treatment of Refractory Meningioma: Human and Orthotopic Xenograft Studies. World Neurosurg 2016;86: 210–9.

41. Grunberg SM, Weiss MH. Lack of efficacy of megestrol acetate in the treatment of unresectable meningioma. J Neuro Oncol 1990;8(1):61–5.

42. Jääskeläinen J, Laasonen E, Kärkkäinen J, et al. Hormone treatment of meningiomas: lack of response to medroxyprogesterone acetate (MPA). A pilot study of five cases. Acta Neurochir 1986; 80(1–2):35–41.

43. Grunberg SM, Weiss MH, Spitz IM, et al. Treatment of unresectable meningiomas with the antiprogesterone agent mifepristone. J Neurosurg 1991; 74(6):861–6.

44. Grunberg SM, Weiss MH, Russell CA, et al. Long-term administration of mifepristone (RU486): clinical tolerance during extended treatment of meningioma. Cancer Invest 2006;24(8):727–33.

45. Touat M, Lombardi G, Farina P, et al. Successful treatment of multiple intracranial meningiomas with the antiprogesterone receptor agent mifepristone (RU486). Acta Neurochir 2014;156(10):1831–5.

46. Lamberts SW, Tanghe HL, Avezaat CJ, et al. Mifepristone (RU 486) treatment of meningiomas. J Neurol Neurosurg Psychiatry 1992;55(6):486–90.

47. de Keizer RJ, Smit JW. Mifepristone treatment in patients with surgically incurable sphenoid-ridge meningioma: a long-term follow-up. Eye 2004; 18(9):954–8.

48. Cossu G, Levivier M, Daniel RT, et al. The role of mifepristone in meningiomas management: a systematic review of the literature. BioMed Res Int 2015;2015:267831.

49. Chamberlain MC. Adjuvant combined modality therapy for malignant meningiomas. J Neurosurg 1996;84(5):733–6.

50. Chamberlain MC, Tsao-Wei DD, Groshen S. Temozolomide for treatment-resistant recurrent meningioma. Neurology 2004;62(7):1210–2.

51. Gupta V, Su YS, Samuelson CG, et al. Irinotecan: a potential new chemotherapeutic agent for atypical or malignant meningiomas. J Neurosurg 2007; 106(3):455–62.

52. Preusser M, Spiegl-Kreinecker S, Lötsch D, et al. Trabectedin has promising antineoplastic activity in high-grade meningioma. Cancer 2012;118(20): 5038–49.

53. Balik V, Sulla I, Park HH, et al. In vitro testing to a panel of potential chemotherapeutics and current concepts of chemotherapy in benign meningiomas. Surg Oncol 2015;24(3):292–9.

54. Rünzi MW, Jaspers C, Windeck R, et al. Successful treatment of meningioma with octreotide. Lancet 1989;1(8646):1074.

55. García-Luna PP, Relimpio F, Pumar A, et al. Clinical use of octreotide in unresectable meningiomas. A report of three cases. J Neurosurg Sci 1993; 37(4):237–41.

56. Jaffrain-Rea ML, Minniti G, Santoro A, et al. Visual improvement during octreotide therapy in a case of episellar meningioma. Clin Neurol Neurosurg 1998;100(1):40–3.

57. Johnson DR, Kimmel DW, Burch PA, et al. Phase II study of subcutaneous octreotide in adults with recurrent or progressive meningioma and meningeal hemangiopericytoma. Neuro Oncol 2011; 13(5):530–5.

58. Simó M, Argyriou AA, Macià M, et al. Recurrent high-grade meningioma: a phase II trial with somatostatin analogue therapy. Cancer Chemother Pharmacol 2014;73(5):919–23.

59. Norden AD, Ligon KL, Hammond SN, et al. Phase II study of monthly pasireotide LAR (SOM230C) for recurrent or progressive meningioma. Neurology 2015;84(3):280–6.

60. Graillon T, Defilles C, Mohamed A, et al. Combined treatment by octreotide and everolimus: Octreotide enhances inhibitory effect of everolimus in aggressive meningiomas. J Neuro Oncol 2015;124(1): 33–43.

61. Louis DN, Perry A, Wesseling P, et al. The 2021 WHO Classification of Tumors of the Central Nervous System: a summary. Neuro Oncol 2021;23(8):1231–51.

62. Aizer AA, Abedalthagafi M, Bi WL, et al. A prognostic cytogenetic scoring system to guide the adjuvant management of patients with atypical meningioma. Neuro Oncol 2016;18(2):269–74.

63. Domingues PH, Sousa P, Otero Á, et al. Proposal for a new risk stratification classification for meningioma based on patient age, WHO tumor grade, size, localization, and karyotype. Neuro Oncol 2014;16(5):735–47.

64. Sahm F, Schrimpf D, Stichel D, et al. DNA methylation-based classification and grading system for meningioma: a multicentre, retrospective analysis. Lancet Oncol 2017;18(5):682–94.

65. Nassiri F, Mamatjan Y, Suppiah S, et al. DNA methylation profiling to predict recurrence risk in

meningioma: development and validation of a nomogram to optimize clinical management. Neuro Oncol 2019;21(7):901–10.

66. Weller M, Roth P, Sahm F, et al. Durable control of metastatic AKT1-mutant WHO Grade 1 meningothelial meningioma by the AKT inhibitor, AZD5363. J Natl Cancer Inst 2017;109(3):1–4.

67. Clark VE, Erson-Omay EZ, Serin A, et al. Genomic analysis of non-NF2 meningiomas reveals mutations in TRAF7, KLF4, AKT1, and SMO. Science 2013;339(6123):1077–80.

68. Bi WL, Zhang M, Wu WW, et al. Meningioma genomics: diagnostic, prognostic, and therapeutic applications. Front Surg 2016;3:40.

69. Youngblood MW, Miyagishima DF, Jin L, et al. Associations of meningioma molecular subgroup and tumor recurrence. Neuro Oncol 2021;23(5): 783–94.

70. Driver J, Hoffman SE, Tavakol S, et al. A molecularly integrated grade for meningioma. Neuro Oncol 2022;24(5):796–808.

71. Choudhury A, Magill ST, Eaton CD, et al. Meningioma DNA methylation groups identify biological drivers and therapeutic vulnerabilities. Nat Genet 2022;54(5):649–59.

72. Loewenstern J, Rutland J, Gill C, et al. Comparative genomic analysis of driver mutations in matched primary and recurrent meningiomas. Oncotarget 2019;10(37):3506–17.

73. Prager BC, Vasudevan HN, Dixit D, et al. The meningioma enhancer landscape delineates novel subgroups and drives druggable dependencies. Cancer Discov 2020;10(11):1722–41.

74. Kannapadi NV, Shah PP, Mathios D, et al. Synthesizing molecular and immune characteristics to move beyond WHO grade in meningiomas: a focused review. Front Oncol 2022;12:892004.

75. Nassiri F, Liu J, Patil V, et al. A clinically applicable integrative molecular classification of meningiomas. Nature 2021;597(7874):119–25.

76. Schmidt M, Mock A, Jungk C, et al. Transcriptomic analysis of aggressive meningiomas identifies PTTG1 and LEPR as prognostic biomarkers independent of WHO grade. Oncotarget 2016;7(12): 14551–68.

77. Pemov A, Dewan R, Hansen NF, et al. Comparative clinical and genomic analysis of neurofibromatosis type 2-associated cranial and spinal meningiomas. Sci Rep 2020;10(1):12563.

78. Goutagny S, Yang HW, Zucman-Rossi J, et al. Genomic profiling reveals alternative genetic pathways of meningioma malignant progression dependent on the underlying NF2 status. Clin Cancer Res 2010;16(16):4155–64.

79. Fèvre-Montange M, Champier J, Durand A, et al. Microarray gene expression profiling in meningiomas: differential expression according to grade or histopathological subtype. Int J Oncol 2009; 35(6):1395–407.

80. Patel AJ, Wan YW, Al-Ouran R, et al. Molecular profiling predicts meningioma recurrence and reveals loss of DREAM complex repression in aggressive tumors. Proc Natl Acad Sci U S A 2019;116(43):21715–26.

81. Sahm F, Schrimpf D, Olar A, et al. TERT promoter mutations and risk of recurrence in meningioma. J Natl Cancer Inst 2016;108(5):djv377.

82. Yesilöz Ü, Kirches E, Hartmann C, et al. Frequent AKT1E17K mutations in skull base meningiomas are associated with mTOR and ERK1/2 activation and reduced time to tumor recurrence. Neuro Oncol 2017;19(8):1088–96.

83. Boetto J, Bielle F, Sanson M, et al. SMO mutation status defines a distinct and frequent molecular subgroup in olfactory groove meningiomas. Neuro Oncol 2017;19(3):345–51.

84. Sievers P, Hielscher T, Schrimpf D, et al. CDKN2A/B homozygous deletion is associated with early recurrence in meningiomas. Acta Neuropathol 2020;140(3):409–13.

85. Bi WL, Wu WW, Santagata S, et al. Checkpoint inhibition in meningiomas. Immunotherapy 2016;8(6): 721–31.

86. Abedalthagafi M, Bi WL, Aizer AA, et al. Oncogenic PI3K mutations are as common as AKT1 and SMO mutations in meningioma. Neuro Oncol 2016;18(5): 649–55.

87. Barbera S, San Miguel T, Gil-Benso R, et al. Genetic changes with prognostic value in histologically benign meningiomas. Clin Neuropathol 2013; 32(4):311–7.

88. Maillo A, Orfao A, Espinosa AB, et al. Early recurrences in histologically benign/grade I meningiomas are associated with large tumors and coexistence of monosomy 14 and del(1p36) in the ancestral tumor cell clone. Neuro Oncol 2007; 9(4):438–46.

89. Pérez-Magán E, Rodríguez de Lope A, Ribalta T, et al. Differential expression profiling analyses identifies downregulation of 1p, 6q, and 14q genes and overexpression of 6p histone cluster 1 genes as markers of recurrence in meningiomas. Neuro Oncol 2010;12(12):1278–90.

90. Ruiz J, Martínez A, Hernández S, et al. Clinicopathological variables, immunophenotype, chromosome 1p36 loss and tumour recurrence of 247 meningiomas grade I and II. Histol Histopathol 2010;25(3):341–9.

91. Serna E, Morales JM, Mata M, et al. Gene expression profiles of metabolic aggressiveness and tumor recurrence in benign meningioma. PLoS One 2013;8(6):e67291.

92. Ho CY, Mosier S, Safneck J, et al. Genetic profiling by single-nucleotide polymorphism-based array

analysis defines three distinct subtypes of orbital meningioma. Brain Pathol 2015;25(2):193–201.

93. Agnihotri S, Suppiah S, Tonge PD, et al. Therapeutic radiation for childhood cancer drives structural aberrations of NF2 in meningiomas. Nat Commun 2017;8(1):186.

94. Paramasivam N, Hübschmann D, Toprak UH, et al. Mutational patterns and regulatory networks in epigenetic subgroups of meningioma. Acta Neuropathol 2019;138(2):295–308.

95. Kalamarides M, Stemmer-Rachamimov AO, Niwa-Kawakita M, et al. Identification of a progenitor cell of origin capable of generating diverse meningioma histological subtypes. Oncogene 2011; 30(20):2333–44.

96. Okano A, Miyawaki S, Hongo H, et al. Associations of pathological diagnosis and genetic abnormalities in meningiomas with the embryological origins of the meninges. Sci Rep 2021;11(1):6987.

97. Morin O, Chen WC, Nassiri F, et al. Integrated models incorporating radiologic and radiomic features predict meningioma grade, local failure, and overall survival. Neurooncol Adv 2019;1(1):vdz011.

98. Shin I, Park YW, Ahn SS, et al. Clinical and diffusion parameters may noninvasively predict TERT promoter mutation status in grade II meningiomas. J Neuroradiol 2022;49(1):59–65.

99. Bayley JCt, Hadley CC, Harmanci AO, et al. Multiple approaches converge on three biological subtypes of meningioma and extract new insights from published studies. Sci Adv 2022;8(5):eabm6247.

100. Behling F, Fodi C, Gepfner-Tuma I, et al. H3K27me3 loss indicates an increased risk of recurrence in the Tübingen meningioma cohort. Neuro Oncol 2021;23(8):1273–81.

101. Berghoff AS, Hielscher T, Ricken G, et al. Prognostic impact of genetic alterations and methylation classes in meningioma. Brain Pathol 2022; 32(2):e12970.

102. Katz LM, Hielscher T, Liechty B, et al. Loss of histone H3K27me3 identifies a subset of meningiomas with increased risk of recurrence. Acta Neuropathol 2018;135(6):955–63.

103. Maas SLN, Stichel D, Hielscher T, et al. Integrated molecular-morphologic meningioma classification: a multicenter retrospective analysis, retrospectively and prospectively validated. J Clin Oncol 2021; 39(34):3839–52.

104. Nassiri F, Wang JZ, Singh O, et al. Loss of H3K27me3 in meningiomas. Neuro Oncol 2021; 23(8):1282–91.

105. Olar A, Wani KM, Wilson CD, et al. Global epigenetic profiling identifies methylation subgroups associated with recurrence-free survival in meningioma. Acta Neuropathol 2017;133(3):431–44.

106. Pérez-Magán E, Campos-Martín Y, Mur P, et al. Genetic alterations associated with progression and recurrence in meningiomas. J Neuropathol Exp Neurol 2012;71(10):882–93.

107. Domingues PH, Teodósio C, Ortiz J, et al. Immunophenotypic identification and characterization of tumor cells and infiltrating cell populations in meningiomas. Am J Pathol 2012;181(5):1749–61.

108. Proctor DT, Huang J, Lama S, et al. Tumor-associated macrophage infiltration in meningioma. Neurooncol Adv 2019;1(1):vdz018.

109. Grund S, Schittenhelm J, Roser F, et al. The microglial/macrophagic response at the tumour-brain border of invasive meningiomas. Neuropathol Appl Neurobiol 2009;35(1):82–8.

110. Li YD, Veliceasa D, Lamano JB, et al. Systemic and local immunosuppression in patients with high-grade meningiomas. Cancer Immunol Immunother 2019;68(6):999–1009.

111. Pinton L, Solito S, Masetto E, et al. Immunosuppressive activity of tumor-infiltrating myeloid cells in patients with meningioma. OncoImmunology 2018;7(7):e1440931.

112. Nidamanuri P, Drappatz J. Immune checkpoint inhibitor therapy for recurrent meningiomas: a retrospective chart review. J Neuro Oncol 2022; 157(2):271–6.

113. Fang L, Lowther DE, Meizlish ML, et al. The immune cell infiltrate populating meningiomas is composed of mature, antigen-experienced T and B cells. Neuro Oncol 2013;15(11):1479–90.

114. Everson RG, Hashimoto Y, Freeman JL, et al. Multiplatform profiling of meningioma provides molecular insight and prioritization of drug targets for rational clinical trial design. J Neuro Oncol 2018; 139(2):469–78.

115. Garzon-Muvdi T, Bailey DD, Pernik MN, et al. Basis for immunotherapy for treatment of meningiomas. Front Neurol 2020;11:945.

116. Han SJ, Reis G, Kohanbash G, et al. Expression and prognostic impact of immune modulatory molecule PD-L1 in meningioma. J Neuro Oncol 2016;130(3):543–52.

117. Rapp C, Dettling S, Liu F, et al. Cytotoxic T cells and their activation status are independent prognostic markers in meningiomas. Clin Cancer Res 2019;25(17):5260–70.

118. Zador Z, Landry AP, Balas M, et al. Landscape of immune cell gene expression is unique in predominantly WHO grade 1 skull base meningiomas when compared to convexity. Sci Rep 2020;10(1): 9065.

119. Kosugi K, Tamura R, Ohara K, et al. Immunological and vascular characteristics in cavernous sinus meningioma. J Clin Neurosci 2019;67: 198–203.

120. Polyzoidis S, Koletsa T, Panagiotidou S, et al. Mast cells in meningiomas and brain inflammation. J Neuroinflammation 2015;12:170.

121. Tirakotai W, Mennel HD, Celik I, et al. Secretory meningioma: immunohistochemical findings and evaluation of mast cell infiltration. Neurosurg Rev 2006; 29(1):41–8.

122. Chen X, Tian F, Lun P, et al. Profiles of immune infiltration and its relevance to survival outcome in meningiomas. Biosci Rep 2020;40(5).

123. Yankova G, Bogomyakova O, Tulupov A. The glymphatic system and meningeal lymphatics of the brain: new understanding of brain clearance. Rev Neurosci 2021;32(7):693–705.

124. Louveau A, Smirnov I, Keyes TJ, et al. Structural and functional features of central nervous system lymphatic vessels. Nature 2015;523(7560):337–41.

125. Eide PK, Vatnehol SAS, Emblem KE, et al. Magnetic resonance imaging provides evidence of glymphatic drainage from human brain to cervical lymph nodes. Sci Rep 2018;8(1):7194.

126. Carare RO, Bernardes-Silva M, Newman TA, et al. Solutes, but not cells, drain from the brain parenchyma along basement membranes of capillaries and arteries: significance for cerebral amyloid angiopathy and neuroimmunology. Neuropathol Appl Neurobiol 2008;34(2):131–44.

127. Gelerstein E, Berger A, Jonas-Kimchi T, et al. Regression of intracranial meningioma following treatment with nivolumab: Case report and review of the literature. J Clin Neurosci 2017;37:51–3.

128. Bi WL, Nayak L, Meredith DM, et al. Activity of PD-1 blockade with nivolumab among patients with recurrent atypical/anaplastic meningioma: phase II trial results. Neuro Oncol 2022;24(1):101–13.

129. Chamberlain MC, Tsao-Wei DD, Groshen S. Salvage chemotherapy with CPT-11 for recurrent meningioma. J Neuro Oncol 2006;78(3):271–6.

130. Kaba SE, DeMonte F, Bruner JM, et al. The treatment of recurrent unresectable and malignant meningiomas with interferon alpha-2B. Neurosurgery 1997;40(2):271–5.

131. Muhr C, Gudjonsson O, Lilja A, et al. Meningioma treated with interferon-alpha, evaluated with [(11) C]-L-methionine positron emission tomography. Clin Cancer Res 2001;7(8):2269–76.

132. Markwalder TM, Seiler RW, Zava DT. Antiestrogenic therapy of meningiomas–a pilot study. Surg Neurol 1985;24(3):245–9.

133. Goodwin JW, Crowley J, Eyre HJ, et al. A phase II evaluation of tamoxifen in unresectable or refractory meningiomas: a Southwest Oncology Group study. J Neuro Oncol 1993;15(1):75–7.

134. Nunes FP, Merker VL, Jennings D, et al. Bevacizumab treatment for meningiomas in NF2: a retrospective analysis of 15 patients. PLoS One 2013; 8(3):e59941.

135. Shih KC, Chowdhary S, Rosenblatt P, et al. A phase II trial of bevacizumab and everolimus as treatment for patients with refractory, progressive intracranial meningioma. J Neuro Oncol 2016;129(2):281–8.

136. Cardona AF, Ruiz-Patiño A, Zatarain-Barrón ZL, et al. Systemic management of malignant meningiomas: A comparative survival and molecular marker analysis between octreotide in combination with everolimus and sunitinib. PLoS One 2019; 14(6):e0217340.

137. Brastianos PK, Kim AE, Giobbie-Hurder A, et al. Phase 2 study of pembrolizumab in patients with recurrent and residual high-grade meningiomas. Nat Commun 2022;13(1):1325.

Advanced Meningioma Imaging

Erik K. Loken, MD, PhD*, Raymond Y. Huang, MD, PhD

KEYWORDS

- Magnetic resonance imaging • Dotatate PET • Radiomic • Diffusion • Perfusion

KEY POINTS

- Due to its high sensitivity and specificity for somastatin receptor abundant in meningiomas, 68GA DOTATATE PET has many potential clinical applications in the diagnosis and management of meningioma.
- Radiomics approach to imaging of meningioma has shown promising results in predicting tumor grade, brain invasion, and tumor recurrence but need validation with multicenter, prospective data sets.
- ADC values in meningiomas show potential for differentiating benign from atypical or malignant tumors, however lack of a validated threshold limits reliability.

INTRODUCTION

The introduction of computed tomography (CT) and MRI greatly improved the use of imaging in the diagnosis and management of meningiomas.[1,2] These technologies, when paired with intravenous contrast, showed patterns of growth of meningiomas, their dural spread, and their variable involvement of adjacent bone. These insights in addition to the resolution between the meningioma and neighboring tissue provided by cross sectional imaging have led to improved surgical planning. CT and MR angiography also allowed for more detailed study of relevant vascular relationships to meningiomas under investigation.[3] Advanced imaging techniques such as nuclear scintigraphy or PET can be used to identify residual or recurrent tumor by using specific characteristics of meningiomas, for example, binding of radiolabeled octreotide to tumor-specific somatostatin receptors.

CT and MRI now frequently allow the incidental discovery of meningiomas in asymptomatic patients. The ability to track tumor growth with these noninvasive methods has increased interest in predicting tumor behavior and grade based on imaging features alone. Conventional imaging techniques and more advanced imaging techniques such as MR spectroscopy and PET are now used to aid in prediction of tumor behavior from imaging characteristics.

The application of machine learning methods to evaluate intracranial tumors including meningiomas has greatly increased during the last decade due to the availability of computing resources and also large clinical, molecular, and imaging database among major cancer centers. These methods generally include computing radiomic feature-derived preoperative MRI, PET, CT, or a combination of these imaging modalities[4] to construct diagnostic or prognostic models that aim to predict tumor characteristics such as tumor grade, tumor consistency, brain invasion, or clinical course such as tumor recurrence or patient survival.

IMAGING FEATURES OF MENINGIOMAS

Meningiomas usually are found as intracranial extra-axial masses that are attached to the dura mater and originate from meningoepithelial cells (arachnoid cap cells), typically occurring where

Department of Radiology, Brigham and Women's Hospital, Harvard Medical School, 75 Francis Street, Boston, MA 02115, USA
* Corresponding author.
E-mail address: eloken@bwh.harvard.edu

Neurosurg Clin N Am 34 (2023) 335–345
https://doi.org/10.1016/j.nec.2023.02.015
1042-3680/23/© 2023 Elsevier Inc. All rights reserved.

they are most numerous, for example, the arachnoid granulations along the dural venous sinuses.[5] Meningiomas are usually solitary, with a case series demonstrating multiple meningiomas occurring in about 8.9% of cases.[6] Approximately half of all intracranial meningiomas are located along the skull base, 40% along the calvarial convexities, 10% along the falx/parasagittal region, and a small proportion within the ventricles or involving multiple areas.[7,8] Meningiomas are mostly found within these locations as primarily intradural tumors; however, approximately 1% to 2% are extradural and occur outside of the dura, including in the calvarium as a primary intraosseous meningioma, scalp, paranasal sinuses, nasopharynx, neck, and skin.[9,10]

APPEARANCE ON COMPUTED TOMOGRAPHY

On CT, meningiomas typically appear as homogeneous, hyperdense masses that enhance homogeneously after contrast administration (**Fig. 1**).[5,11] They typically have sharply circumscribed borders with a broad-based dural attachment.[5] Meningiomas are classically associated with intratumoral calcification, with some subtypes showing dystrophic or metaplastic calcification giving a more speckled hyperdense appearance in 15% to 20% of cases.[12] Bony changes such as hyperostosis, osteolysis, and pneumosinus dilatans, which can be seen in anterior skull base meningiomas. The most common of the bony findings in meningioma is hyperostosis, seen as bony thickening on CT, which is seen in up to 25% to 49% of meningiomas.[13] Hyperostosis may be reactive or a result of tumor invasion, with tumor invasion more likely if there is strong enhancement within the hyperostotic bone.

APPEARANCE ON MAGNETIC RESONANCE IMAGING

Meningiomas are typically hypointense to isointense on T1-weighted MRI sequences and isointense to hyperintense on T2-weighted sequences (**Fig. 2**).[5,14] Most meningiomas demonstrate avid enhancement on MRI, and a dural tail will be seen in up to 72% of meningiomas.[11] The dural tail itself may only represent reactive changes; however, a study has shown that nearly two-thirds of dural tails show invasion by tumor cells.[15,16] Although dural tails are not entirely specific to meningioma, the feature can be used to confirm extra-axial location for meningiomas that appear inseparable from brain parenchyma on imaging. Moreover, some extra-axial tumors such as schwannomas and pituitary adenomas do not typically show a dural tail.

As meningiomas increase in size, they will cause inward displacement of the underlying brain tissue.[5] The presence of a cleft of cerebrospinal fluid (CSF) between the tumor and the brain can help define the tumor as extra-axial, although it should be noted that these CSF clefts may be absent, for example, when there is brain parenchymal invasion. Less typical findings, which have been described in meningioma include tumor necrosis, cystic change, hemorrhage, and fatty infiltration.[17] Edema in the brain adjacent to a meningioma is seen in slightly over half of meningiomas and this finding is not well correlated with tumor size.[18,19] Edema may be secondary to brain parenchymal invasion by the tumor; however, it is also seen in WHO grade 1 meningiomas that are not showing invasion and, therefore, is not a reliable distinguishing feature between benign and atypical or malignant meningiomas. Multiple proposed causes may explain the presence of edema without invasion, for example, compressive ischemia with compromise of the blood–brain barrier, vascular shunting due to parasitization of pial microvessels, mechanical venous obstruction, elevated hydrostatic pressure within the tumor, and secretory-excretory phenomena within the tumor cells.[12,20,21]

The typical findings on MR spectroscopy are elevated choline and alanine with diminished N-acetylaspartate.[22,23] The finding of elevated alanine is relatively specific for meningioma; however, this is of more limited utility because the alanine peak can be difficult to identify.

MR perfusion typically demonstrates high relative cerebral blood flow (rCBF) and high relative cerebral blood volume (rCBV; see **Fig. 2**). In dynamic susceptibility contrast technique, less than 50% return to baseline signal intensity has been described in meningiomas, limiting rCBV quantitation.[24,25] Arterial spin labeling (ASL) perfusion and dynamic contrast-enhanced perfusion techniques have also been investigated, and rCBF has been shown to be increased with ASL, particularly the angiomatous histological subtype.[26–28]

Atypical and malignant meningiomas have a more compact architecture with smaller and tightly packed cells with a high nucleus-to-cytoplasm ratio, which is expected to decrease water diffusivity resulting in lower apparent diffusion coefficient (ADC) values on diffusion-weighted imaging.[29–31] Several studies have evaluated the ability of ADC values to differentiate benign from atypical/malignant meningiomas but their conclusions vary. Some studies found no statistically significant difference in ADC values between benign and atypical/malignant meningiomas,[29,32–35] whereas others found that atypical/malignant meningiomas

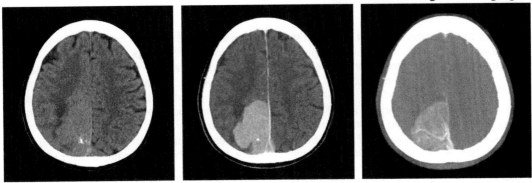

Fig. 1. CT imaging demonstrating calcification within a parasagittal meningioma. It demonstrates avid enhancement. Angiography for surgical planning shows prominent draining vessels with invasion of the superior sagittal sinus.

have lower ADC values. Some limitations that may account for the variability in findings are histological criteria and imaging methodology.[24,30,31,36–39] ADC cutoff values have been suggested to categorize meningiomas by grade.[30,31] Although an inverse correlation between ADC values and tumor microstructure of meningiomas was established, a review of ADC and meningioma found no validated threshold for ADC to reliably distinguish benign from high-grade meningiomas.[40] A limitation of ADC is that it can be altered to a lower than expected value due to calcification, a typical finding in meningioma and one which is also associated with a more indolent clinical course, possibly causing misclassifications by analysis of ADC and limiting the predictive value.[41]

POSITRON EMISSION TOMOGRAPHY

Although MRI provides exquisite structural details that are critical for the diagnosis and management of meningiomas, PET imaging methods with

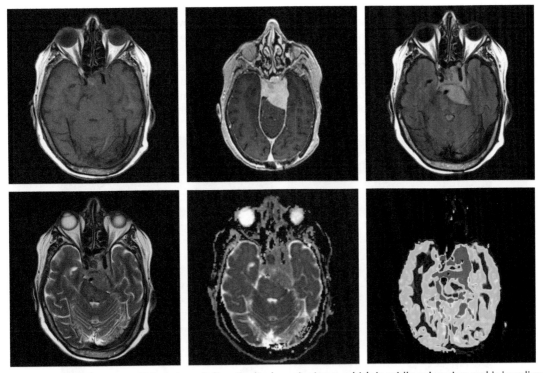

Fig. 2. MRI demonstrates a T1 isointense left petroclival meningioma, which is avidly enhancing and is invading the bilateral cavernous sinuses and the sella with encasement of the pituitary. It is moderately hyperintense on FLAIR imaging and isointense to slightly hyperintense on T2-weighted images. Intermediate signal on ADC suggests the meningioma may be of more moderate grade. The corrected rCBV map shows increased blood volume in the areas of the mass.

radiotracers that specifically target somatostatin receptors are increasingly utilized for diagnosis and treatment planning of meningiomas. Because most meningiomas express somatostatin receptors,[42,43] radiotracers based on somatostatin such as 68Ga-DOTATOC and 68Ga-DOTATATE are sensitive in detecting meningiomas[44,45] (**Fig. 3**). Compared with 68Ga-DOTATOC, 68Ga-DOTATATE has 10 times the affinity to somatostatin receptor 2[46] and is recommended for the applications of meningioma imaging.[47] 68Ga-DOTATATE PET can improve the sensitivity of detecting intracranial meningiomas compared to MRI.[48] For small lesions and in certain anatomic locations such as those near the petroclival ligament, MRI has much lower sensitivity than 68Ga-DOTATATE PET.[49]

An important differential diagnosis for meningioma with similar structural MRI appearances is dural-based metastasis. Although follow-up imaging should allow one to differentiate meningiomas from metastases because the latter typically grow at a much higher rate, earlier diagnosis of meningioma can confirm staging of systemic cancer. In a retrospective study of patients with meningiomas and dural metastases using 68Ga DOTA-NOC PET/CT, intense tracer uptake was observed in almost all the cases, whereas dural metastases showed much lower uptake that is visually discernible.[50] Although this promising result needs further validation with larger trials, it is important to consider a number of other intracranial tumors, including glioma, pituitary adenoma, medulloblastoma, primitive neuroectodermal tumors, solitary fibrous tumor, and hemangioblastoma that express SSTR2 and can confound the diagnosis of meningioma[51,52] (**Figs. 4** and **5**).

Although uptake of 68Ga-DOTATATE has not been shown to correlate with WHO grades of meningioma, growth rates in grade-1 and grade-2 meningiomas have been associated with radiotracer uptake.[53] This may provide guidance for how meningioma should be managed, with those more likely to have a greater growth rate being treated earlier.

DIFFERENTIAL DIAGNOSIS

The imaging appearance of meningiomas or suspected meningiomas informs the differential diagnosis, and findings can be used to narrow the differential diagnosis. There are several conditions that can mimic meningiomas, such as metastasis of tumors, lymphoma and leukemia, solitary fibrous tumors, and hemangiopericytoma. Solitary fibrous tumor and hemangiopericytoma are part of a spectrum of tumors that can be difficult to distinguish from angiomatous meningiomas.[54] Texture analysis of magnetic resonance images has been shown to be potentially useful in distinguishing solitary fibrous tumors from meningioma.[54] Moreover, normalized ADC values from diffusion-weighted imaging and ADC histogram analysis have been shown to be potentially reliable tools to differentiate solitary fibrous tumors from meningioma.[55,56]

Sarcoidosis and tuberculosis may also cause enhancing dural masses, more likely to be multiple than meningioma. Diffuse dural thickening may be seen in idiopathic hypertrophic pachymeningitis,

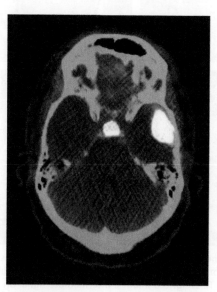
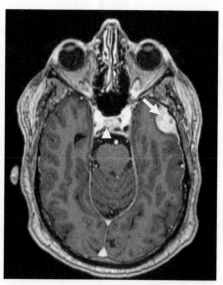

Fig. 3. 68Ga-DOTATATE PET/CT and MRI. 68Ga-DOTATATE uptake in a left middle cranial fossa meningioma (*arrow*), and in a normal pituitary gland (*arrowhead*).

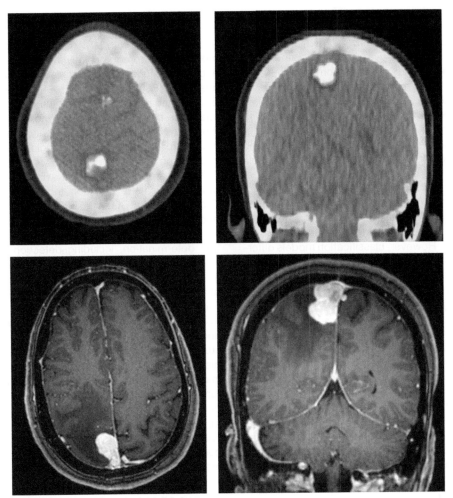

Fig. 4. 68Ga-DOTATATE PET/CT and MRI. 68Ga-DOTATATE uptake in a solitary fibrous tumor (also known as hemangiopericytoma).

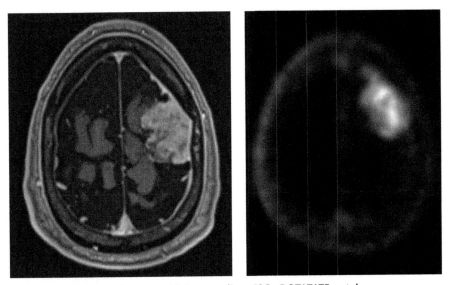

Fig. 5. Recurrent extra-axial glioblastoma with intermediate 68Ga-DOTATATE uptake.

extranodal sinus histiocytosis,[57] and IgG4-related disease, which may seem similar to en plaque and multiple meningioma.[11] Particular findings suggestive of alternative diagnoses rather than meningioma could include homogeneous T2 signal, which is hyperintense or hypointense to what is expected, findings of osseous destruction, leptomeningeal disease, and the absence of a dural tail.[58]

Chakrabarty and colleagues developed a deep learning model based on MRI data from multiple public and internal databases to differentiate meningiomas from other different intracranial tumor types.[59] Although such classification models may be helpful clinically, differentiating intra-axial versus extra-axial tumors tend not to be clinically challenging. However, classification models differentiating intracranial hemangiopericytoma from angiomatous meningioma may improve preoperative planning.[60]

GRADING OF MENINGIOMA

Prediction of WHO grades of meningioma based on preoperative MRI can provide prognosis and guide management. Tumor grading models that divide low grade (WHO grade 1) versus high grades (WHO grade 2 and 3) may be valuable in deciding surgical versus nonsurgical treatment.[61–65] Morin and colleagues[66] trained an integrated model that classifies WHO grade 1 from grade 2 and grade 3 meningiomas and also provides prediction for local failure and overall survival.

TREATMENT PLANNING

Meningiomas are considered slow-growing lesions often with an indolent clinical course.[67] Meningiomas are often discovered incidentally, and for an asymptomatic tumor where treatment is not mandatory, it has been recommended that linear growth be documented in at least 3 serial MRI scans during period greater than 1.5 years.[68] Prospective studies have shown that the tendency of meningiomas is to grow but that over half of meningiomas show a self-limited growth pattern.[68,69]

68Ga-DOTATATE PET provides additional advantages in delineating the extent of tumor boundary, thus has potential clinical utilities in treatment planning and treatment monitoring for meningiomas. For meningiomas that involve osseous structures or dural venous sinuses, defining extent of tumor can be challenging using MRI techniques. Such difficulties can be much more exacerbated in postoperative or postradiotherapy settings with distorted anatomy and presence of scarring.

68Ga-DOTATATE PET/CT has been shown to improve the detection of transosseous meningiomas compared with MRI[70] and help discover tumor remnants predominantly in Simpson grade 1 and 2 resections that are not visible in intraoperative MRI.[71] 68Ga-DOTATATE PET/CT can reliably discriminate between recurrent tumor and scar tissue after previous surgery or radiotherapy and thus may have utilities as a monitoring imaging marker for posttreatment meningiomas that are challenging to evaluate with MRI[72,73] (Fig. 6).

Accurate delineation of the extent of meningioma is critical for radiation treatment planning. The use of 68Ga-DOTATATE PET/CT in the preradiation treatment planning of meningiomas can improve the accuracy of tumor volume and location determination, including detection of tumor not visible on MRI and avoiding nontumor tissues from treatment field, leading to more precise radiation delivery and potentially better outcomes.[74–79]

Diagnosis of brain invasion based on radiomic features derived from the interface between tumor and brain can also help surgical planning.[80,81] A study using an MRI nomogram showed potential discriminatory ability for predicting brain invasion in meningioma with tumor shape, boundary, peritumoral edema, and maximum diameter as independent predictors for brain invasion.[82] Finally, tumor consistency can affect the extent of resection and various surgical outcomes,[83] and has been correlated with radiomic features for preoperative prediction.[84]

RESPONSE PREDICTION AND RESPONSE ASSESSMENT

High expression of somatostatin receptor has been associated with longer progression-free survival after therapy.[85] The somatostatin receptor-expression pattern identified by 68Ga-DOTATOC/DOTATATE PET can help predict the response of a meningioma to somatostatin analog therapy.[85]

Following radiation treatment, mean total lesion activity 68 Ga-DOTATATE PET decreased 14.7%, whereas meningioma volumes based on MRI measurements did not significantly change.[86] Similarly, following gamma knife radiosurgery the 68Ga-DOTATOC PET SUV (standardized uptake value) of meningiomas was reduced in 7 out of 12 patients (58%), stable in 2 out of 12 (17%), and increased in 3 out of 12 (25%).[87] The measurable response by 68Ga-DOTATOC and 68Ga-DOTATATE PET needs to be correlated with longer term endpoints to confirm if they can be valuable tools in assessing clinically meaningful treatment response.

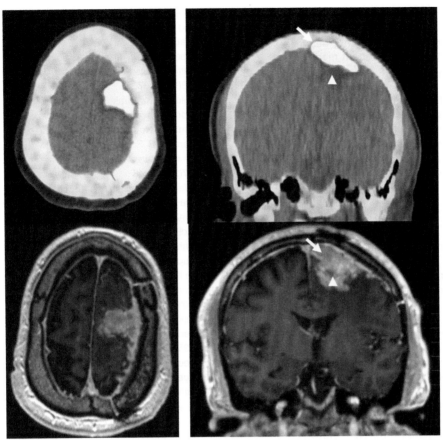

Fig. 6. 68Ga-DOTATATE PET/CT and MRI. 68Ga-DOTATATE uptake in active recurrent meningioma (*arrow*). Enhancing tissues from radiation treatment do not demonstrate 68Ga-DOTATATE uptake (*arrowhead*).

FUTURE DIRECTIONS

Although there are numerous studies reporting results supporting the clinical use of machine learning approach to facilitate meningioma management, most of these studies are limited by their cohort size and lack of sufficient validation with independent data sets. For clinical translation of these machine learning models, there is a need to validate their reproducibility and generalizability using large data set from multi-institutional sources as well as prospective validation.

SUMMARY

CT and MRI continue to have a central role in treatment and management of meningioma, with their usefulness in determining location, growth, and relationship to adjacent tissue and structures. 68Ga-DOTATATE PET has increasingly important roles for the diagnosis and treatment planning of intracranial meningiomas. It can complement structural MRI by increasing specificity of diagnosis, outlining regions of tumors for more precise surgical and radiation planning, and detecting residual or recurrent tumor. Considered together, these techniques may be used in the prediction of tumor grade and prediction of tumor behavior, allowing improved clinical management of meningioma.

CLINICS CARE POINTS

- Typical appearance of meningiomas on CT: homogeneous, hyperdense mass with sharply circumscribed borders and a broad-based dural attachment.

- Typical apperance of meningiomas on MRI: hypo- to isointense on T1-weighted sequences, iso- to hyperintense on T2-weighted sequences, and avid enhancement with a dural tail in up to 72% of cases.

- The dural tail is not entirely specific to meningioma and cannot be solely relied upon for diagnosis.

- Edema in the brain adjacent to a meningioma is not well correlated with tumor size and is not a reliable distinguisher between benign and atypical or malignant meningiomas.
- PET imaging methods with radiotracers targeting somatostatin receptors (e.g., 68Ga-DOTATOC and 68Ga-DOTATATE) are increasingly used for meningioma diagnosis and treatment planning.
- 68Ga-DOTATAE PET can help delineate tumor boundaries, aiding in treatment planning and monitoring.

DISCLOSURE

E.K. Loken: No disclosures. R.Y. Huang: Vysioneer, Paid scientific advisory. Nuvation Bio, paid consultant. Bristol Myers Squibb: Research support paid to institution.

REFERENCES

1. Lauterbur PC. Image formation by induced local interactions: examples employing nuclear magnetic resonance. Nature 1973;242(5394):190–1.
2. Hounsfield GN. Computerized transverse axial scanning (tomography): Part 1. Description of system. Br J Radiol 1973;46(552):1016–22.
3. Bi WL, Brown PA, Abolfotoh M, et al. Utility of dynamic computed tomography angiography in the preoperative evaluation of skull base tumors. J Neurosurg 2015;123(1):1–8.
4. Galldiks N, Angenstein F, Werner J, et al. Use of advanced neuroimaging and artificial intelligence in meningiomas. Brain Pathol 2022;32(2):e13015.
5. Buetow MP, Buetow PC, Smirniotopoulos J. Typical, atypical, and misleading features in meningioma. Radiographics 1991;11(6):1087–106.
6. Lusins JO, Nakagawa H. Multiple meningiomas evaluated by computed tomography. Neurosurgery 1981;9(2):137–41.
7. Magill ST, Young JS, Chae R, et al. Relationship between tumor location, size, and WHO grade in meningioma. Neurosurg Focus 2018;44(4):E4.
8. Wang D jun, Xie Q, Gong Y, et al. Histopathological classification and location of consecutively operated meningiomas at a single institution in China from 2001 to 2010. Chin Med J (Engl) 2013;126(3):488–93.
9. Chen TC. Primary intraosseous meningioma. Neurosurg Clin 2016;27(2):189–93.
10. Lang FF, Macdonald OK, Fuller GN, et al. Primary extradural meningiomas: a report on nine cases and review of the CT-era literature. J Neurosurg 2000;93(6):940–50.
11. O'leary S, Adams W, Parrish R, et al. Atypical imaging appearances of intracranial meningiomas. Clin Radiol 2007;62(1):10–7.
12. Sheporaitis L, Osborn A, Smirniotopoulos J, et al. Intracranial meningioma. Am J Neuroradiol 1992;13(1):29–37.
13. Bikmaz K, Mrak R, Al-Mefty O. Management of bone-invasive, hyperostotic sphenoid wing meningiomas. J Neurosurg 2007;107(5):905–12.
14. Tamrazi B, Shiroishi MS, Liu CSJ. Advanced imaging of intracranial meningiomas. Neurosurg Clin 2016;27(2):137–43.
15. Wen M, Jung S, Moon KS, et al. Immunohistochemical profile of the dural tail in intracranial meningiomas. Acta Neurochir 2014;156(12):2263–73.
16. Aoki S, Sasaki Y, Machida T, et al. Contrast-enhanced MR images in patients with meningioma: importance of enhancement of the dura adjacent to the tumor. Am J Neuroradiol 1990;11(5):935–8.
17. Russell EJ, George AE, Kricheff II, et al. Atypical computed tomography features of intracranial meningioma: radiological-pathological correlation in a series of 131 consecutive cases. Radiology 1980;135(3):673–82.
18. Lee KJ, Joo WI, Rha HK, et al. Peritumoral brain edema in meningiomas: correlations between magnetic resonance imaging, angiography, and pathology. Surg Neurol 2008;69(4):350–5.
19. Yoshioka H, Hama S, Taniguchi E, et al. Peritumoral brain edema associated with meningioma: influence of vascular endothelial growth factor expression and vascular blood supply. Cancer Interdiscip Int J Am Cancer Soc 1999;85(4):936–44.
20. Tamiya T, Ono Y, Matsumoto K, et al. Peritumoral brain edema in intracranial meningiomas: effects of radiological and histological factors. Neurosurgery 2001;49(5):1046–52.
21. Go GK, Wilmink JT, Molenaar WM. Peritumoral brain edema associated with meningiomas. Neurosurgery 1988;23(2):175–9.
22. Kousi E, Tsougos I, Fountas K, et al. Distinct peak at 3.8 ppm observed by 3T MR spectroscopy in meningiomas, while nearly absent in high-grade gliomas and cerebral metastases. Mol Med Rep 2012;5(4):1011–8.
23. Demir MK, Iplikcioglu AC, Dincer A, et al. Single voxel proton MR spectroscopy findings of typical and atypical intracranial meningiomas. Eur J Radiol 2006;60(1):48–55.
24. Hakyemez B, Yildirim N, Erdoðan C, et al. Meningiomas with conventional MRI findings resembling intra-axial tumors: can perfusion-weighted MRI be helpful in differentiation? Neuroradiology 2006;48(10):695–702.
25. Cha S, Knopp EA, Johnson G, et al. Intracranial mass lesions: dynamic contrast-enhanced susceptibility-weighted echo-planar perfusion MR imaging. Radiology 2002;223(1):11–29.

26. Keil VC, Pintea B, Gielen GH, et al. Meningioma assessment: kinetic parameters in dynamic contrast-enhanced MRI appear independent from microvascular anatomy and VEGF expression. J Neuroradiol 2018;45(4):242–8.

27. Koizumi S, Sakai N, Kawaji H, et al. Pseudo-continuous arterial spin labeling reflects vascular density and differentiates angiomatous meningiomas from non-angiomatous meningiomas. J Neuro Oncol 2015;121(3):549–56.

28. Qiao XJ, Kim HG, Wang DJ, et al. Application of arterial spin labeling perfusion MRI to differentiate benign from malignant intracranial meningiomas. Eur J Radiol 2017;97:31–6.

29. Sanverdi SE, Ozgen B, Oguz KK, et al. Is diffusion-weighted imaging useful in grading and differentiating histopathological subtypes of meningiomas? Eur J Radiol 2012;81(9):2389–95.

30. Tang Y, Dundamadappa SK, Thangasamy S, et al. Correlation of apparent diffusion coefficient with Ki-67 proliferation index in grading meningioma. AJR Am J Roentgenol 2014;202(6):1303–8.

31. Nagar V, Ye J, Ng W, et al. Diffusion-weighted MR imaging: diagnosing atypical or malignant meningiomas and detecting tumor dedifferentiation. Am J Neuroradiol 2008;29(6):1147–52.

32. Yamasaki F, Kurisu K, Satoh K, et al. Apparent diffusion coefficient of human brain tumors at MR imaging. Radiology 2005;235(3):985–91.

33. Ginat DT, Mangla R, Yeaney G, et al. Correlation of diffusion and perfusion MRI with Ki-67 in high-grade meningiomas. Am J Roentgenol 2010;195(6):1391–5.

34. Pavlisa G, Rados M, Pazanin L, et al. Characteristics of typical and atypical meningiomas on ADC maps with respect to schwannomas. Clin Imaging 2008; 32(1):22–7.

35. Santelli L, Ramondo G, Della Puppa A, et al. Diffusion-weighted imaging does not predict histological grading in meningiomas. Acta Neurochir 2010; 152(8):1315–9.

36. Watanabe Y, Yamasaki F, Kajiwara Y, et al. Preoperative histological grading of meningiomas using apparent diffusion coefficient at 3T MRI. Eur J Radiol 2013;82(4):658–63.

37. Filippi CG, Edgar MA, Uluğ AM, et al. Appearance of meningiomas on diffusion-weighted images: correlating diffusion constants with histopathologic findings. Am J Neuroradiol 2001;22(1):65–72.

38. Toh CH, Castillo M, Wong AC, et al. Differentiation between classic and atypical meningiomas with use of diffusion tensor imaging. Am J Neuroradiol 2008;29(9):1630–5.

39. Yin B, Liu L, Zhang BY, et al. Correlating apparent diffusion coefficients with histopathologic findings on meningiomas. Eur J Radiol 2012;81(12):4050–6.

40. Meyer HJ, Wienke A, Surov A. ADC values of benign and high grade meningiomas and associations with tumor cellularity and proliferation–A systematic review and meta-analysis. J Neurol Sci 2020;415: 116975.

41. Schwyzer L, Berberat J, Remonda L, et al. Susceptibility changes in meningiomas influence the apparent diffusion coefficient in diffusion-weighted MRI. J Neuroradiol 2015;42(6):332–7.

42. Menke JR, Raleigh DR, Gown AM, et al. Somatostatin receptor 2a is a more sensitive diagnostic marker of meningioma than epithelial membrane antigen. Acta Neuropathol 2015;130(3):441–3.

43. Dutour A, Kumar U, Panetta R, et al. Expression of somatostatin receptor subtypes in human brain tumors. Int J Cancer 1998;76(5):620–7.

44. Poeppel TD, Binse I, Petersenn S, et al. 68Ga-DOTATOC versus 68Ga-DOTATATE PET/CT in functional imaging of neuroendocrine tumors. J Nucl Med 2011;52(12):1864–70.

45. Reubi JC, Schär JC, Waser B, et al. Affinity profiles for human somatostatin receptor subtypes SST1–SST5 of somatostatin radiotracers selected for scintigraphic and radiotherapeutic use. Eur J Nucl Med 2000;27(3):273–82.

46. Soto-Montenegro ML, Peña-Zalbidea S, Mateos-Pérez JM, et al. Meningiomas: a comparative study of 68Ga-DOTATOC, 68Ga-DOTANOC and 68Ga-DOTATATE for molecular imaging in mice. PLoS One 2014;9(11):e111624.

47. Galldiks N, Albert NL, Sommerauer M, et al. PET imaging in patients with meningioma—report of the RANO/PET Group. Neuro Oncol 2017;19(12):1576–87.

48. Afshar-Oromieh A, Giesel FL, Linhart HG, et al. Detection of cranial meningiomas: comparison of 68Ga-DOTATOC PET/CT and contrast-enhanced MRI. Eur J Nucl Med Mol Imaging 2012;39(9):1409–15.

49. Einhellig HC, Siebert E, Bauknecht HC, et al. Comparison of diagnostic value of 68 Ga-DOTATOC PET/MRI and standalone MRI for the detection of intracranial meningiomas. Sci Rep 2021;11(1):1–9.

50. Purandare NC, Puranik A, Shah S, et al. Differentiating dural metastases from meningioma: role of 68Ga DOTA-NOC PET/CT. Nucl Med Commun 2020;41(4):356–62.

51. Cleary JO, Yeung J, McMeekin H, et al. The significance of incidental brain uptake on 68Ga-DOTATATE PET-CT in neuroendocrine tumour patients. Nucl Med Commun 2016;37(11):1197–205.

52. Bashir A, Broholm H, Clasen-Linde E, et al. Pearls and pitfalls in interpretation of 68Ga-DOTATOC PET imaging. Clin Nucl Med 2020;45(6):e279–80.

53. Sommerauer M, Burkhardt JK, Frontzek K, et al. 68Gallium-DOTATATE PET in meningioma: A reliable predictor of tumor growth rate? Neuro Oncol 2016; 18(7):1021–7.

54. Kanazawa T, Minami Y, Jinzaki M, et al. Preoperative prediction of solitary fibrous tumor/hemangiopericytoma and angiomatous meningioma using magnetic

resonance imaging texture analysis. World Neurosurg 2018;120:e1208–16.

55. Liu X., Deng J., Sun Q., et al., Differentiation of intracranial solitary fibrous tumor/hemangiopericytoma from atypical meningioma using apparent diffusion coefficient histogram analysis, Neurosurg Rev, 45(3), 2022, 2449–2456.

56. Chen T, Jiang B, Zheng Y, et al. Differentiating intracranial solitary fibrous tumor/hemangiopericytoma from meningioma using diffusion-weighted imaging and susceptibility-weighted imaging. Neuroradiology 2020;62(2):175–84.

57. Prayson RA, Rowe JJ. Dural-based Rosai–Dorfman disease. Differential diagnostic considerations. J Clin Neurosci 2014;21(11):1872–3.

58. Starr C, Cha S. Meningioma mimics: five key imaging features to differentiate them from meningiomas. Clin Radiol 2017;72(9):722–8.

59. Chakrabarty S, Sotiras A, Milchenko M, et al. MRI-based identification and classification of major intracranial tumor types by using a 3D convolutional neural network: A retrospective multi-institutional analysis. Radiol Artif Intell 2021;3(5):e200301.

60. Fan Y, Liu P, Li Y, et al. Non-invasive preoperative imaging differential diagnosis of intracranial hemangiopericytoma and angiomatous meningioma: a novel developed and validated multiparametric mri-based clini-radiomic model. Front Oncol 2022; 11:792521.

61. Ke C, Chen H, Lv X, et al. Differentiation between benign and nonbenign meningiomas by using texture analysis from multiparametric MRI. J Magn Reson Imaging 2020;51(6):1810–20.

62. Chen C, Guo X, Wang J, et al. The diagnostic value of radiomics-based machine learning in predicting the grade of meningiomas using conventional magnetic resonance imaging: a preliminary study. Front Oncol 2019;9:1338.

63. Coroller TP, Bi WL, Huynh E, et al. Radiographic prediction of meningioma grade by semantic and radiomic features. PLoS One 2017;12(11):e0187908.

64. Hamerla G, Meyer HJ, Schob S, et al. Comparison of machine learning classifiers for differentiation of grade 1 from higher gradings in meningioma: a multicenter radiomics study. Magn Reson Imaging 2019;63:244–9.

65. Zhu Y, Man C, Gong L, et al. A deep learning radiomics model for preoperative grading in meningioma. Eur J Radiol 2019;116:128–34.

66. Morin O, Chen WC, Nassiri F, et al. Integrated models incorporating radiologic and radiomic features predict meningioma grade, local failure, and overall survival. Neuro-Oncol Adv. 2019;1(1): vdz011.

67. Goldbrunner R, Minniti G, Preusser M, et al. EANO guidelines for the diagnosis and treatment of meningiomas. Lancet Oncol 2016;17(9):e383–91.

68. Strømsnes TA, Lund-Johansen M, Skeie GO, et al. Growth dynamics of incidental meningiomas: a prospective long-term follow-up study. Neuro-Oncol Pract 2022;npac088.

69. Behbahani M, Skeie GO, Eide GE, et al. A prospective study of the natural history of incidental meningioma—Hold your horses. Neuro-Oncol Pract 2019;6(6):438–50.

70. Kunz WG, Jungblut LM, Kazmierczak PM, et al. Improved detection of transosseous meningiomas using 68Ga-DOTATATE PET/CT compared with contrast-enhanced MRI. J Nucl Med 2017;58(10): 1580–7.

71. Ueberschaer M, Vettermann FJ, Forbrig R, et al. Simpson grade revisited–intraoperative estimation of the extent of resection in meningiomas versus postoperative somatostatin receptor positron emission tomography/computed tomography and magnetic resonance imaging. Neurosurgery 2021; 88(1):140–6.

72. Ivanidze J, Roytman M, Lin E, et al. Gallium-68 DOTATATE PET in the evaluation of intracranial meningiomas. J Neuroimaging 2019;29(5):650–6.

73. Rachinger W, Stoecklein VM, Terpolilli NA, et al. Increased 68Ga-DOTATATE uptake in PET imaging discriminates meningioma and tumor-free tissue. J Nucl Med 2015;56(3):347–53.

74. Mahase SS, Roth O'Brien DA, No D, et al. [68Ga]-DOTATATE PET/MRI as an adjunct imaging modality for radiation treatment planning of meningiomas. Neuro-Oncol Adv. 2021;3(1):vdab012.

75. Nyuyki F, Plotkin M, Graf R, et al. Potential impact of 68Ga-DOTATOC PET/CT on stereotactic radiotherapy planning of meningiomas. Eur J Nucl Med Mol Imaging 2010;37(2):310–8.

76. Combs SE, Welzel T, Habermehl D, et al. Prospective evaluation of early treatment outcome in patients with meningiomas treated with particle therapy based on target volume definition with MRI and 68Ga-DOTATOC-PET. Acta Oncol 2013;52(3): 514–20.

77. Graf R, Nyuyki F, Steffen IG, et al. Contribution of 68Ga-DOTATOC PET/CT to target volume delineation of skull base meningiomas treated with stereotactic radiation therapy. Int J Radiat Oncol Biol Phys 2013;85(1):68–73.

78. Pelak MJ, Flechl B, Mumot M, et al. The value of SSTR2 receptor-targeted PET/CT in proton irradiation of grade I meningioma. Cancers 2021;13(18): 4707.

79. Perlow H.K., Siedow M., Gokun Y., et al., 68Ga-DOTATATE PET-based radiation contouring creates more precise radiation volumes for meningioma patients, Int J Radiat Oncol Biol Phys, 113(4). 2022. 859-865.

80. Zhang J, Yao K, Liu P, et al. A radiomics model for preoperative prediction of brain invasion in

meningioma non-invasively based on MRI: a multi-centre study. EBioMedicine 2020;58:102933.

81. Li N, Mo Y, Huang C, et al. A clinical semantic and radiomics nomogram for predicting brain invasion in WHO Grade II meningioma based on tumor and tumor-to-brain interface features. Front Oncol 2021; 11:4362.

82. Zhang J., Cao Y., Zhang G., et al., Nomogram based on MRI can preoperatively predict brain invasion in meningioma, *Neurosurg Rev*, 45(6),2022, 1–9.

83. Itamura K, Chang KE, Lucas J, et al. Prospective clinical validation of a meningioma consistency grading scheme: association with surgical outcomes and extent of tumor resection. J Neurosurg 2018;131(5):1356–60.

84. Zhai Y, Song D, Yang F, et al. Preoperative prediction of meningioma consistency via machine learning-based radiomics. Front Oncol 2021;11:1519.

85. Seystahl K, Stoecklein V, Schüller U, et al. Somatostatin receptor-targeted radionuclide therapy for progressive meningioma: benefit linked to 68Ga-DOTATATE/-TOC uptake. Neuro Oncol 2016;18(11): 1538–47.

86. Kowalski ES, Khairnar R, Gryaznov AA, et al. 68Ga-DOTATATE PET-CT as a tool for radiation planning and evaluating treatment responses in the clinical management of meningiomas. Radiat Oncol 2021; 16(1):1–10.

87. Barone F, Inserra F, Scalia G, et al. 68Ga-DOTATOC PET/CT follow up after single or hypofractionated gamma knife ICON radiosurgery for meningioma patients. Brain Sci 2021;11(3):375.

Incidental Meningiomas
Potential Predictors of Growth and Current State of Management

Natalie Mahgerefteh, HSD[a], Khashayar Mozaffari, BS[a], Zoe Teton, MD[a],
Yelena Malkhasyan, BS[a], Kihong Kim, MD[a], Isaac Yang, MD[a,b,c,d,e,f,g],*

KEYWORDS

- Incidental meningioma • Stereotactic radiosurgery • Neuroimaging • Brain tumors
- Surgical resection

KEY POINTS

- Because of more frequent use of brain imaging for patients with nonspecific neurologic symptoms, the rate of incidentally discovered meningiomas has increased.
- Large initial tumor size, hyperintensity on T2-weighted MRI, absence of calcification, and peritumoral edema are all associated with higher growth rate.
- Incidental meningiomas can be managed with active surveillance, stereotactic radiosurgery, fractionated stereotactic radiotherapy, or surgery.
- Optimal management for incidental meningiomas is controversial, but most clinicians recommend observation with serial imaging, unless further intervention is deemed necessary owing to concern for impending mass effect.
- Prognostic models such as IMPACT and AIMSS are under development for assessing progression risk based on a variety of radiological and clinical characteristics.

INTRODUCTION

Meningiomas are the most common primary brain tumors, accounting for approximately 37% of all intracranial neoplasms.[1–4] They are thought to arise from arachnoid cap cells of the meninges surrounding the brain and spinal cord.[5] The World Health Organization (WHO) stratifies meningiomas into 3 groups based on histologic criteria.[6] Most of these tumors are WHO grade 1, meaning they are benign, well-circumscribed, and slow-growing.[7,8] Less common are WHO grade 2 tumors, also known as atypical meningiomas, which have a higher propensity for recurrence, and WHO grade 3 tumors, which display malignant histology with a more aggressive course.[6,9,10] Meningiomas are more common among women and the elderly, increasing significantly in incidence after the age of 65 years.[11–14]

Although meningiomas may typically present with symptoms such as headaches, dizziness, hearing loss, changes in vision, and seizures, they are often detected without any accompanying symptoms.[5] In fact, approximately 38.9% of newly diagnosed intracranial meningiomas are incidentally discovered.[14,15] Because of advances in neuroimaging and increased use of diagnostic screening, more cases of asymptomatic meningiomas are being reported.[16–18] Among patients with incidental meningioma, the risk of developing

[a] Department of Neurosurgery, University of California, 300 Stein Plaza, Suite 562, Los Angeles, CA 90095-1761, USA; [b] Department of Radiation Oncology, 300 Stein Plaza, Suite 562, Los Angeles, CA 90095-1761, USA; [c] Department of Head and Neck Surgery, 300 Stein Plaza, Suite 562, Los Angeles, CA 90095-1761, USA; [d] Jonsson Comprehensive Cancer Center, 300 Stein Plaza, Suite 562, Los Angeles, CA 90095-1761, USA; [e] Los Angeles Biomedical Research Institute, 300 Stein Plaza, Suite 562, Los Angeles, CA 90095-1761, USA; [f] Harbor–UCLA Medical Center, 300 Stein Plaza, Suite 562, Los Angeles, CA 90095-1761, USA; [g] David Geffen School of Medicine, Los Angeles, 100 West Carson Street, Torrance, CA 90502, USA
* Corresponding author. University of California, 300 Stein Plaza, Suite 562, Los Angeles, CA 90095-1761.
E-mail address: iyang@mednet.ucla.edu

Neurosurg Clin N Am 34 (2023) 347–369
https://doi.org/10.1016/j.nec.2023.02.009
1042-3680/23/© 2023 Elsevier Inc. All rights reserved.

tumor-related signs and symptoms is relatively low because of the indolent nature of the lesion.[7] As these tumors tend to be asymptomatic, there is a low level of evidence to support guidelines for diagnosis and treatment, especially compared with other tumors, such as high-grade gliomas.[19,20] However, studies have shown that 24% to 44% of small to moderately sized meningiomas will display growth within 4 to 5 years after diagnosis.[21–25] Any growth of intracranial lesions carries risk of compression to the surrounding neurovasculature and brain parenchyma.[18,26] If this growth occurs near eloquent regions, tumor progression may lead to permanent neurologic deficits.[18,27,28] Although these risks are real, treatment is not without potential complication, especially for elderly patients. The growing elderly population in our country calls attention to the need to address this clinical challenge.[29–31]

Management options for incidental meningioma include surgery, stereotactic radiosurgery (SRS), fractionated stereotactic radiotherapy (FSRT), and active surveillance.[27,32] Although gross total resection is typically the treatment of choice for large and symptomatic meningiomas, the approach for asymptomatic patients is not as straightforward.[29,31] In most cases, surgery is not recommended upon diagnosis, or even after the first sign of radiological progression, as such measures may lead to overtreatment.[17,21,29,33,34] Depending on the patient's medical history and health status, as well as the location and size of the tumor, there can be notable risks associated with surgical intervention.[22,35,36] These risks, along with postoperative complications, must be weighed against long-term benefits of tumor resection.[22,35,36] Recent international guidelines have recommended conservative management with serial monitoring as the most appropriate therapeutic strategy for patients with smaller asymptomatic tumors.[19] However, several studies have shown that, compared with active surveillance, SRS can be more effective in preventing tumor progression and reducing symptoms for patients with small or moderately sized incidental meningiomas.[21,27,37,38] For incidental meningiomas found in locations considered to be unfavorable surgically, SRS has become increasingly recommended as a safe and effective treatment option owing to its ability to confer both tumor control and neurologic preservation.[7,22,23,37,39]

Although incidental meningioma has become an increasingly prevalent issue, there still is no consensus on optimal management, as its natural history remains highly variable.[19,40] A recent study surveying neurosurgeons on incidental meningioma management demonstrated wide heterogeneity and

revealed a lack of evidence-based guidelines to steer decision making.[7,20,41] Although multiple clinical and radiological risk factors associated with tumor progression have been identified, there remains high variability among studies, so results are often conflicting and difficult to draw conclusions from.[33,36,40] Those that have been identified include young age,[23,33] absence of calcification,[23,25,33,40,42] MRI signal hyperintensity,[23,34,41,42] and peritumoral edema.[23,40] Fortunately, development of prognostic models using these known risk factors is underway in an effort to introduce standardization to management of this heterogenous disease.[20,26,43] This article aims to encapsulate where we are in this moment of evolving practice patterns.

EPIDEMIOLOGY

Many studies have attempted to elucidate the relationship between meningioma and various clinical risk factors.[32] For instance, studies have found that, owing to a loss of function mutation in a tumor-suppressor protein, individuals with neurofibromatosis type 2 are very likely to develop meningiomas as well as other benign proliferative tumors.[44,45] Other documented risks include female sex and exposure to ionizing radiation.[46–48] Other factors, such as exposure to female hormones[49–55] and elevated body mass index (BMI),[49,56,57] are possible risk factors of which impacts on tumor growth remain debated. It is important to identify the validity and reliability of potential risk factors, so that patients and clinicians can make informed decisions about appropriate management of these tumors.[27]

Age

Both the prevalence and the relative size of meningiomas are known to increase with age.[15,31,58] Many studies have attempted to discern whether age is an independent risk factor for tumor growth.[7,20,27,36,38,59] Pikis and colleagues[59] found that advancing age was predictive of tumor progression. In addition, a study conducted by Behbahani and colleagues[20] observed tumor growth rates of 0.10 cm^3 per year among patients younger than 55 years, 0.24 cm^3 per year among patients between the ages of 55 and 75 years, and 0.86 cm^3 per year among patients older than 75 years. However, the investigators did not identify a statistically significant relationship between age and tumor growth.[20] On the contrary, Thomann and colleagues[36] actually found that older age at diagnosis had a negative predictive value for tumor progression. This finding was supported by a series of 354 patients by Kim and colleagues[38] that found that age was significantly correlated with clinical progression and poor prognosis, and by Romani and colleagues,[7] whose work revealed a significant correlation between age and tumor stability in patients with incidental meningioma older than 65 years. Many other studies support the idea that younger age predicts faster tumor growth.[23,24,33,60–63] These mixed findings may be attributable to heterogeneity across studies.[20] Larger studies with longer follow-up and greater statistical power are necessary to accurately discern the relationship between age and tumor growth rate, as it is difficult to draw conclusions at this point.

Sex

There is a strong consensus in the literature that incidental meningiomas are significantly more common in women.[11–14,49] Although many investigators have identified an association between female sex and increased risk for the presence of incidental meningioma,[49] there does not appear to be a correlation between female sex and tumor progression or growth rate.[7,20,24,33,38] Multiple recent retrospective studies by Romani and colleagues,[7] Kim and colleagues,[38] and Behbahani and colleagues[20] have concluded that sex does not have a significant effect on clinical or radiological progression, and this has been consistently supported by other investigators in the field.[24,33] It appears that, although female sex may be a risk factor for incidental meningioma, it is not necessarily correlated with a particular growth rate or pattern of clinical progression.

Metabolic and Hormonal Factors

Along with female sex, elevated BMI has also been noted as a potential risk factor for presence of meningioma, as observed by Cerhan and colleagues.[49,57] It has been suggested that these 2 findings may reflect the existence of metabolic and hormone-related influences in tumor progression.[49–54] BMI is known to be connected to several types of cancer, and some think this may explain its association with meningioma.[49,56] However, more research is necessary to elucidate the mechanism in question.[49] It is important to note that, although obesity has been associated with meningioma, there is no consensus as to whether diabetes is also a risk factor.[64–68]

An additional conjecture that has been proposed to explain the increased incidence of meningioma in women is the increased use of oral contraceptives and hormone replacement therapy (HRT) in the modern day.[11,69] A large European multicenter study of more than 270,000 women identified a higher risk of meningioma

development in HRT users as well as women on oral contraceptives.[55] These findings are supported by 2 other large studies that also found a positive association between HRT usage and meningioma presence.[52,54] However, few studies have attempted to examine the role of estrogen in meningioma growth risk. Behbahani's series on 102 patients with meningioma did not find any correlation between tumor volume or growth rate and exposure to female hormones.[20] Larger studies with data on individual hormones are warranted to clarify this potential relationship.

RADIOGRAPHIC STUDIES

The increase in prevalence of incidental brain findings is largely due to advancements in neuroimaging, along with increased use of radiological screenings for brain injuries and nonspecific neurologic symptoms.[16–18,27] In population-based studies, incidental meningiomas have been detected in up to 2.5% of brain MRIs.[15,70] One study of more than 10,000 autopsies discovered incidental meningioma in 2.3% of cases.[58] This effect has likely been magnified by more advanced imaging techniques. For example, a systematic review including data from 16 cohorts reported a higher likelihood of encountering an incidental brain finding when using high-resolution MRI compared with standard resolution sequences alone (4.3% and 1.7%, respectively).[16] The most common presenting symptoms to prompt neuroimaging that lead to an incidental meningioma diagnosis are unrelated neurologic deficit, headache, audiovestibular symptoms, and head injury (**Fig. 1**).[32]

In addition to broadening diagnostic capabilities, radiological examination has provided valuable insight into tumor growth potential. Several predictive factors for progression have been identified in incidental meningioma, including tumor size, location, hyperintensity on T2-weighted MRI, absence of calcification, and peritumoral edema (**Table 1**).[7,18,23–27,33,34,36,38,40–42,71–75]

Tumor Size and Location

It is well-documented that larger tumors tend to have higher growth potential.[23,24,42] This is consistent with findings from a systematic review by Zhang and Zhang[27] as well as a large retrospective study by Lee and colleagues.[26] Others have noted that growth potential seems to be predicted by location as well, with skull base tumors generally growing slower than their convexity counterparts.[71–73] Generally, tumor location is more predictive of difficulty of resection and risk of complications as opposed to growth rate.[27,76]

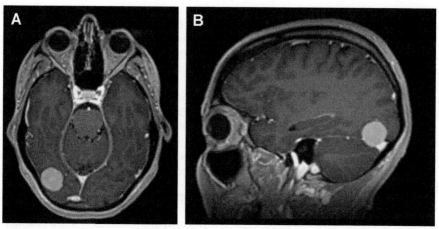

Fig. 1. Brain MRI demonstrates a homogenously enhancing mass in the right occipital lobe. This was diagnosed in an adult woman who had undergone radiographic studies following craniofacial trauma (*A*: axial plane; *B*: sagittal plane).

Proximity to eloquent structures is also known to result in increased adverse events, and these findings are reflected in literature surrounding radiosurgery as well.[27]

Relative Tumor Intensity on MRI

Various patterns on imaging have been identified that may correlate with propensity for tumor progression. Chief among them are T2 and T2 fluid-attenuated inversion recovery (FLAIR) hyperintensity seen on MRI.[75,77,78] It is thought that these are associated with high microvascularity and axonal loss, and they have been indicated as strong predictors of tumor progression.[77] Lee and colleagues[26] and Zhang and Zhang[27] found that T2 hyperintensity predicted rapid tumor growth, whereas Romani and colleagues[7] found that T2 and FLAIR hyperintensity was strongly correlated with tumor progression. This was supported by Kim and colleagues,[38] who found that T2 hyperintensity also correlated with poor prognosis. These findings align with those of earlier reports[23,34,42,74] and establish high T2 signal as a valid predictive factor for progression.

Tumor Calcification

Although T2 hyperintensity suggests increased tumor aggression, evidence of calcification in meningiomas actually portends slower tumor growth.[79] This was demonstrated in a multivariate analysis by Romani and colleagues,[7] where they found calcification to be the strongest radiological predictive factor for nonprogression and tumor stability. Results from studies by Zhang and Zhang,[27] Lee and colleagues,[26] and Kim and colleagues,[38] among others,[18,40,80] support this finding.

Presence of Peritumoral Edema

The degree of invasion for any given meningioma is denoted by the extent of peritumoral edema, a sign associated with increased intracranial pressure, higher seizure risk, and increased likelihood of tumor recurrence.[81] In line with previous studies,[23,40] Romani and colleagues' multivariate analysis distinguished edema as the strongest radiological factor for tumor progression,[7] and Kim and colleagues[38] found a correlation between edema and clinical progression. These conclusions are supported by Lee and colleagues' finding that peritumoral edema was also strongly associated with a higher labeling index for the cell proliferation marker MIB-1.[26] Although edema is widely associated with progression of meningioma, its pathogenesis is not well understood.[82,83] Future studies on the development of peritumoral edema in meningioma may be helpful in identifying related biomarkers and predictive factors and guiding clinicians on appropriate treatment strategies to maximize prevention.

MANAGEMENT

Although many incidental meningiomas remain stable and asymptomatic, some may develop an aggressive growth pattern and compress surrounding neurovascular structures.[7] Thus, the recommended approach for managing incidental meningioma largely depends on the individual case. Management options for incidental meningioma include active surveillance, SRS, fractionated radiotherapy, and surgery, with most clinicians preferring a conservative approach until further intervention is deemed absolutely necessary (**Table 2**).[27,29,32]

Table 1
Literature review of studies evaluating prognostic factors for incidental meningioma

First Author, Publication Year	Total Patients (n)	Male (n)	Age at Dx (Mean), y	Follow-up Period (Mean)	Initial Tumor Volume (Mean)	Definition of Tumor Growth	Progression	Prognostic Factors
Thomann et al,[36] 2022	188	39	59.5 ± 15.0	46.9 ± 30.1 mo	0.51 cm³ (median)	Volume increase of 14.35%	159/240 (66.3%, TG)	Tumor growth: young age, absence of calcification, T2W hyperintensity, T2W isointensity
Pikis et al,[59] 2022	98 (SRS) 98 (AS)	22 (22.45%, SRS) 20 (20.41%, AS)	56.46 ± 12.61 (SRS) 58.05 ± 11.07 (AS)	48 mo radiological, 46 mo clinical (median, SRS) 40 mo radiological, 40 mo clinical (median, AS)	4.06 ± 3.9 cm³ (SRS) 3.99 ± 8.32 cm³ (AS)	Progression (?)	1 (1.02%, SRS, TG) 30 (30.61%, AS, TG)	Tumor growth: old age, AS policy Local tumor control: higher KPS at diagnosis, initial tumor volume
Ikawa, 2021	6628	2040 (30.78%)	54 (<65 y) 69 (65–74 y) 78 (≥75 y) (all median)					BI deterioration: old age In-hospital mortality: midline and posterior fossa location, diabetes mellitus, chronic heart disease

(continued on next page)

Table 1
(continued)

First Author, Publication Year	Total Patients (n)	Male (n)	Age at Dx (Mean), y	Follow-up Period (Mean)	Initial Tumor Volume (Mean)	Definition of Tumor Growth	Progression	Prognostic Factors
Li et al,[117] 2020	80 (<65 y) 70 (≥65 y)	33 (41.2%, <65 y) 32 (45.7%, ≥65 y)	55.2 ± 4.1 (<65 y) 71.6 ± 4.3 (≥65 y)					Length of stay and lower KPS at discharge: old age Postoperative complications: blood loss, BMI
Behbahani et al,[20] 2019	64 (PA) 38 (RA)	17 (26.56%, PA) 8 (21.05%, RA)	64 (PA) 61 (RA)		4.9 cm³ (PA, mean) 5.4 cm³ (RA, mean)	A more than 15%, and more than 8.2%, respectively, increase in tumor volume	48 (75%, PA, TG 15% cutoff) 55 (85.9%, PA, TG 8.2% cutoff) 24 (63.2%, RA, TG 15% cutoff), 26 (68.4%, RA, TG 8.2% cutoff)	Tumor growth: old age
Cerhan et al,[49] 2019	52	19 (36.5%)	75					Meningioma presence: BMI, NSAIDs, aspirin, blood pressure–lowering medication, female sex, absence of CAD, lower self-reported anxiety

	N	Growth n (%)	Age	Follow-up	Size	Growth definition	Growth/progression	Poor prognosis
Kim et al,[38] 2018	354	77 (21.8%)	57.6 ± 9.3 (mean)	57 mo (clinical) 47 mo (radiological)	1.7 cm³	Volume increase of more than 30%	150 (42.4%, RP) 77 (21.75%, CP) 43 (55.8%, SP)	Poor prognosis: young age, absence of calcification, T2W hyperintensity, peritumoral edema
Romani et al,[7] 2018	136	34 (25%)	65 (mean)	43 mo		Increase in maximum intracranial diameter by a minimum of 3 mm	RP: 37 (27.2%) CP: 27 (19.8%)	Tumor growth: edema, hyperintensity in T2W and FLAIR T2W, absence of isointensity in FLAIR T2W, absence of calcification, young age
Lee et al,[26] 2017	232	40 (17.2%)	60 ± 10	47 mo (mean)	11.5 ± 19.3 cm³	≥2 cm³/y (rapid growth)	59 (25.4%, rapid growth)	Tumor growth: initial tumor size, absence of calcification, peritumoral edema, T2W hyperintensity, T2W isointensity

Abbreviations: AS, active surveillance; BI, Barthel index; CAD, coronary artery disease; CP, clinical progression; NSAIDs, nonsteroidal anti-inflammatory drugs; PA, prospective arm; RA, retrospective arm; RP, radiological progression; SP, symptomatic progression; T2W, T2-weighted; TG, tumor growth.

Table 2
Summary of outcomes of studies assessing treatment options for incidental meningioma

First Author, y	Treatment	Total Patients, n	Male, n	Age at Dx (Mean), y	Baseline Tumor Volume (Median)	Follow-up Period (Median)	Treatment Conditions (Median)	Postoperative Complications	Clinical Outcomes
Islim et al,[98] 2022	AS, SRS	28 (AS) 84 (SRS) 25 (AS) 25 (SRS)	27 (24.1%) (AS) 9 (32.1%) (AS) 18 (21.4%) (SRS) 8 (32%) (AS) 4 (16%) (SRS)	58.8 ± 12.8 (AS) 62.1 ± 13.3 (AS) 57.6 ± 12.5 (SRS) 60.8 ± 11.3 (AS) 59.7 ± 9.9 (SRS)	2.0 cm³ 1.7 cm³ (AS) 2.0 cm³ (SRS) 1.7 cm³ (AS) 2.0 cm³ (SRS)	Clinical: 42 mo (AS) 44 mo (SRS) Radiologic: 42 mo (AS) 36 mo (SRS) Clinical: 42 mo (AS) 38 mo (SRS) Radiologic: 42 mo (AS) 36 mo (SRS)	Margin: 12 Gy Maximum: 25 Gy Isocenters: 9 Treatment volume: 3.0 cm³ Margin: 12 Gy Maximum: 24 Gy Isocenters: 7 Treatment volume: 3.0 cm³	Treatment-related complications: 5/84 (6%) (SRS) 0/28 (0%) (AS) Treatment-related complications: 0 (0%) of AS 0 (0%) of SRS	Tumor progression: 13 (46.4%) (AS), 0 (0%) (SRS) Further intervention for tumor growth (after mean of 30 mo): 3 (10.7%) (AS), 0 (0%) (SRS) Tumor progression: 13 (52%) (AS), 0 (0%) (SRS) Further intervention for tumor growth (after mean of 30 mo): 3 (12%) (AS), 0 (0%) (SRS)
Pikis et al,[59] 2022	AS, SRS	140 (AS) 99 (SRS) Matched: 98 (AS) 98 (SRS)	30 (21.43%) (AS) 22 (22.22%) (SRS) 20 (20.41%, AS) 22 (22.45%, SRS)	61.22 ± 11.07 (AS) 56.52 ± 12.56 (SRS) 58.05 ± 11.07 (AS) 56.46 ± 12.61 (SRS)	3.74 cm³ (AS) 4.06 cm³ (SRS) 3.99 cm³ (AS) 4.06 cm³ (SRS)	Clinical: 36 mo (AS) 46 mo (SRS) Radiologic: 36 mo (AS) 48 mo (SRS) Clinical: 40 mo (AS) 46 mo (SRS) Radiologic:	Margin: 13.26 ± 1.76 Gy Maximum: 26.49 ± 5.00 Gy Isocenters: 8 Treatment volume: 4.59 ± 3.90 cm³		Tumor progression: 41 (29.29%) (AS), 1 (1.01%) (SRS) Further intervention for tumor growth: 18 (12.9%) (AS), 0 (0%) (SRS) New neurologic deficits:

Study	Treatment	N	(%)	Age	Tumor volume	Follow-up	Dose	Outcomes
						40 mo (AS) 48 mo (SRS)	Margin: 13.26 ± 1.77 Gy Maximum: 26.48 ± 5.03 Gy Isocenters: 8 Treatment volume: 4.62 ± 3.90 cm³	3 (2.14%) (AS), 2 (2.02%) (SRS) Tumor progression: 30 (30.61%) (AS), 1 (1.02%) (SRS) Further intervention for tumor growth: 14 (14.3%) (AS), 0 (0%) (SRS) New neurologic deficits: 2 (2.04%) (AS), 2 (2.04%) (SRS)
Pikis et al,[59] 2021	SRS	37	29 (78.4%)	55.05 ± 11.56	5.73 ± 4.36 cm³	Clinical: 66 mo Radiologic: 72 mo	Margin: 12.27 ± 2.3 Gy Maximum: 24.03 ± 5.59 Gy Isocenters: 11	Tumor control: 37 (100%) Tumor progression: 0 (100%) Tumor regression: 19 (51.35%) Tumor stability: 18 (48.65%) New neurologic deficits: 1 (2.7%) Treatment-related complications: 2 (5.4%)
Sheehan et al,[22] 2022	AS, SRS	388 (AS) 727 (SRS) 311 (AS) 311 (SRS)	82 (21.1%) (AS) 160 (22.1%) (SRS) 63 (20.3%) (AS) 72 (23.2%) (SRS)	62.6 ± 12 (AS) 56.9 ± 13.7 (SRS) 60.7 ± 11.7 (AS) 61.1 ± 12.9 (SRS)	3.7 cm³ (AS) 4.3 cm³ (SRS) (mean) 3.9 cm³ (AS) 3.8 cm³ (SRS) (mean)	(median) Clinical: 36 mo (AS) 45 mo (SRS) Radiologic: 36 mo (AS) 48 mo (SRS) Clinical: 42 mo (AS) 36 mo (SRS) Radiologic: 42 mo (AS) 36 mo (SRS)	Margin (mean): 13.0 ± 1.9 Gy Maximum (mean): 26.0 ± 5.1 Gy Isocenters: 9 Treatment volume (mean): 5.4 ±	Tumor control: 249 (64.2%) (AS), 713 (99.0%) (SRS) Tumor progression: 141 (36.3%) (AS), 7 (1.0%) (SRS) Tumor regression: 3 (0.8%) (AS), 327 (45.4%) (SRS) New neurologic deficits:

(continued on next page)

Table 2
(continued)

First Author, y	Treatment	Total Patients, n	Male, n	Age at Dx (Mean), y	Baseline Tumor Volume (Median)	Follow-up Period (Median)	Treatment Conditions (Median)	Postoperative Complications	Clinical Outcomes
							4.7 cm^3 Margin (mean): 12.9 ± 1.8 Gy Maximum (mean): 26.0 ± 4.7 Gy Isocenters: 9 Treatment volume (mean): 4.9 ± 4.1 cm^3		11 (2.8%) (AS), 18 (2.5%) (SRS) Tumor control: 193 (62.1%) (AS), 309 (99.4%) (SRS) Tumor progression: 118 (37.9%) (AS), 2 (1.0%) (SRS) Tumor regression: 3 (1.0%) (AS), 138 (44.4%) (SRS) New neurologic deficits: 10 (3.2%) (AS), 7 (2.3%) (SRS)
Li et al,[117] 2020	Surgery	80 (<65 y) 70 (≥65 y)	33 (41.2%) (<65 y) 32 (45.7%) (≥65 y)	55.2 ± 4.1 (<65 y) 71.6 ± 4.3 (≥65 y)	NR	NR	Surgery length (mean): 336.1 ± 80.0 min (<65 y) 345.9 ± 88.2 min (≥65 y) Estimated blood loss (mean): 760.6 ± 210.4 mL (<65 y) 778.6 ±	Postoperative cranial nerve palsy: 32 (40.0%) (<65 y) 20 (28.6%) (≥65 y) Postoperative cognitive change: 8 (10.0%) (<65 y) 4 (5.7%) (≥65 y) Postoperative CNS infection: 2 (2.5%) (<65 y) 4 (5.7%) (≥65 y) Postoperative infarction or	

							244.7 mL (≥65 y) Blood transfusion: 35 (43.8%) (<65 y) 37 (52.9%) (≥65 y)	hemorrhage: 5 (6.3%) (<65 y) 3 (4.3%) (≥65 y) Postoperative seizure: 4 (5%) (<65 y) 6 (8.6%) (≥65 y) Postoperative CSF fistula: 1 (1.3%) (<65 y) 2 (2.9%) (≥65 y)
Islim et al,[98] 2020	Surgery, radiotherapy	441 (IMPACT) 44 (Treatment)	93 (21.1%) (IMPACT) 9 (20.5%) (Treatment)	64 (median) (IMPACT) 56.1 (median) (Treatment)	1.6 cm³ (IMPACT) 4.55 cm³ (Treatment)	55 mo (Treatment)	Postoperative surgical complications: 11/40 (27.5%) Surgical complications requiring treatment: 6/40 (15%)	Tumor regression: 100% Early and late moderate adverse events limiting activities of daily living: 126 (28.6%) Recurrence rate after surgery: 2.5%
Näslund et al,[29] 2020	Surgery	45	14 (31.1%)	56.1 ± 11.5	9.3 cm³		Complications within 30 d: 16 (35.6%) Postoperative hematoma: 3 (6.7%) Infection: 3 (6.7%) Seizure: 3 (6.7%) Significant edema: 1 (2.2%) Reoperation due to complication: 3 (6.7%)	Recurrence: 4 (9.5%) New/worsened focal deficit: 4 (8.9%) Postoperative rehabilitation: 8 (18.6%)

(continued on next page)

Table 2
(continued)

First Author, y	Treatment	Total Patients, n	Male, n	Age at Dx (Mean), y	Baseline Tumor Volume (Median)	Follow-up Period (Median)	Treatment Conditions (Median)	Postoperative Complications	Clinical Outcomes
Kim et al,[82] 2018	AS, Gamma Knife surgery (SRS)	201 (AS) 153 (SRS)	43(21.4%) (AS) 34 (22.2%) (SRS)	58.3 ± 10.4 (mean) (AS) 56.6 ± 7.4 (mean) (SRS)	1.0 cm³ (AS) 2.5 cm³ (SRS)	Clinical: 62 mo (AS) 53 mo (SRS) Radiologic: 47 mo (AS) 46 mo (SRS)	Median dose: 14 Gy		Radiological progression: 141 (70.1%) (AS) 9 (5.9%) (SRS) Clinical progression: 73 (36.3%) (AS) 4 (2.6%) (SRS) Symptomatic progression: 40 (19.9%) (AS) 3 (2%) (SRS)

Abbreviations: CNS, central nervous system; CSF, cerebrospinal fluid.

Conservative Management

According to recent guidelines by the European Association of Neuro-Oncology, the best management strategy for asymptomatic meningiomas is observation with serial imaging.[19] This is supported by data from Behbahani and colleagues' 5-year study on 64 patients with untreated incidental meningioma, in which none of the patients developed tumor-related symptoms and 61.1% of the tumors displayed a self-limiting growth pattern.[20] From 2004 to 2014, the decision to observe benign meningiomas and refrain from surgical intervention has increased by 13%.[84] It is generally held that WHO grade 1 meningiomas should receive annual MRI monitoring for 5 years, because incidental meningiomas with growth potential will typically show some radiological progression within this period.[7,19,29] In fact, a systematic review by Islim and colleagues[32] observed that 94% of asymptomatic meningiomas that eventually require intervention will receive it within the first 5 years following diagnosis. Although observation delays costly, unnecessary procedures and their associated risks, there is always the possibility that a conservatively managed meningioma can suddenly display rapid growth, leaving surgery the only management option.[34,85] Future studies should aim to establish recommendations regarding appropriate follow-up intervals for small, asymptomatic tumors, as this would help clinicians identify growth, reach accurate histopathologic diagnosis, and refer their patients to intervention when needed.[29]

Radiation Treatment

An alternative, noninvasive treatment option is radiation, primarily either FSRT or SRS, also known as Gamma Knife surgery.[27,32,86] These options are particularly useful when surgery would introduce additional risk, owing to either inaccessible location of the tumor, elevated surgical morbidity, or older age.[86] Prophylactic radiation can also be used for tumors in areas that are especially prone to symptom development secondary to mass effect, such as the petroclival junction or cavernous sinus.[34,37,85] FSRT and SRS are difficult to directly compare owing to confounding factors, such as tumor size and location, although they have largely been found to demonstrate similar rates of local tumor control.[86,87]

FSRT divides radiation doses into several fractions and treatments, targeting meningioma cells when they are least hypoxic and most radiosensitive in order to maximize treatment delivery.[88] Typically, benign tumors receive FSRT doses of 50 to 54 Gy and 5 subsequent fractions of 1.8 to 2 Gy each week.[86,89] Among patients with grade 1 meningioma treated with FSRT, 93% to 95% have achieved progression-free survival (PFS) at 5 years, and nearly 88% maintain that status at 10 years.[90,91] FSRT is usually preferred over SRS for meningiomas that may reside near critical structures.[86,92] For example, it is the optimal intervention strategy for optic nerve sheath meningioma, which has been shown to achieve post-FSRT tumor stability or reduction in nearly 100% of cases with symptom control or improvement in 80% to 90% of those.[93–97]

Single-fraction SRS delivers a high dose of radiation and targets meningioma cells with great precision, damaging their DNA and reducing tumor volume.[92] SRS has been shown to achieve tumor control in 90% to 100% of cases without increasing risk of symptom development or morbidity.[22,37,39,98,99] Several large retrospective studies comparing active surveillance with SRS observed minimal to no tumor progression among their SRS cohorts, with similar rates of new neurologic deficits between both groups.[22,38,59,98] SRS is typically only recommended for lesions less than 10 cm^3 in volume, as it tends to demonstrate higher efficacy in smaller masses.[86,100,101] For example, one study demonstrated 91% 5-year PFS among patients with tumors measuring up to 10 cm^3, and 68% 5-year PFS among patients with tumors larger than 10 cm^3.[100] There is also some concern that larger tumors may carry a higher risk of developing SRS-related toxicities.[86,102] In a 22-year study, post-SRS complication rates were reported at 4.8% for patients with tumors smaller than 3.2 cm^3 and nearly 5 times that for patients with tumors greater than 9.6 cm^3.[102] Along with size limitations, SRS intervention is also limited to tumors distant from critical structures.[86,103] SRS tends to be more common than FSRT in the treatment of incidental meningioma, likely owing to the typically small size of the tumor at diagnosis.[85,86]

Risks associated with radiation treatment include cognitive impairment, cranial nerve palsy, and peritumoral edema.[59,98,104] Prior studies noted these complication rates as high as 7% to 13%, although it is important to note that these cohorts consisted of symptomatic patients who had undergone previous surgical intervention.[98,105,106] Among 153 Gamma Knife surgeries reviewed by Kim and colleagues,[38] only one patient experienced severe edema requiring surgery, and all other adverse outcomes were either transient or resolved with steroid treatment. In another cohort of 84 patients reviewed by Islim and colleagues,[98] only 5 experienced SRS-related headache, blurred vision, or seizure about 6 months after treatment. These symptoms also resolved after treatment with corticosteroids.[98] As with any treatment, the possibility of radiation-related complications must be weighed against the risk of tumor growth and symptomatic development. Although SRS appears to have an acceptable rate of complications, studies with longer follow-up are needed to better understand the late sequelae of radiosurgery.

Surgery

Persistent clinical progression or radiological growth of more than 1 cm^3 a year typically warrants surgical intervention.[33] When possible, it is usually optimal to completely excise the lesion in order to reduce the likelihood of recurrence.[86] Extent of resection (EOR) is described by the Simpson grading scale, which classifies resections on a scale from 1 to 5.[86,107] Simpson grade I and II resections, which constitute near-gross total removal of tumor, have demonstrated higher rates of median survival compared with resections of lesser grade.[108,109] One study reported that 92% of patients with incidental meningioma who received Simpson grade I resections achieved good recovery.[110] Because Simpson grade is based on intraoperative visual assessment, it has generated controversy owing to concerns regarding interrater reliability.[111] However, in the modern day, clearer visualization of EOR can be achieved with the assistance of intraoperative imaging technologies, such as intraoperative MRI (iMRI), intraoperative CT (iCT), augmented reality, and ultrasonography (**Table 3**).[112–115] These technologies provide real-time imaging of the surgical field, which can help surgeons avoid critical neurovascular structures and achieve optimal EOR while avoiding adverse events.[112–115]

Although surgery is considered a reasonable option to prevent tumor progression in younger patients, the situation is slightly more complicated in older patients. Elderly patients tend to be more prone to postoperative complications, have lower tolerance to withstand surgery, and generally exhibit poorer outcomes.[116–122] Yano and colleagues[78] observed a morbidity rate greater than 9% for patients older than the age of 70 years compared with just half that for younger patients. In a study by Kuratsu and colleagues,[14] patients older than the age of 70 years demonstrated nearly an eight-fold increase in morbidity compared with that of younger patients (23% vs 3.5%). This was supported by another study that identified a strong negative correlation between Glasgow Outcome Score and age.[123] Although these statistics may be disconcerting for older patients, there is some evidence that this initial morbidity risk may be overcome with time. Li and colleagues[117] observed that patients

older than the age of 65 years with incidentally discovered anterior cranial fossa meningiomas had longer hospital stays and lower Karnofsky Performance Status (KPS) scores at discharge, but most of them recovered 1 year after surgery.

Regardless of patient age, the decision of whether to operate on an incidentally discovered meningioma is a difficult one, especially if the location of the tumor presents additional risks. The middle and posterior fossae overlie vital vessels and cranial nerves deep within the skull base, and gross total resection of these tumors tends to be more difficult for surgeons and more morbid for patients.[124,125] Even ostensibly straightforward convexity and parasagittal tumors may reside by essential motor, sensory, or language cortical areas, and be more susceptible to postoperative edema.[126] Nonetheless, tumors in anatomically precarious locations can be especially imperative to remove.[127] For example, a recent case report highlighted an incidental grade 1 posterior clinoid meningioma that was not surgically resected until after it displayed growth. As a result, the tumor recurred significantly and caused substantial neurologic deficit.[127] In another case report, a patient with an incidentally discovered grade 1 intraventricular meningioma treated with early surgical intervention was able to fully recover with complete resection of the tumor.[128]

Early or unnecessary surgical intervention may contribute to the widely discussed concern of overtreatment in management.[17,21,29,129] Some surgeons prefer removing incidental meningiomas before they grow and become more difficult to resect, and as a result, many patients are operated on before they even develop symptoms.[29] According to Islim and colleagues,[32] who observed a 25% risk of postoperative complications requiring treatment, this approach appears unreasonable, especially because only 10% to 25% of patients will demonstrate growth requiring intervention.[80,126] In any case, surgical excision of meningioma can be challenging owing to postoperative complications and adverse events.[130] As expressed by Näslund and colleagues,[29] because incidental meningiomas can remain asymptomatic even with growth, the deciding factor for surgical intervention should be the extent of clinical progression.[117,126]

Ultimately, the natural history of incidental meningioma is unpredictable, and outcomes from large-scale studies do not always reflect the individual needs of patients.[17,127] The decision to surgically resect an incidental meningioma should be carefully assessed and discussed with each patient, with factors such as growth potential, tumor location, age, and risk of morbidity taken into consideration.[29,117]

Table 3
Summary of various neuroimaging techniques used for diagnosis and management of incidental meningiomas

Neuroimaging Technique	Purpose of Imaging Modality	Mechanism and Role of Imaging Modality	Utility of Imaging Modality	Additional Notes or Limitations
MRI	Diagnostic imaging	MRI uses strong magnetic fields to provide nonionizing multiplanar neuroimaging. It is the gold-standard imaging technique for meningioma detection and serial monitoring	MRI monitoring allows clinicians to assess tumor growth pattern, progression, and operative risk. MRI can display valuable information, such as relative intensity to cerebral cortex, tumor heterogeneity, enhancement, and presence of dural tail, calcification, en plaque meningioma, or edema	Although dural tails are known to be associated with meningioma, the finding could indicate a variety of other dural neoplasms. MRI is not as good at outlining calcifications
Computed tomography (CT)	Diagnostic imaging	CT uses radiographs to display brain tissue, liquid flow, and osseous or calcified structures. It is commonly used to track tumor progression and monitor the brain for effects of treatment	CT scans are commonly used to assess tumor enhancement, presence of calcification, tumor-induced bony changes (hyperostosis, osteolysis), and relative tumor density	CT presents the risk of exposure to radiation; hence, serial monitoring is typically conducted with MRI. However, CT is lower cost than MRI and more accessible.
Diffusion tensor imaging (DTI)	Diagnostic imaging	DTI demonstrates the magnitude and direction of water diffusion in the brain, which can be helpful in assessing meningioma grade and consistency	High-grade meningiomas have shown lower apparent diffusion coefficient values. Most studies have found higher fractional anisotropy values in hard meningiomas	Many DTI parameters have not been shown to be helpful with regards to meningioma differentiation. Studies have demonstrated variable and contrasting findings
Magnetic resonance (MR) spectroscopy	Diagnostic imaging	Spectroscopy reveals metabolite concentration in a particular region. It can be used to differentiate meningiomas from other cerebral metastases	Meningioma is associated with increased choline and alanine levels and decreased N-acetylaspartate and creatinine levels. An elevated metabolite peak at 3.8 parts per million is expected	Studies have shown that MR spectroscopy is unable to differentiate typical meningiomas from atypical ones. Also, relative alanine levels are difficult to assess

(continued on next page)

Table 3
(continued)

Neuroimaging Technique	Purpose of Imaging Modality	Mechanism and Role of Imaging Modality	Utility of Imaging Modality	Additional Notes or Limitations
MR perfusion	Diagnostic imaging	Perfusion imaging can provide data on meningioma vascularity, which helps with differential diagnosis between benign and malignant tumors	High cerebral blood flow (CBF) and cerebral blood volume are expected in meningioma. Also, the time-intensity curve typically demonstrates <50% return to baseline	MR perfusion cannot be used to differentiate meningiomas from hypervascular masses. A recently identified correlation between CBF and VEGF expression suggests the possible utility of MR perfusion to predict tumor response to antiangiogenic treatments
PET with 2-[18F]-fluoro-2-deoxy-D-glucose (18F-FDG)	Diagnostic imaging	PET is a molecular imaging method that reveals biochemical and metabolic information about meningiomas	Meningioma is associated with elevated somatostatin receptor II (SSTR II) expression	Diagnostic accuracy of 18F-FDG-PET is limited in high-grade tumors due to elevated metabolic activity and 18F-FDG accumulation in inflammatory tissue
Frameless stereotactic neuronavigation devices	Biopsy or resection	Frameless stereotaxy displays multiplanar and 3D visualization of perioperative MR or CT images	Frameless stereotaxy has been helpful for planning incisions preoperatively, marking areas of interest, and navigating difficult regions in the brain	Because this method relies on preoperative images, navigation accuracy is hampered by brain shift. Errors with patient registration can increase operating time, navigation errors, and frequency of resections
Intraoperative magnetic resonance imaging (iMRI)	Biopsy or resection	iMRI provides real-time MR imaging during surgery	iMRI helps surgeons determine the extent of resection as well as avoid postoperative complications. The technology may be especially helpful for microsurgical resection of meningiomas close to vital regions or dural sinuses	Intraoperative imaging offers superior navigation accuracy due to automatic registration. However, usage of the equipment requires costly changes in operating room (OR) infrastructure to allow for smooth workflow

Technique	Indication	Description	Advantages	Comments
Intraoperative CT (iCT)	Biopsy or resection	iCT provides real-time CT imaging during surgery	iCT offers high-resolution visualization of soft tissue and osseous landmarks. Like iMRI, the method provides greater control of resection and helps surgeons avoid adverse events, especially for tumors in difficult locations	Intraoperative imaging offers superior navigation accuracy due to automatic registration. However, usage of the equipment requires costly changes in OR infrastructure to allow for smooth workflow. Also, iCT carries the risk of exposure to radiation
Microscope-based augmented reality (AR)	Biopsy or resection	AR superimposes preoperative images onto the surgical field. AR visualization helps surgeons assess the 3D anatomy and orientation during operation	AR can improve depth perception, provide early identification of critical neurovascular structures, increase the rate of extent of resection, and result in less adverse events	Few cases of AR use in skull base meningioma resection have been reported in the literature to support its use
Intraoperative ultrasonography	Biopsy or resection	Intraoperative ultrasonography allows surgeons to assess tumor location, size, and surrounding arteries	Intraoperative ultrasonography can provide valuable information about tumor-supplying vessels. It can help surgeons improve surgical planning, achieve optimal extent of resection, and reduce risk of injury, and postoperative morbidity	Ultrasound image quality is relatively low and tends to decrease during surgery. However, it is a cost-effective and flexible imaging technique
Intraoperative 5-aminolevulinic acid (5-ALA) fluorescence	Biopsy or resection	Fluorescence-guided surgery is an optical imaging method that provides real-time visualization and comprehensive molecular profiling during surgical operation	5-ALA fluorescence provides information about tumor location and instrument placement with high precision, which can help surgeons identify tumor remnants and dural tails and maximize extent of resection	Fluorescence-guided meningioma resection is currently an experimental procedure that is only recommended for long-term studies; its utility and cost-efficiency remain unclear

CLINICAL IMPLICATIONS

In general, incidental meningiomas are not associated with particularly poor clinical outcomes, regardless of intervention.[126] In a large systematic review by Islim and colleagues,[32] only 10% of 608 untreated incidental meningioma patients developed symptoms, including seizures, cranial nerve palsies, or motor, cognitive, and visual deficits. Despite this, 220 patients were referred for further intervention, largely because of radiological progression or symptom development.[32] Although it is unlikely that patients with incidental meningioma develop symptoms, the risk of growth is reported to range between 10% and 70%, and tumor progression increases susceptibility to symptom onset.[20,32,98] Lack of predictability with regards to symptom development and radiological progression is often the primary obstacle to identifying appropriate measures for intervention.[32] Certain clinician groups are working to design predictive modeling methods to make more informed decisions with regards to the most appropriate course of action.[32] Islim and colleagues[32] have been working on validating their prognostic model, Incidental Meningioma: Prognostic Analysis Using Patient Comorbidity and MRI Tests (IMPACT).[43,80] IMPACT is a retrospective multicenter study that categorizes patients into groups of either low, medium, or high risk based on a variety of clinical and radiological characteristics, including tumor volume, hyperintensity, peritumoral signal change, proximity to vital neurovascular structures, age, comorbidity, and WHO performance status.[43,80] The model aims to determine active surveillance management strategies based on risk of progression.[43,80] Another model developed by Lee and colleagues,[26] the Asian Intracranial Meningioma Scoring System (AIMSS), calculates growth potential by taking into account meningioma size, calcification, edema, and T2-MRI intensity, and assigns a different weight to each parameter. AIMSS has been validated by Brugada-Bellsolà and colleagues,[30] who observed rapid growth in 0% of patients in the low-risk group, 12% of patients in the intermediate-risk group, and 25% of patients in the high-risk group. Such risk assessment tools can be useful in identifying patients that may be in need of early intervention as well as in limiting costly long-term follow-up for patients who are unlikely to progress.[7]

SUMMARY

With the increase in technological advancements and neuroimaging accessibility, the rate of incidental meningioma detection has increased significantly.

Incidental meningiomas are much more common among women and the elderly, and higher growth rate is associated with factors such as absence of calcification, MRI T2 hyperintensity, peritumoral edema, and large initial tumor volume. There is no clear consensus on optimal management, with each treatment strategy having unique advantages and disadvantages. Active surveillance is best for small tumors that have yet to demonstrate growth, whereas SRS and FSRT are best for slow-growing small tumors. Surgical intervention is pursued for larger tumors and in cases whereby further growth is particularly dangerous. As most incidental meningiomas are WHO grade 1, a conservative approach is typically recommended. This strategy would involve initial observation with serial monitoring, and then the addition of radiation if the tumor has grown or demonstrates high growth potential. It is agreed that surgical intervention should only be used when proven necessary. In efforts to establish a systematic approach to management of incidental meningiomas, researchers have been developing prognostic models, such as IMPACT and AIMSS, that use known predictive factors to assess growth potential and prescribe different treatment strategies based on estimated risk of progression. Validating these models and conducting larger prospective studies are necessary to definitively reach a conclusion on this controversial, yet important topic.

CLINICS CARE POINTS

- Incidental meningiomas are generally asymptomatic and slow-growing tumors that are more prevalent among women and the elderly.
- Active surveillance remains the preferred management option, unless radiation or surgical resection is deemed necessary.
- Several radiographic predictive factors for tumor growth have been identified for usage in prognostic models for risk assessment.

DECLARATIONS

Funding: K. Mozaffari is supported by the Gurtin Skull Base Research Fellowship. Isaac Yang is supported by the UCLA Visionary Ball Fund Grant, Eli and Edythe Broad UCLA Center of Regenerative Medicine and Stem Cell Research Scholars in Translational Medicine Program Award, Jason Dessel Memorial Seed Grant, UCLA Honberger

Endowment Brain Tumor Research Seed Grant, and Stop Cancer (US) Research Career Development Award.

CONFLICTS OF INTEREST

All authors declare that they have no conflicts of interest.

ACKNOWLEDGMENTS

None.

REFERENCES

1. Nakamura H, Makino K, Yano S, et al, Kumamoto Brain Tumor Research Group. Epidemiological study of primary intracranial tumors: a regional survey in Kumamoto prefecture in southern Japan–20-year study. Int J Clin Oncol 2011;16(4):314–21.
2. Bondy M, Ligon BL. Epidemiology and etiology of intracranial meningiomas: a review. J Neuro Oncol 1996;29(3):197–205.
3. Whittle IR, Smith C, Navoo P, et al. Meningiomas. Lancet Lond Engl 2004;363(9420):1535–43.
4. Claus EB, Bondy ML, Schildkraut JM, et al. Epidemiology of intracranial meningioma. Neurosurgery 2005;57(6):1088–95 [discussion: 1088-1095].
5. Ogasawara C, Philbrick BD, Adamson DC. Meningioma: A Review of Epidemiology, Pathology, Diagnosis, Treatment, and Future Directions. Biomedicines 2021;9(3):319.
6. Louis DN, Perry A, Wesseling P, et al. The 2021 WHO Classification of Tumors of the Central Nervous System: a summary. Neuro Oncol 2021; 23(8):1231–51.
7. Romani R, Ryan G, Benner C, et al. Non-operative meningiomas: long-term follow-up of 136 patients. Acta Neurochir 2018;160(8):1547–53.
8. Reinert M, Babey M, Curschmann J, et al. Morbidity in 201 patients with small sized meningioma treated by microsurgery. Acta Neurochir 2006; 148(12):1257–65 [discussion: 1266].
9. Kshettry VR, Ostrom QT, Kruchko C, et al. Descriptive epidemiology of World Health Organization grades II and III intracranial meningiomas in the United States. Neuro Oncol 2015;17(8):1166–73.
10. Violaris K, Katsarides V, Karakyriou M, et al. Surgical Outcome of Treating Grades II and III Meningiomas: A Report of 32 Cases. Neurosci J 2013; 2013:706481.
11. Klaeboe L, Lonn S, Scheie D, et al. Incidence of intracranial meningiomas in Denmark, Finland, Norway and Sweden, 1968-1997. Int J Cancer 2005; 117(6):996–1001.
12. Cea-Soriano L, Wallander MA, García Rodríguez LA. Epidemiology of meningioma in the United Kingdom. Neuroepidemiology 2012;39(1):27–34.
13. Ostrom QT, Gittleman H, Farah P, et al. CBTRUS statistical report: Primary brain and central nervous system tumors diagnosed in the United States in 2006-2010. Neuro Oncol 2013;15(Suppl 2):ii1–56.
14. Kuratsu J, Kochi M, Ushio Y. Incidence and clinical features of asymptomatic meningiomas. J Neurosurg 2000;92(5):766–70.
15. Bos D, van der Lugt A, Ikram MA, et al. [Incidental findings on brain MRIPrevalence, clinical management and natural course]. Ned Tijdschr Geneeskd 2017;161:D1051.
16. Morris Z, Whiteley WN, Longstreth WT, et al. Incidental findings on brain magnetic resonance imaging: systematic review and meta-analysis. BMJ 2009;339:b3016.
17. Chamoun R, Krisht KM, Couldwell WT. Incidental meningiomas. Neurosurg Focus 2011;31(6):E19.
18. Nakasu S, Nakasu Y. Natural History of Meningiomas: Review with Meta-analyses. Neurol Med-Chir 2020;60(3):109–20.
19. Goldbrunner R, Minniti G, Preusser M, et al. EANO guidelines for the diagnosis and treatment of meningiomas. Lancet Oncol 2016;17(9):e383–91.
20. Behbahani M, Skeie GO, Eide GE, et al. A prospective study of the natural history of incidental meningioma-Hold your horses. Neuro-Oncol Pract 2019;6(6):438–50.
21. Jo KW, Kim CH, Kong DS, et al. Treatment modalities and outcomes for asymptomatic meningiomas. Acta Neurochir 2011;153(1):62–7 [discussion: 67].
22. Sheehan J, Pikis S, Islim AI, et al. An international multicenter matched cohort analysis of incidental meningioma progression during active surveillance or after stereotactic radiosurgery: the IMPASSE study. Neuro Oncol 2021;24(1):116–24.
23. Oya S, Kim SH, Sade B, et al. The natural history of intracranial meningiomas. J Neurosurg 2011; 114(5):1250–6.
24. Yoneoka Y, Fujii Y, Tanaka R. Growth of incidental meningiomas. Acta Neurochir 2000;142(5):507–11.
25. Jadid KD, Feychting M, Höijer J, et al. Long-term follow-up of incidentally discovered meningiomas. Acta Neurochir 2015;157(2):225–30 [discussion: 230].
26. Lee EJ, Kim JH, Park ES, et al. A novel weighted scoring system for estimating the risk of rapid growth in untreated intracranial meningiomas. J Neurosurg 2017;127(5):971–80.
27. Zhang C, Zhang H. Stereotactic Radiosurgery Versus Observation for Treating Incidental Meningiomas: A Systematic Review and Meta-Analysis. Turk Neurosurg 2021;31(2):151–60.
28. Chuang CC, Chang CN, Tsang NM, et al. Linear accelerator-based radiosurgery in the management of skull base meningiomas. J Neuro Oncol 2004;66(1–2):241–9.

29. Näslund O, Skoglund T, Farahmand D, et al. Indications and outcome in surgically treated asymptomatic meningiomas: a single-center case-control study. Acta Neurochir 2020;162(9):2155–63.

30. Brugada-Bellsolà F, Teixidor Rodríguez P, Rodríguez-Hernández A, et al. Growth prediction in asymptomatic meningiomas: the utility of the AIMSS score. Acta Neurochir 2019;161(11): 2233–40.

31. Nassiri F, Zadeh G. How should we manage incidental meningiomas? Neuro Oncol 2020;22(2): 173–4.

32. Islim AI, Mohan M, Moon RDC, et al. Incidental intracranial meningiomas: a systematic review and meta-analysis of prognostic factors and outcomes. J Neuro Oncol 2019;142(2):211–21.

33. Nakamura M, Roser F, Michel J, et al. The natural history of incidental meningiomas. Neurosurgery 2003;53(1):62–70 [discussion: 70-72].

34. Sughrue ME, Rutkowski MJ, Aranda D, et al. Treatment decision making based on the published natural history and growth rate of small meningiomas. J Neurosurg 2010;113(5):1036–42.

35. Nassiri F, Price B, Shehab A, et al. Life after surgical resection of a meningioma: a prospective cross-sectional study evaluating health-related quality of life. Neuro Oncol 2019;21(Suppl 1): i32–43.

36. Thomann P, Häni L, Vulcu S, et al. Natural history of meningiomas: a serial volumetric analysis of 240 tumors. J Neurosurg 2022;1(aop):1–11.

37. Salvetti DJ, Nagaraja TG, Levy C, et al. Gamma Knife surgery for the treatment of patients with asymptomatic meningiomas. J Neurosurg 2013; 119(2):487–93.

38. Kim KH, Kang SJ, Choi JW, et al. Clinical and radiological outcomes of proactive Gamma Knife surgery for asymptomatic meningiomas compared with the natural course without intervention. J Neurosurg 2018;1–10.

39. Pikis S, Mantziaris G, Samanci Y, et al. Stereotactic Radiosurgery for Incidentally Discovered Cavernous Sinus Meningiomas: A Multi-institutional Study. World Neurosurg 2021. S1878-8750(21)01738-1.

40. Hashiba T, Hashimoto N, Izumoto S, et al. Serial volumetric assessment of the natural history and growth pattern of incidentally discovered meningiomas. J Neurosurg 2009;110(4):675–84.

41. Mohammad MH, Chavredakis E, Zakaria R, et al. A national survey of the management of patients with incidental meningioma in the United Kingdom. Br J Neurosurg 2017;31(4):459–63.

42. Niiro M, Yatsushiro K, Nakamura K, et al. Natural history of elderly patients with asymptomatic meningiomas. J Neurol Neurosurg Psychiatry 2000; 68(1):25–8.

43. Islim AI, Millward CP, Piper RJ, et al. External validation and recalibration of an incidental meningioma prognostic model – IMPACT: protocol for an international multicentre retrospective cohort study. BMJ Open 2022;12(1):e052705.

44. Bachir S, Shah S, Shapiro S, et al. Neurofibromatosis Type 2 (NF2) and the Implications for Vestibular Schwannoma and Meningioma Pathogenesis. Int J Mol Sci 2021;22(2):E690.

45. Selvanathan SK, Shenton A, Ferner R, et al. Further genotype–phenotype correlations in neurofibromatosis 2. Clin Genet 2010;77(2):163–70.

46. Braganza MZ, Kitahara CM, Berrington de González A, et al. Ionizing radiation and the risk of brain and central nervous system tumors: a systematic review. Neuro Oncol 2012;14(11): 1316–24.

47. Anzalone CL, Glasgow AE, Van Gompel JJ, et al. Racial Differences in Disease Presentation and Management of Intracranial Meningioma. J Neurol Surg Part B Skull Base 2019;80(6):555–61.

48. Sadetzki S, Modan B, Chetrit A, et al. An iatrogenic epidemic of benign meningioma. Am J Epidemiol 2000;151(3):266–72.

49. Cerhan JH, Butts AM, Syrjanen JA, et al. Factors Associated with Meningioma Detected in a Population-Based Sample. Mayo Clin Proc 2019; 94(2):254–61.

50. Andersen L, Friis S, Hallas J, et al. Hormone replacement therapy increases the risk of cranial meningioma. Eur J Cancer 2013;49(15):3303–10.

51. Fan ZX, Shen J, Wu YY, et al. Hormone replacement therapy and risk of meningioma in women: a meta-analysis. Cancer Causes Control 2013; 24(8):1517–25.

52. Benson VS, Kirichek O, Beral V, et al. Menopausal hormone therapy and central nervous system tumor risk: large UK prospective study and meta-analysis. Int J Cancer 2015;136(10):2369–77.

53. Jay JR, MacLaughlin DT, Riley KR, et al. Modulation of meningioma cell growth by sex steroid hormones in vitro. J Neurosurg 1985;62(5):757–62.

54. Blitshteyn S, Crook JE, Jaeckle KA. Is there an association between meningioma and hormone replacement therapy? J Clin Oncol Off J Am Soc Clin Oncol 2008;26(2):279–82.

55. Michaud DS, Gallo V, Schlehofer B, et al. Reproductive factors and exogenous hormone use in relation to risk of glioma and meningioma in a large European cohort study. Cancer Epidemiol Biomark Prev Publ Am Assoc Cancer Res Cosponsored Am Soc Prev Oncol 2010;19(10):2562–9.

56. Lauby-Secretan B, Scoccianti C, Loomis D, et al. Body Fatness and Cancer–Viewpoint of the IARC Working Group. N Engl J Med 2016;375(8):794–8.

57. Niedermaier T, Behrens G, Schmid D, et al. Body mass index, physical activity, and risk of adult

meningioma and glioma: A meta-analysis. Neurology 2015;85(15):1342–50.

58. Nakasu S, Hirano A, Shimura T, et al. Incidental meningiomas in autopsy study. Surg Neurol 1987; 27(4):319–22.

59. Pikis S, Mantziaris G, Islim AI, et al. Stereotactic radiosurgery versus active surveillance for incidental, convexity meningiomas: a matched cohort analysis from the IMPASSE study. J Neuro Oncol 2022; 157(1):121–8.

60. Herscovici Z, Rappaport Z, Sulkes J, et al. Natural history of conservatively treated meningiomas. Neurology 2004;63(6):1133–4.

61. Olivero WC, Lister JR, Elwood PW. The natural history and growth rate of asymptomatic meningiomas: a review of 60 patients. J Neurosurg 1995; 83(2):222–4.

62. Rubin G, Herscovici Z, Laviv Y, et al. Outcome of untreated meningiomas. Isr Med Assoc J IMAJ 2011;13(3):157–60.

63. Nakasu S, Nakasu Y, Fukami T, et al. Growth curve analysis of asymptomatic and symptomatic meningiomas. J Neuro Oncol 2011;102(2):303–10.

64. Brenner AV, Linet MS, Fine HA, et al. History of allergies and autoimmune diseases and risk of brain tumors in adults. Int J Cancer 2002;99(2):252–9.

65. Schneider B, Pülhorn H, Röhrig B, et al. Predisposing conditions and risk factors for development of symptomatic meningioma in adults. Cancer Detect Prev 2005;29(5):440–7.

66. Schwartzbaum J, Jonsson F, Ahlbom A, et al. Prior Hospitalization for Epilepsy, Diabetes, and Stroke and Subsequent Glioma and Meningioma Risk. Cancer Epidemiol Biomarkers Prev 2005;14(3): 643–50.

67. Schlehofer B, Blettner M, Preston-Martin S, et al. Role of medical history in brain tumour development. Results from the international adult brain tumour study. Int J Cancer 1999;82(2):155–60.

68. Bernardo BM, Orellana RC, Weisband YL, et al. Association between prediagnostic glucose, triglycerides, cholesterol and meningioma, and reverse causality. Br J Cancer 2016;115(1):108–14.

69. Topo P, Køster A, Holte A, et al. Trends in the use of climacteric and postclimacteric hormones in Nordic countries. Maturitas 1995;22(2):89–95.

70. Vernooij MW, Ikram MA, Tanghe HL, et al. Incidental findings on brain MRI in the general population. N Engl J Med 2007;357(18):1821–8.

71. Hashimoto N, Rabo CS, Okita Y, et al. Slower growth of skull base meningiomas compared with non-skull base meningiomas based on volumetric and biological studies. J Neurosurg 2012;116(3): 574–80.

72. Kasuya H, Kubo O, Tanaka M, et al. Clinical and radiological features related to the growth potential of meningioma. Neurosurg Rev 2006;29(4):293–7.

73. McGovern SL, Aldape KD, Munsell MF, et al. A comparison of World Health Organization tumor grades at recurrence in patients with non-skull base and skull base meningiomas. J Neurosurg 2010;112(5):925–33.

74. Sun C, Dou Z, Wu J, et al. The Preferred Locations of Meningioma According to Different Biological Characteristics Based on Voxel-Wise Analysis. Front Oncol 2020;10:1412.

75. Wang M, Wang Z, Ren P, et al. Meningioma with ring enhancement on MRI: a rare case report. BMC Med Imaging 2021;21(1):22.

76. Uchida H, Hirano H, Moinuddin F, et al. Radiologic and histologic features of the T2 hyperintensity rim of meningiomas on magnetic resonance images. NeuroRadiol J 2017;30(1):48–56.

77. Watts J, Box G, Galvin A, et al. Magnetic resonance imaging of meningiomas: a pictorial review. Insights Imaging 2014;5(1):113–22.

78. Yano S, Kuratsu J, Kumamoto Brain Tumor Research Group. Indications for surgery in patients with asymptomatic meningiomas based on an extensive experience. J Neurosurg 2006;105(4):538–43.

79. Schneider JR, Kulason KO, White T, et al. Management of Tiny Meningiomas: To Resect or Not Resect. Cureus 2017;9(7):e1514.

80. Islim AI, Kolamunnage-Dona R, Mohan M, et al. A prognostic model to personalize monitoring regimes for patients with incidental asymptomatic meningiomas. Neuro Oncol 2020;22(2):278–89.

81. Simis A, Pires de Aguiar PH, Leite CC, et al. Peritumoral brain edema in benign meningiomas: correlation with clinical, radiologic, and surgical factors and possible role on recurrence. Surg Neurol 2008;70(5):471–7 [discussion: 477].

82. Kim BW, Kim MS, Kim SW, et al. Peritumoral Brain Edema in Meningiomas : Correlation of Radiologic and Pathologic Features. J Korean Neurosurg Soc 2011;49(1):26–30.

83. Toh CH, Siow TY, Castillo M. Peritumoral Brain Edema in Meningiomas May Be Related to Glymphatic Dysfunction. Front Neurosci. 2021;15. Accessed 4 August, 2022. Available at: https://www.frontiersin.org/articles/10.3389/fnins.2021.674898.

84. Dutta SW, Peterson JL, Vallow LA, et al. National care among patients with WHO grade I intracranial meningioma. J Clin Neurosci Off J Neurosurg Soc Australas 2018;55:17–24.

85. Spasic M, Pelargos PE, Barnette N, et al. Incidental Meningiomas: Management in the Neuroimaging Era. Neurosurg Clin N Am 2016;27(2):229–38.

86. Day SE, Halasz LM. Radiation therapy for WHO grade I meningioma. Chin Clin Oncol 2017;6(1):5.

87. Huang SH, Wang CC, Wei KC, et al. Treatment of intracranial meningioma with single-session and fractionated radiosurgery: a propensity score matching study. Sci Rep 2020;10(1):18500.

88. Tomé WA, Mehta MP, Meeks SL, et al. Fractionated Stereotactic Radiotherapy: A Short Review. Technol Cancer Res Treat 2002;1(3):153–72.

89. Maclean J, Fersht N, Short S. Controversies in Radiotherapy for Meningioma. Clin Oncol 2014; 26(1):51–64.

90. Soldà F, Wharram B, De Ieso PB, et al. Long-term efficacy of fractionated radiotherapy for benign meningiomas. Radiother Oncol 2013;109(2):330–4.

91. Combs SE, Adeberg S, Dittmar JO, et al. Skull base meningiomas: Long-term results and patient self-reported outcome in 507 patients treated with fractionated stereotactic radiotherapy (FSRT) or intensity modulated radiotherapy (IMRT). Radiother Oncol 2013;106(2):186–91.

92. Shaw E, Scott C, Souhami L, et al. Single dose radiosurgical treatment of recurrent previously irradiated primary brain tumors and brain metastases: final report of RTOG protocol 90-05. Int J Radiat Oncol Biol Phys 2000;47(2):291–8.

93. Lesser RL, Knisely JPS, Wang SL, et al. Long-term response to fractionated radiotherapy of presumed optic nerve sheath meningioma. Br J Ophthalmol 2010;94(5):559–63.

94. Saeed P, Blank L, Selva D, et al. Primary radiotherapy in progressive optic nerve sheath meningiomas: a long-term follow-up study. Br J Ophthalmol 2010;94(5):564–8.

95. Soldà F, Wharram B, Gunapala R, et al. Fractionated Stereotactic Conformal Radiotherapy for Optic Nerve Sheath Meningiomas. Clin Oncol 2012; 24(8):e106–12.

96. Paulsen F, Doerr S, Wilhelm H, et al. Fractionated Stereotactic Radiotherapy in Patients With Optic Nerve Sheath Meningioma. Int J Radiat Oncol 2012;82(2):773–8.

97. Abouaf L, Girard N, Lefort T, et al. Standard-Fractionated Radiotherapy for Optic Nerve Sheath Meningioma: Visual Outcome Is Predicted by Mean Eye Dose. Int J Radiat Oncol 2012;82(3):1268–77.

98. Islim AI, Mantziaris G, Pikis S, et al. Comparison of Active Surveillance to Stereotactic Radiosurgery for the Management of Patients with an Incidental Frontobasal Meningioma—A Sub-Analysis of the IMPASSE Study. Cancers 2022;14(5):1300.

99. Pinzi V, Biagioli E, Roberto A, et al. Radiosurgery for intracranial meningiomas: A systematic review and meta-analysis. Crit Rev Oncol Hematol 2017; 113:122–34.

100. DiBiase SJ, Kwok Y, Yovino S, et al. Factors predicting local tumor control after gamma knife stereotactic radiosurgery for benign intracranial meningiomas. Int J Radiat Oncol Biol Phys 2004; 60(5):1515–9.

101. Kollová A, Liscák R, Novotný J, et al. Gamma Knife surgery for benign meningioma. J Neurosurg 2007; 107(2):325–36.

102. Pollock BE, Stafford SL, Link MJ, et al. Single-fraction radiosurgery for presumed intracranial meningiomas: efficacy and complications from a 22-year experience. Int J Radiat Oncol Biol Phys 2012;83(5):1414–8.

103. Biau J, Khalil T, Verrelle P, et al. Fractionated radiotherapy and radiosurgery of intracranial meningiomas. Neurochirurgie 2018;64(1):29–36.

104. Kan P, Liu JK, Wendland MM, et al. Peritumoral edema after stereotactic radiosurgery for intracranial meningiomas and molecular factors that predict its development. J Neuro Oncol 2007;83(1): 33–8.

105. Gande A, Kano H, Bowden G, et al. Gamma Knife radiosurgery of olfactory groove meningiomas provides a method to preserve subjective olfactory function. J Neuro Oncol 2014;116(3):577–83.

106. Sheehan JP, Starke RM, Kano H, et al. Gamma Knife radiosurgery for sellar and parasellar meningiomas: a multicenter study. J Neurosurg 2014; 120(6):1268–77.

107. Simpson D. The recurrence of intracranial meningiomas after surgical treatment. J Neurol Neurosurg Psychiatry 1957;20(1):22–39.

108. Zaher A, Abdelbari Mattar M, Zayed DH, et al. Atypical meningioma: a study of prognostic factors. World Neurosurg 2013;80(5):549–53.

109. Hammouche S, Clark S, Wong AHL, et al. Long-term survival analysis of atypical meningiomas: survival rates, prognostic factors, operative and radiotherapy treatment. Acta Neurochir 2014; 156(8):1475–81.

110. Zeng L, Wang L, Ye F, et al. Clinical characteristics of patients with asymptomatic intracranial meningiomas and results of their surgical management. Neurosurg Rev 2015;38(3):481–8 [discussion: 488].

111. Schwartz TH, McDermott MW. The Simpson grade: abandon the scale but preserve the message. J Neurosurg 2020;1(aop):1–8.

112. Tuleasca C, Aboukais R, Vannod-Michel Q, et al. Intraoperative MRI for the microsurgical resection of meningiomas close to eloquent areas or dural sinuses: patient series. J Neurosurg Case Lessons 2021;1(8):CASE20149.

113. Mao Y, Zhou L, Du G, et al. Image-guided resection of cerebral cavernous malformations. Chin Med J (Engl). 2003;116(10):1480–3.

114. Cannizzaro D, Zaed I, Safa A, et al. Augmented Reality in Neurosurgery, State of Art and Future Projections. A Systematic Review. Front Surg 2022;9: 864792.

115. Tang H, Sun H, Xie L, et al. Intraoperative ultrasound assistance in resection of intracranial meningiomas. Chin J Cancer Res 2013;25(3):339–45.

116. Boviatsis EJ, Bouras TI, Kouyialis AT, et al. Impact of age on complications and outcome in meningioma

surgery. Surg Neurol 2007;68(4):407–11 [discussion: 411].

117. Li Y, Lu D, Feng D, et al. Management of incidental anterior skull base large and giant meningiomas in elderly patients. J Neuro Oncol 2020;148(3):481–8.

118. Nosova K, Nuño M, Mukherjee D, et al. Urinary tract infections in meningioma patients: analysis of risk factors and outcomes. J Hosp Infect 2013; 83(2):132–9.

119. Konglund A, Rogne SG, Lund-Johansen M, et al. Outcome following surgery for intracranial meningiomas in the aging. Acta Neurol Scand 2013;127(3): 161–9.

120. Pirracchio R, Resche-Rigon M, Bresson D, et al. One-year outcome after neurosurgery for intracranial tumor in elderly patients. J Neurosurg Anesthesiol 2010;22(4):342–6.

121. Poon MTC, Fung LHK, Pu JKS, et al. Outcome of elderly patients undergoing intracranial meningioma resection–a systematic review and meta-analysis. Br J Neurosurg 2014;28(3):303–9.

122. Bateman BT, Pile-Spellman J, Gutin PH, et al. Meningioma resection in the elderly: nationwide inpatient sample, 1998-2002. Neurosurgery 2005;57(5): 866–72 [discussion: 866-872].

123. Nishizaki T, Ozaki S, Kwak T, et al. Clinical features and surgical outcome in patients with asymptomatic meningiomas. Br J Neurosurg 1999;13(1): 52–5.

124. Meling TR, Da Broi M, Scheie D, et al. Skull base versus non-skull base meningioma surgery in the elderly. Neurosurg Rev 2019;42(4):961–72.

125. Sharma M, Ugiliweneza B, Boakye M, et al. Feasibility of Bundled Payments in Anterior, Middle, and Posterior Cranial Fossa Skull Base Meningioma Surgery: MarketScan Analysis of Health Care Utilization and Outcomes. World Neurosurg 2019; 131:e116–27.

126. Islim AI, Mohan M, Moon RDC, et al. Treatment Outcomes of Incidental Intracranial Meningiomas: Results from the IMPACT Cohort. World Neurosurg 2020;138:e725–35.

127. Young IM, Yeung J, Glenn C, et al. Aggressive Progression of a WHO Grade I Meningioma of the Posterior Clinoid Process: An Illustration of the Risks Associated With Observation of Skull Base Meningiomas. Cureus 2021;13(3):e14005.

128. Raguž M, Rotim A, Sajko T, et al. Microsurgical management of a rare incidental intraventricular meningioma: a case report and relevant literature review. Acta Clin Croat 2021;60(1):156–60.

129. Born KB, Levinson W. Choosing Wisely campaigns globally: A shared approach to tackling the problem of overuse in healthcare. J Gen Fam Med 2018;20(1):9–12.

130. da Silva CE, de Freitas PEP. Surgical Removal of Skull Base Meningiomas in Symptomatic Elderly Patients. World Neurosurg 2018;120:e1149–55.

Endovascular Embolization of Intracranial Meningiomas

Michelle Lin, MD, Vincent Nguyen, MD, William J. Mack, MD*

KEYWORDS:

- Meningioma • Embolization • Skull base • Anastomoses

KEY POINTS

- In appropriately selected patients with large tumors, anatomically challenging skull base lesions, or robust parasitic arterial supply encountered late in the surgical approach, preoperative embolization may be beneficial.
- Studies have demonstrated decreased intraoperative blood loss and transfusion requirements in patients with completed preoperative devascularization.
- Postcontrast MRI should be considered to evaluate the extent of devascularization even in the setting of completed angiographic devascularization.
- Superselective provocative testing and thorough evaluation for dangerous anastomoses is critical for preventing ischemic complications.
- A periprocedural course of steroids can decrease tumoral edema and its associated neurologic symptoms.

INTRODUCTION

Meningiomas are common primary intracranial neoplasms arising from arachnoid cap cells. They comprise roughly one-third (37.6%) of primary central nervous system neoplasms [1] with a predilection for women and the elderly. These lesions are classified as the WHO Grade I–III dependent on histopathologic features of atypia and proliferative index, with higher grade lesions corresponding to an increased risk of recurrence and local invasion. Although these lesions are considered benign, mass effect can result in presenting symptoms of headache, seizure, and neurologic deficit secondary to involvement of local structures, especially when such lesions arise from the skull base.

Small, asymptomatic lesions in elderly patients may be managed expectantly with serial imaging and observation, whereas, larger, progressively enlarging lesions, or those with associated neurologic deficits, may necessitate intervention. Stereotactic radiosurgery can be considered for lesions less than 3 cm, lesions in challenging anatomic regions that preclude safe resection, or for patients who are poor surgical candidates. In rare instances, palliative embolization has been considered for patients whose medical comorbidities prohibit safe surgical intervention; however, no large series have validated the benefits of this approach. Most of the symptomatic meningiomas are treated with first-line surgical resection.

Given the extraaxial nature of these lesions, they often grow to considerable size undetected before symptomatic presentation. In addition, they often parasitize the surrounding vascular supply, rendering surgical resection more challenging, particularly when the major vascular pedicles are encountered late along the surgical corridor. Therefore, preoperative embolization may be used as an adjunct to decrease intraoperative bleeding and soften lesions through necrosis,

Department of Neurological Surgery, Keck School of Medicine, University of Southern California, 1200 North State Street Suite 3300, Los Angeles, CA 90033, USA
* Corresponding author.
E-mail address: William.mack@med.usc.edu

Neurosurg Clin N Am 34 (2023) 371–380
https://doi.org/10.1016/j.nec.2023.02.008
1042-3680/23/© 2023 Elsevier Inc. All rights reserved.

enabling improved mobilizing of the tumor and decreased retraction on the surrounding neural tissue.

DISCUSSION
Imaging/Diagnostic Cerebral Angiography

On MRI, meningiomas are classically homogeneously contrast-enhancing lesions with an associated dural tail. This uniform, avid contrast enhancement is thought to correlate with the hypervascular tumor blush appreciated on catheter angiogram. Meningiomas characteristically fill in the early arterial phase through the late venous phase in a sunburst pattern, with smaller vascular supplies emanating from larger vascular pedicles.[2]

Advancement of the microcatheter into such vascular pedicles allows for superselective angiography, which can detect distal perfusion to normal brain tissue and aid in identifying dangerous anastomoses. Provocative testing can be performed in awake patients via selective injection of sodium amytal to determine if a vascular pedicle to eloquent territory can be sacrificed (WADA Test). Alternatively, lidocaine may be preferred, given its ability to test vascular supply to cranial nerves.[2] A combination of both provocative agents has been proposed to increase sensitivity before irreversible embolization.[3]

Embolization

Preoperative embolization of meningiomas was first reported by Manelfe and colleagues [4] in 1986. Early descriptions of adjunctive embolization included direct intraoperative puncture of feeding dural pedicles.[5] Advancements in minimally invasive endovascular and microcatheter technologies now allow the superselection of distal arterial feeding pedicles through transfemoral and transradial approaches. Embolization is often performed under general anesthesia so that patients can safely undergo chemical paralysis to permit adequate visualization of embolic agents at high magnification. Although older 4-French (Fr) catheters only allowed access to the proximal middle meningeal artery (MMA), occipital artery, or superficial temporal artery (STA),[5] innovations in hydrophilic catheter and microwire development have facilitated progressively more selective procedures without significant risk of vasospasm or arterial injury to fragile distal vasculature. Larger bore triaxial systems with improved proximal support allow for increased navigability to distal targets, even through tortuous anatomy. Dual lumen balloon microcatheters such as the Scepter and Scepter Mini (MicroVention Terumo,

Aliso Viejo, CA, USA) provide a backstop to minimize liquid embolic agent reflux during embolization. As the navigability and other adjunctive features of microcatheters continue to improve along with an increased temporal and spatial resolution of digital subtraction fluoroscopy, cannulation of tortuous and small dural branches is increasingly feasible and safe.[3]

Arterial access is first obtained via a transfemoral or transradial approach, and a guide catheter (typically 5 Fr or greater) is placed in the proximal cerebral arterial vasculature. A diagnostic cerebral angiogram is performed to assess the feasibility of accessing the feeding vascular pedicles and potentially dangerous anastomoses to uninvolved eloquent structures. Digital subtraction fluoroscopy roadmaps are used to navigate a triaxial system composed of an intermediate catheter, microcatheter, and micro-guidewire through the guide catheter into the vascular pedicle of interest. Superselective diagnostic angiography is subsequently performed to confirm the absence of supply to normal neural tissue. Injection of the desired embolic agent is then performed under live fluoroscopic visualization. Given the risks associated with the embolization of pial feeders, it is less commonly performed, and embolization is targeted toward dural branches.

Frequently used particulate embolic agents included polyvinyl alcohol (PVA) particles and gelatin spheres. PVA particles are an older technology, and their irregular shape and generally larger size can result in early proximal aggregation with poor distal penetration. Smaller PVA particles permit deeper penetration and improved devascularization, but they are also associated with a higher risk of cranial nerve palsies.[6,7] Therefore, the use of PVA particles 150 microns or larger is generally recommended to avoid penetration into the vasa nervorum.[8] The radiolucency of PVA particles makes real-time visualization challenging, and reflux into the parent vessel may go undetected. Furthermore, because of PVA's high coefficient of friction, substantial injection pressures can be needed, resulting in a less controlled embolization.[9] Alternatively, trisacryl gelatin microspheres, which have a more uniform shape, have been used. In one study out of Germany, the investigators found a lower estimated blood loss after surgical resection in 30 patients treated with gelatin microspheres compared with 30 patients treated with PVA particles of various sizes.[10] The addition of platinum coils or gelfoam in the parent vessel can be used as an adjunct to particle embolization to prevent unintended recanalization.[11]

Liquid agents such as n-butyl cyanoacrylate and Onyx have also been successfully used. However, careful preparation is required to allow for polymerization at the desired rate. Prepared with ethiodized Lipiodol, N-butyl-2-cyanoacrylate (n-BCA)'s radiologic visibility allows the operator to monitor its migration in real time. Similar to smaller particles, the liquid nature of n-BCA allows for deeper penetration. With this property also comes the risk of injection into nearby dural venous structures. Onyx (Medtronic, Minneapolis, MN, USA) is a liquid embolic agent that comes premixed and polymerizes on contact with blood, as its delivery vehicle dimethyl sulfoxide (DMSO) dissipates. The microcatheter is first primed with DMSO, and then Onyx is injected under live blank roadmap guidance. Various strategies to facilitate distal penetration without reflux include a "plug and push" technique where adequate time is allowed for a proximal plug of Onyx to form between injections. DMSO-compatible dual lumen balloon microcatheters can also be used to establish a proximal backstop to avoid unintended reflux more readily. General anesthesia is typically used given the caustic nature of DMSO. The inner core of the onyx column remains liquid for a longer period than n-BCA. It is less adherent to vessel walls or the catheter, decreasing the risks associated with catheter removal at the end of the procedure; this can also affect the rate of vessel occlusion. Beyond these standard agents of choice, the investigators have also described the use of ethyl alcohol with balloon assistance,[12] fibrin glue,[13] or even lyophilized dura.[14]

Clinical Effectiveness

Complete endovascular devascularization of meningiomas is not always feasible. Aihara and colleagues reported an 89% tumor penetration rate but obtained completed devascularization in only 51% of patients.[15] Among patients in whom complete angiographic devascularization had been achieved, Borg and colleagues found a significantly lower rate of intraoperative blood transfusion ($P = .035$, n = 117).[16] Comparably, in a single-institution retrospective chart review, Raper and colleagues found lower estimated blood loss in patients who had undergone preoperative embolization ($P = .0074$, n = 224).[17] However, on multivariate analysis, the categorical presence or absence of preoperative embolization was no longer associated with the extent of blood loss, suggesting that variables such as patient selection and extent of devascularization are important in determining efficacy. In a meta-analysis that pooled 34 studies encapsulating a total of 1782 meningiomas, Jumah and colleagues found no clear benefit of preoperative embolization on reduction of intraoperative blood loss, operative duration, the extent of resection, or complication rates.[18] Most investigators conclude that the literature remains equivocal regarding the benefits of preoperative embolization when weighed against the potential risks of embolization and radiation exposure.[19] Preoperative embolization may offer greater benefit in selected patients with particularly large lesions or skull base involvement where access to the main vascular supply occurs late in the surgical approach.[20]

Recent studies suggest that diagnostic cerebral angiography may overestimate the extent of devascularization, prompting comparisons between the fraction of devascularization evaluated on diagnostic angiogram to values estimated from postcontrast MRI. Gruber and colleagues found strong correlations between angiographic devascularization and MRI devascularization, as represented by decreased relative cerebral blood volume and tumor enhancement.[21] Contrary to this, Wakhloo reported complete angiographic devascularization in 14 patients treated with 50 to 150 micron PVA particles; however contrast-enhanced MRIs demonstrated a reduction in enhancement in only 2 of these patients.[7] Similarly, Catapano and colleagues found that angiography overestimated the embolization fraction by approximately 10% more than MRI. These investigators found that only lesions with estimated embolization fractions of greater than 50% on MRI were associated with less than half a liter of intraoperative blood loss, a correlation not observed with 50% embolization fraction as estimated by catheter angiogram.[22] Ali and colleagues found an association between increased embolization fractions on MRI and improved postoperative Karnofsky performance status score and decreased intraoperative blood loss, a finding not observed in the corollary catheter angiogram cohort. These studies indicate that this discrepancy may be due to the improved sensitivity of postcontrast MRI in demonstrating pial vasculature parasitized by tumors.[23]

Postembolization MRI spectroscopy may also be used to demonstrate lactate peaks indicative of ischemia as early as 4 hours postprocedure.[7] Developments in intraarterial MRI perfusion and new gradient echo sequences, such as the susceptibility-weighted principles of echo shifting with a train of observations (SW-PRESTO), may further aid in determining the extent of necrosis following embolization. Histopathologic analysis of embolized meningiomas has validated the presence of necrosis, ischemic changes, and intravascular embolic agents.[24]

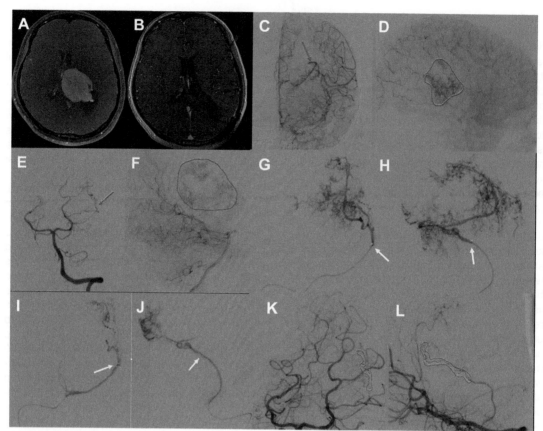

Fig. 1. A woman in her 40s presented with chronic headaches, and post-gadolinium contrast MRI demonstrated an avidly enhancing left intraventricular atrial meningioma (*A*). Long-term follow-up MRI at 18 months postresection demonstrated gross total resection with no evidence of recurrence (*B*). Left ICA injection: feeder from the left anterior choroidal artery (*red arrow*) with tumor blush outlined (*C, D*). Left vertebral artery injection: left lateral posterior choroidal artery feeder (*red arrow*) with tumor blush outlined (*E, F*). Superselective microcatheter (Headway Duo, DMSO compatible, *yellow arrow*) injection of left lateral posterior choroidal artery demonstrated tumor blush without any en-passage vessels identified (*G, H*). Embolization with 200 to 355 micron particles was performed. Follow-up microcatheter injection demonstrated significantly reduced tumor blush (*I, J*). Subsequently, DMSO was used to prime the microcatheter, followed by Onyx 18 injection to embolize the proximal aspect of the left lateral posterior choroidal feeding vessel. Final magnified left vertebral artery angiogram with Onyx cast outlined in red (*K, L*).

Timing of Preoperative Embolization

There is no consensus regarding the optimal timing of surgical resection following preoperative embolization.[25] A retrospective analysis of 50 patients demonstrated a statistically significant increase in estimated blood loss and transfusion requirements for patients undergoing immediate resection (<24 hours after embolization) compared with those who underwent delayed (>24 hours) operative intervention, but there was no association found with the duration of surgery nor hospital length of stay. Studies have demonstrated similar benefits of decreased transfusion requirements when delaying surgical intervention by 7 days after embolization.[26]

Complications

Complication rates reported in the literature range from 0% to 20%.[23,27,28] A meta-analysis from 2021 found a pooled complication rate of 4.3%.[18] Patients with embolization-associated complications have higher rates of operative complications and worse functional outcomes.[23] Some known complications include scalp necrosis, unintended embolization with resultant ischemia, arteriovenous fistulas from arterial perforation, and dural venous sinus embolization. Higher rates of deep venous thrombosis and pulmonary embolism were also identified on multivariate analysis for patients who had undergone preoperative embolization.[29]

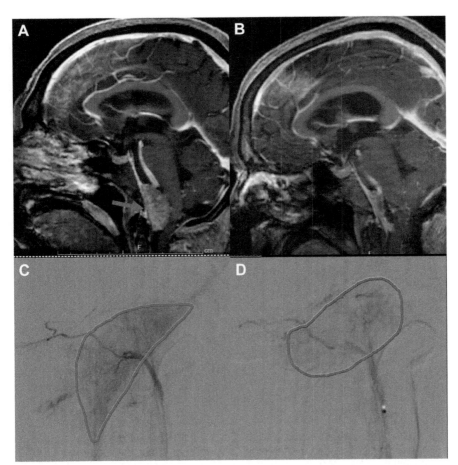

Fig. 2. A woman in her 70s presented with headaches, and post-gadolinium contrast MRI demonstrated an enhancing meningioma centered at the clivus/anterior foramen magnum (*A*). Follow-up MRI at 12 months post-resection imaging revealed good decompression of the brainstem with residual tumor left at surgery due to significant adherence to the brainstem (*B*). Superselective right ascending pharyngeal artery injection (Echelon 10 microcatheter) demonstrates tumor blush consistent with the clival meningioma (*C*). Bilateral ascending pharyngeal arteries supplied the tumor. Following injection of 250 to 350 micron particles through bilateral ascending pharyngeal arteries, there is a greater than 50% reduction in tumor blush, indicating a significant reduction in tumor vascularity (*D*). The *red arrow* indicated the location of the tumor on MRI. The *red color outline* demonstrates the tumor blush on superselective angiography

The most frequently discussed morbidities involve ischemic complications from inadvertent embolization of functionally critical regions.[30] Liquid and smaller particulate embolic agents are associated with higher rates of complete intratumoral devascularization but higher postprocedure cranial nerve palsies.[15] Clinically significant strokes, including a hemispheric stroke, have been reported following embolization, highlighting the importance of careful evaluation of dangerous anastomoses to the intracranial and pial circulation as well as vigilant real-time monitoring for reflux during embolization.[2,23] Vision loss from ophthalmic artery embolization is another important potential ischemic complication, especially given the anastomoses between the ophthalmic artery and MMA seen in both patients and cadaveric models.[8,31–33] Proximal reflux of liquid embolic agents to the petrosal branch of the MMA can result in permanent facial paresis or palsy given its supply to the vasa nervorum of the seventh cranial nerve. Careful study of the diagnostic angiogram and selective provocative testing can assist in detecting dangerous anastomoses or supply to eloquent territory to prevent subsequent ischemic neurologic complications.[2]

Another feared postembolization complication is tumoral hemorrhage.[16] Although a rare complication, when present, it often requires emergent craniotomy for tumor resection and hematoma evacuation.[6,34] It is postulated that postembolization hemorrhage may be secondary to a series of

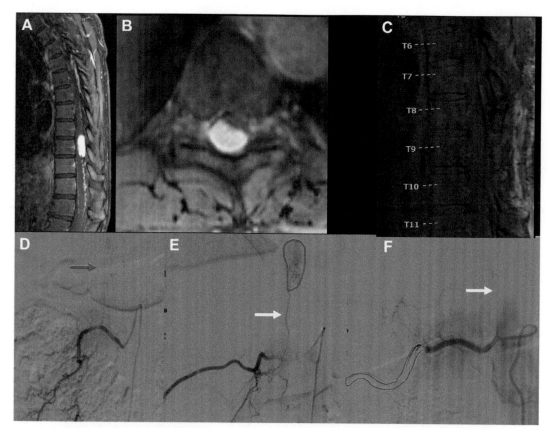

Fig. 3. A middle-aged man presented with sudden onset of lower extremity weakness. He was transferred to our center after an aborted laminectomy at an outside institution because the meningioma was highly vascular at surgery. Post-gadolinium contrast MRI demonstrated an enhancing meningioma centered at T9 (*A, B*). Follow-up MRI at 12 months postresection imaging demonstrated gross total resection with good spinal cord decompression (*C*). Superselective Right T7 intercostal artery demonstrates the artery of Adamkiewicz supplying the anterior spinal artery, marked by the red arrow (*D*). Superselective injection of the Right T11 intercostal artery (Headway Duo microcatheter) demonstrates an arterial pedicle (*yellow arrow*) to a tumor blush at the T9 level outlined in red (*E*). Following flushing of the microcatheter with DMSO and Onyx 18 and Onyx 34 embolization (Onyx cast outlined in red), no further filling of the pedicle feeding the tumor was visualized (*yellow arrow*) (*F*).

pathologic processes including obstruction of venous outflow, forceful embolic injections, tumor necrosis and reperfusion, and the presence of fragile tumor vessels.[9,16] There are some investigators who believe that more cystic lesions are at higher risk for postembolization hemorrhage due to the higher ratio of necrotic tumor and associated fragile vasculature.[34]

Neurologic deficits following embolization can occur secondary to tumoral and peritumoral edema with compression of adjacent structures or acute inflammatory responses. Postembolization tumor edema can result in as great as a 25% increase in tumor volume.[7] A specific delayed (24–72 hours) postembolization neurologic syndrome with associated headache, nausea/emesis, fevers, and malaise has also been described. This syndrome is thought to be self-limiting and best treated with a course of periprocedural steroids.[28]

Dangerous Anastomoses

Orbital region and olfactory groove meningiomas

Lesions in this region carry potential meningo-ophthalmic anastomoses. Inadvertent embolization of the ophthalmic artery carries a risk for monocular blindness, as the central retinal artery is the first branch from the ophthalmic artery. The absence of a choroidal blush, an identifying feature of the ophthalmic artery, on an internal carotid artery (ICA) injection should raise suspicions for a potential aberrant ophthalmic artery origin. The presence of a choroidal blush on an external carotid artery (ECA) run may not be detected until

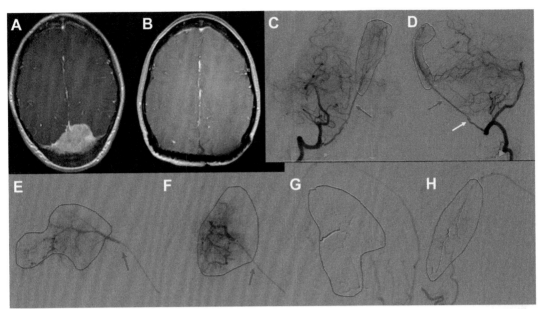

Fig. 4. A woman in her 30s presented with progressive occipital tenderness, and post-gadolinium contrast MRI demonstrated an enhancing midline posterior parasagittal meningioma with invasion of bone, soft tissue, and the venous sinuses/torcula (*A*). Follow-up MRI at 3 years postresection demonstrated gross total resection (*B*). Right vertebral artery injection demonstrates posterior meningeal supply (*red arrow*) with tumor blush outlined in red (*C, D*). A significant tortuosity (*yellow arrow*) precluded microcatheter advancement (*D*). Superselective injection of the left middle meningeal artery (Headway Duo, *red arrow*) demonstrates tumor blush (*E, F*). After flushing the microcatheter with DMSO and Onyx-34, a significant reduction in tumor blush was demonstrated (*outlined in red*) (*G, H*). The right middle meningeal artery was embolized in a similar fashion.

after embolization once pressure dynamics have been altered.[8] There may also be an accessory ophthalmic artery coursing through a duplicate optic canal or superior orbital fissure.[32] In an anatomic study of 14 cadaveric ophthalmic arteries, most of them carried anastomoses with the MMA[33]; this includes possible anastomoses between the recurrent meningeal branch of the middle meningeal and lacrimal artery at the apex of the superior orbital fissure. Similarly, potential anastomoses between the internal maxillary branch of the ECA and the ophthalmic artery have been described. For olfactory groove meningiomas, there are potential connections between the sphenopalatine artery and the ethmoidal branches of the ophthalmic artery.

Parasellar, cavernous, sphenoid wing meningiomas

Sellar, parasellar, cavernous, and sphenoid wing meningiomas have potential anastomoses between the ECA with the cavernous segment of the ICA.[8] The first primary branch of the cavernous ICA is McConnell capsular artery, which supplies the sellar dura as well as the pituitary capsule. Sphenoid wing meningiomas may be supplied by the second branch of the cavernous ICA, the meningohypophyseal trunk. The meningohypophyseal trunk may also share anastomoses with the petrosquamous or posterior MMA. An accessory meningeal artery arising from the internal maxillary artery (IMA) carries potential anastomoses with the final branch of the cavernous ICA, the inferolateral trunk (ILT). Furthermore, the artery of the foramen rotundum connects the IMA with the ILT, which supplies cranial nerves IV and V.[35]

Petroclival, tentorial, cerebellopontine angle meningiomas

For meningiomas in the petroclival, tentorial, and cerebellopontine space, the following anastomoses with the petrous ICA and cranial nerve arterial supply are of clinical importance.[8] The ascending pharyngeal artery gives rise to the neuromeningeal trunk that forms the hypoglossal and jugular branches. These branches travel through the hypoglossal and jugular foramen, supplying cranial nerves IX to XII. In addition, the hypoglossal and jugular arteries give rise to the medial and lateral clival branches, respectively. Jacobson canal transmits the inferior tympanic branch of the ascending pharyngeal that anastomoses with the

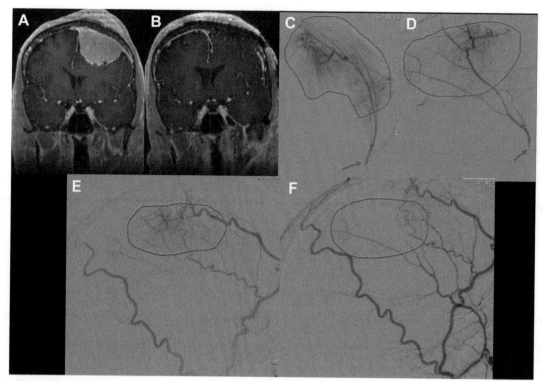

Fig. 5. A middle-aged man presented with word-finding difficulty, and post-gadolinium contrast MRI demonstrated an enhancing giant intra- and extracranial left frontal meningioma with invasion of bone, soft tissue, and mass effect on the underlying cortex (*A*). Follow-up MRI at 12 months postresection demonstrated gross total resection (*B*). Superselective injection of the left middle meningeal artery (Echelon 10 microcatheter, *red arrow*) demonstrates a significant contribution to the tumor's vascularity outlined in red (*C*, *D*). Lateral views of the left external carotid injection demonstrate the tumor blush outlined in red (*E*) with a significant reduction in tumor blush postembolization with 250 to 350 micron particles (*F*).

caroticotympanic branch of the petrous ICA. The distal IMA gives rise to the vidian artery that travels through the vidian canal, followed by the foramen lacerum, in a characteristic horizontal trajectory culminating in a connection with the mandibulovidian branch of the petrous ICA. The distal IMA also has a known anastomoses with the petrous ICA via the pterygovaginal artery. In addition, cranial nerves VII and VIII receive arterial supply both from the labyrinthine artery intracranially and the stylomastoid artery from either the posterior auricular or occipital arteries, an important facial arcade to understand.

Cervicomedullary meningiomas
A musculospinal branch of the ascending pharyngeal curves anteriorly along the odontoid arch to connect with the vertebral artery's C3 radicular anastomotic artery, placing the spinal cord and brainstem at risk. The stylomastoid arising from either the posterior auricular or occipital artery supplies the posterior fossa meninges in additional to cranial nerves VII and VIII as discussed earlier. The thyrocervical and costocervical trunks of the

subclavian artery give rise to the ascending and posterior deep cervical arteries, respectively, which may connect to the vertebral artery.

SUMMARY

Meningiomas are frequently encountered benign intracranial lesions. The hypervascularity, size, and deep location at the skull base in a subset of these tumors can make them surgically challenging. Preoperative embolization may aid in decreasing intraoperative blood loss and transfusion requirements. This clinical benefit is best observed following complete devascularization as evidenced by angiography or postcontrast MRIs. These potential benefits should be weighed against known ischemic and hemorrhagic complications, which can be minimized with provocative preembolization testing and a thorough understanding of potentially dangerous anastomoses. A periprocedural course of steroids may also be considered to minimize tumoral edema and compressive symptoms (**Figs. 1–5**).

CLINICS CARE POINTS

- Preoperative embolization of meningiomas can be beneficial in decreasing intraoperative blood loss and transfusion requirements in appropriately selected patients (often with large skull base tumors that have vascular pedicles encountered late in the operative corridor). This decreased transfusion requirement has not been proved to correlate with improved postoperative functional outcomes nor decreased hospital length of stay.

- Smaller particles and liquid embolic agents are more efficacious in distal tumor vasculature penetration and complete devascularization. However, these agents are also associated with higher rates of ischemic complications and potential postprocedural cranial nerve palsies. Provocative testing and vigilant evaluation of anastomoses can be beneficial in minimizing such complications.

- All patients should be monitored closely following embolization; potential complications include worsening tumor edema and intratumoral hemorrhage, which may necessitate emergent operative intervention.

- A course of prophylactic and postprocedural steroids may be beneficial in minimizing neurologic symptoms associated with embolization.

DISCLOSURES

The authors of this article have no financial or industry connections relevant to the contents of this article.
Clinical Case Presentation #1.
Clinical Case Presentation #2.
Clinical Case Presentation #3.
Clinical Case Presentation #4.
Clinical Case Presentation #5.

REFERENCES

1. Ostrom QT, Gittleman H, Xu J, et al. CBTRUS Statistical Report: Primary Brain and Other Central Nervous System Tumors Diagnosed in the United States in 2009-2013. Neuro Oncol 2016;18(suppl_5):v1–75.

2. Dowd CF, Halbach VV, Higashida RT. Meningiomas: the role of preoperative angiography and embolization. Neurosurg Focus 2003;15(1):E10.

3. Hirohata M, Abe T, Morimitsu H, et al. Preoperative selective internal carotid artery dural branch embolisation for petroclival meningiomas. Neuroradiology 2003;45(9):656–60.

4. Manelfe C, Lasjaunias P, Ruscalleda J. Preoperative embolization of intracranial meningiomas. AJNR American journal of neuroradiology 1986;7(5):963–72.

5. Gruber A, Killer M, Mazal P, et al. Preoperative embolization of intracranial meningiomas: a 17-years single center experience. Minimally invasive neurosurgery : MIN 2000;43(1):18–29.

6. Carli DF, Sluzewski M, Beute GN, et al. Complications of particle embolization of meningiomas: frequency, risk factors, and outcome. AJNR American journal of neuroradiology 2010;31(1):152–4.

7. Wakhloo AK, Juengling FD, Van Velthoven V, et al. Extended preoperative polyvinyl alcohol microembolization of intracranial meningiomas: assessment of two embolization techniques. AJNR American journal of neuroradiology 1993;14(3):571–82.

8. Geibprasert S, Pongpech S, Armstrong D, et al. Dangerous extracranial-intracranial anastomoses and supply to the cranial nerves: vessels the neurointerventionalist needs to know. AJNR American journal of neuroradiology 2009;30(8):1459–68.

9. Fang QR, He XY, Li XF, et al. Comparative efficacy of Glubran and polyvinyl-alcohol particles in the embolization of meningiomas. Int J Neurosci 2016;126(12):1112–9.

10. Bendszus M, Klein R, Burger R, et al. Efficacy of trisacryl gelatin microspheres versus polyvinyl alcohol particles in the preoperative embolization of meningiomas. AJNR American journal of neuroradiology 2000;21(2):255–61.

11. Guglielmi G. Use of the GDC crescent for embolization of tumors fed by cavernous and petrous branches of the internal carotid artery. Technical note. J Neurosurg 1998;89(5):857–60.

12. Jungreis CA. Skull-base tumors: ethanol embolization of the cavernous carotid artery. Radiology 1991;181(3):741–3.

13. Probst EN, Grzyska U, Westphal M, et al. Preoperative embolization of intracranial meningiomas with a fibrin glue preparation. AJNR American journal of neuroradiology 1999;20(9):1695–702.

14. Richter HP, Schachenmayr W. Preoperative embolization of intracranial meningiomas. Neurosurgery 1983;13(3):261–8.

15. Aihara M, Naito I, Shimizu T, et al. Preoperative embolization of intracranial meningiomas using n-butyl cyanoacrylate. Neuroradiology 2015;57(7):713–9.

16. Borg A, Ekanayake J, Mair R, et al. Preoperative particle and glue embolization of meningiomas: indications, results, and lessons learned from 117 consecutive patients. Neurosurgery 2013;73(2 Suppl Operative):ons244–251 [discussionons: 252].

17. Raper DM, Starke RM, Henderson F Jr, et al. Preoperative embolization of intracranial meningiomas:

efficacy, technical considerations, and complications. AJNR American journal of neuroradiology 2014;35(9):1798–804.

18. Jumah F, AbuRmilah A, Raju B, et al. Does preoperative embolization improve outcomes of meningioma resection? A systematic review and meta-analysis. Neurosurg Rev 2021;44(6):3151–63.

19. Iacobucci M, Danieli L, Visconti E, et al. Preoperative embolization of meningiomas with polyvinyl alcohol particles: The benefits are not outweighed by risks. Diagnostic and interventional imaging 2017;98(4):307–14.

20. Ellis JA, D'Amico R, Sisti MB, et al. Pre-operative intracranial meningioma embolization. Expert Rev Neurother 2011;11(4):545–56.

21. Gruber P, Schwyzer L, Klinger E, et al. Longitudinal Imaging of Tumor Volume, Diffusivity, and Perfusion After Preoperative Endovascular Embolization in Supratentorial Hemispheric Meningiomas. World neurosurgery 2018;120:e357–64.

22. Catapano JS, Whiting AC, Mezher AW, et al. Post-embolization Change in Magnetic Resonance Imaging Contrast Enhancement of Meningiomas Is a Better Predictor of Intraoperative Blood Loss Than Angiography. World neurosurgery 2020;135:e679–85.

23. Ali R, Khan M, Chang V, et al. MRI Pre- and Post-Embolization Enhancement Patterns Predict Surgical Outcomes in Intracranial Meningiomas. J Neuroimaging 2016;26(1):130–5.

24. Ng HK, Poon WS, Goh K, et al. Histopathology of post-embolized meningiomas. Am J Surg Pathol 1996;20(10):1224–30.

25. Singla A, Deshaies EM, Melnyk V, et al. Controversies in the role of preoperative embolization in meningioma management. Neurosurg Focus 2013;35(6):E17.

26. Nania A, Granata F, Vinci S, et al. Necrosis score, surgical time, and transfused blood volume in patients treated with preoperative embolization of intracranial meningiomas. Analysis of a single-centre

experience and a review of literature. Clin Neuroradiol 2014;24(1):29–36.

27. Chun JY, McDermott MW, Lamborn KR, et al. Delayed surgical resection reduces intraoperative blood loss for embolized meningiomas. Neurosurgery 2002;50(6):1231–5 [discussion 1235-1237].

28. Tanaka Y, Hashimoto T, Watanabe D, et al. Post-embolization neurological syndrome after embolization for intracranial and skull base tumors: transient exacerbation of neurological symptoms with inflammatory responses. Neuroradiology 2018;60(8):843–51.

29. Wirsching HG, Richter JK, Sahm F, et al. Post-operative cardiovascular complications and time to recurrence in meningioma patients treated with versus without pre-operative embolization: a retrospective cohort study of 741 patients. Journal of neuro-oncology 2018;140(3):659–67.

30. Rosen CL, Ammerman JM, Sekhar LN, et al. Outcome analysis of preoperative embolization in cranial base surgery. Acta neurochirurgica 2002;144(11):1157–64.

31. Friconnet G, Espíndola Ala VH, Lemnos L, et al. Presurgical embolization of intracranial meningioma with Onyx: A safety and efficacy study. Journal of neuroradiology = Journal de neuroradiologie 2020;47(5):353–7.

32. Hayreh SS. Orbital vascular anatomy. Eye 2006;20(10):1130–44.

33. Perrini P, Cardia A, Fraser K, et al. A microsurgical study of the anatomy and course of the ophthalmic artery and its possibly dangerous anastomoses. J Neurosurg 2007;106(1):142–50.

34. Yu SC, Boet R, Wong GK, et al. Postembolization hemorrhage of a large and necrotic meningioma. AJNR American journal of neuroradiology 2004;25(3):506–8.

35. Lasjaunias P, Moret J, Mink J. The anatomy of the inferolateral trunk (ILT) of the internal carotid artery. Neuroradiology 1977;13(4):215–20.

Open Surgical Approaches for Meningiomas

Xiaochun Zhao, MD, Sherwin A. Tavakol, MD, MPH, Panayiotis E. Pelargos, MD, Ali H. Palejwala, MD, Ian F. Dunn, MD*

KEYWORDS

- Cadaveric dissection • Craniotomy • Meningioma • Surgery

KEY POINTS

- Open craniotomies remain the main stream treatment modality in managing meningiomas.
- Exposure that offered by craniotomies and osteotomies is the key for Simpson 1 resection.
- Each craniotomy or approach should be tailored based on individual pathology.

INTRODUCTION

Surgical exposure is of utmost importance in any skull base procedure. A suitable operative corridor will allow for more facile access to the underlying pathology, enable adequate vascular control, limit the need for brain retraction, and reduce the need to traverse healthy parenchyma. Optimal exposure is particularly essential when managing meningiomas, which can be firm in texture and not amenable to significant retraction. In such cases, any additional extent of exposure gained from the approach itself can directly contribute to limiting brain retraction and improving visualization. Since Dr Harvey Cushing described his series of 313 meningiomas in his 1938 monograph,[1] there has been an attempt to refine techniques in open craniotomy for resection of meningiomas. In this article, major open craniotomies and their nuances in managing various meningiomas are demonstrated, along with illustrative case examples.

The authors summarize different approaches or trajectories that can be employed using each craniotomy, and also describe adjunctive osteotomies that offer additional exposure (**Table 1**). The authors believe that pairing the ideal approach and appropriate osteotomy with the proper craniotomy is of paramount importance to optimizing surgical management of meningiomas.

FRONTOTEMPORAL CRANIOTOMY AND ITS VARIANTS

The most widely used open craniotomies are the frontotemporal craniotomy and its variants, which had been used and modified since the dawn of modern neurosurgery by Cushing, Heuer, and Dandy.[2] This craniotomy was optimized and standardized by Yasargil and became the workhorse of neurosurgeons in accessing the anterior, middle, and posterior fossae. Variants include removal of the superior and/or lateral orbital rims, the zygomatic arch, and a number of other modifications including the removal of the clinoid and even the middle fossa floor to access the posterior or infratemporal fossae.

The frontotemporal craniotomy (**Fig. 1**) classically starts with a curvilinear incision behind the hairline, usually 1 cm anterior to the tragus, and curves superiorly and medially, ending at the midline (see **Fig. 1**A). The cutaneous flap, consisting of the dermis, subcutaneous fat, and galea, is reflected anteriorly, and the temporalis muscle is reflected inferiorly. An interfascial or subfascial technique can be used to avoid injuring the temporal branch of the facial nerve (see **Fig. 1**B).[3] The initial burr hole is usually placed posterior to the frontozygomatic suture, exposing the frontal dura. The MacCarty keyhole is designed to provide access to both the orbit and anterior fossa,

Department of Neurosurgery, University of Oklahoma Health Sciences Center, HHDC 4000, 1000 N Lincoln Boulevard, Oklahoma City, OK, 73104, USA
* Corresponding author.
E-mail address: Ian-Dunn@ouhsc.edu

Neurosurg Clin N Am 34 (2023) 381–391
https://doi.org/10.1016/j.nec.2023.02.004
1042-3680/23/© 2023 Elsevier Inc. All rights reserved.

Table 1
Summary of various craniotomies in meningiomas

Craniotomy	Approach/Trajectory	Additional Osteotomies	Meningioma Location	Examples
Frontotemporal (and variants including cranio-orbital, cranio-orbital zygomatic)	Subfrontal	± Orbit removal	Anterior fossa	Olfactory groove, planum, tuberculum sellae, anterior clinoid meningiomas
	Trans-sylvian Pretemporal	Sphenoid wing removal Orbit removal Anterior clinoidectomy	Sphenoid wing Spheno-orbital Cavernous sinus	Sphenoid wing meningioma Spheno-orbital meningioma Cavernous sinus, sphenoid wing meningiomas
	Subtemporal	± Zygoma removal	Middle fossa	Sphenoid wing, middle fossa, cavernous sinus meningiomas
Bicoronal	Transbasal	± Bilateral orbit removal	Midline anterior fossa	Olfactory groove, tuberculum sellae meningiomas
Middle fossa zygomatic	Subtemporal	± Zygoma removal Anterior petrosectomy	Middle fossa Clivus, petroclival region	Middle fossa meningioma Petroclival meningioma
Temporal bone: anterior, posterior, combined petrosal	Presigmoid Subtemporal + presigmoid	Posterior petrosectomy Anterior and posterior petrosectomies	Petroclival region High clivus, dorsum sellae	Petroclival meningioma Dorsum sellae, petroclival meningiomas
Retrosigmoid	Retrosigmoid	± Suprameatal tubercle removal	Petrosal face	Petrosal face meningioma
Transcondylar	Far/extreme lateral	± Jugular tubercle removal	Low clivus, foramen magnum	Foramen magnum meningioma
Supracerebellar	Supracerebellar	Not applicable	Tentorium, pineal region	Tentorial, falco-tentorial meningiomas
Occipital	Occipital transtentorial	Not applicable	Falx, pineal region	Falcine, falco-tentorial meningiomas
Location based	Interhemispheric	Not applicable	Falx	Falcine meningioma

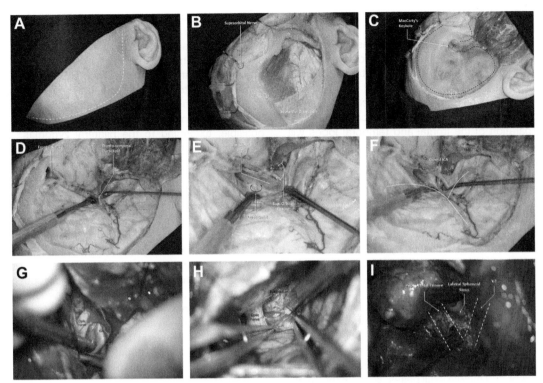

Fig. 1. Illustration of a right fronto-orbital craniotomy representing the frontotemporal craniotomy and its variants. (*A*) The incision starts at the tragus and courses to midline behind the hairline. (*B*) A subfascial dissection is performed to preserve the temporal branch of the facial nerve. (*C*) The MacCarty keyhole is placed, and a one-piece fronto-orbital craniotomy is planned. (*D*) The fronto-temporal dural fold is isolated, deep to which locates the anterior clinoid process; the frontal sinus is entered for illustration purposes. (*E*) Anatomic relationship of the optic canal, anterior clinoid process, and superior orbital fissure is demonstrated. (*F*) After an extradural clinoidectomy, the clinoid segment of the ICA, which is between the proximal and distal dural rings, can be exposed and reserved in proximal vascular control. (*G*) The optic nerve and ICA are demonstrated after proximal sylvian fissure dissection, right-sided approach. (*H*) The lateral subfrontal trajectory is demonstrated in a case of tuberculum sellae meningioma, left-sided approach. (*I*) Illustration of exposure to periorbita and lateral sphenoid sinus pathologies, right-sided approach. Ant, anterior; ICA, internal carotid artery; Proc, process; Sup, superior; V2, maxillary nerve.

with the orbital roof separating the keyhole (see **Fig. 1**C); this is especially useful in the 1-piece cranio-orbital craniotomy[4,5] where the superior orbital rim is removed to facilitate orbital access or an upward view. Then, additional burr holes can be placed along the posterior margin of the bone flap and a craniotomy can be completed depending on the necessity for exposure to the frontal region, the temporal region, or both. The soft tissue dissection and craniotomy should be tailored based on the expected trajectory and exposure.

Additional osteotomies can be carried out to enhance exposure and improve access to the meningioma. Removal of the superior and lateral orbit (eg, cranio-orbital approach) increases the upward accessing angle and superior exposure in anterior skull base meningiomas. Removal of the zygoma

(eg, cranio-orbitozygomatic) permits inferior retraction of the temporalis muscle, and the craniotomy could expose as low as the middle fossa floor.[6] A frontotemporal craniotomy can be considered to be the unmodified version, whereas removal of the orbit or zygoma (or both) is an alteration that provides additional target-based exposure.

Extensive sphenoid wing removal is key to obtaining direct access to the ventral pretemporal dura, which serves as the vascular supply in sphenoid wing meningiomas. The sphenoid wing can be drilled until the fronto-temporal dural fold is exposed (see **Fig. 1**D),[5] and excision of this serves as the gateway to performing the extradural anterior clinoidectomy. The anterior clinoid process (see **Fig. 1**E) is located at the medial end of the sphenoid wing, and an anterior clinoidectomy (see **Fig. 1**F) can unlock the oculomotor triangle, which roofs the cavernous sinus.

Before approaching the skull base, to expand the visualization of the opticocarotid recesses, one may choose to perform a distal to proximal Sylvian fissure split. The arachnoid in the Sylvian cistern is opened with sharp dissection. Arteries and veins should be spared as much as possible. Separation of the frontal and temporal lobes will allow access to the lateral view of the carotid and optic nerve and ease access to the internal carotid artery terminus (see **Fig. 1**G); it also allows for access to the intraoptic triangle, opticocarotid triangle, and the carotid-oculomotor triangle.

Various access trajectories are afforded by this versatile craniotomy. Pure anterior skull base meningiomas can be accessed by the lateral supraorbital approach, which is advocated for by Hernesniemi and colleagues.[7] The lateral supraorbital variant primarily uses the subfrontal trajectory. Anterior skull base pathologies, including some tuberculum sellae, planum sphenoidale, and anterior clinoid meningiomas (see **Fig. 1**H), can be well managed with less exposure of the temporal area. Meningiomas involving both the anterior and middle skull bases, such as the sphenoid wing meningioma and spheno-orbital meningioma, require exposure to both the frontal and temporal areas. In these cases, a full frontotemporal or pterional craniotomy is warranted.

The pretemporal approach can be used through a frontotemporal craniotomy. This approach reduces the distance to the cavernous sinus by way of extensive sphenoid wing drilling, anterior clinoidectomy, and pretemporal dura dissection. This approach provides direct access to the cavernous sinus and posterior fossa pathologies via a transcavernous route. The pretemporal approach was initially proposed by Dolenc[8] and popularized by Krisht,[9] and is less commonly used given the degree of invasiveness. If needed, the superior and lateral orbital walls can be opened in the management of intraorbital pathologies; the area between the first and second branches of the trigeminal nerve can be opened to permit access to the lateral sphenoid sinus (see **Fig. 1**I).

BICORONAL CRANIOTOMY

The bifrontal, or bicoronal, craniotomy is a versatile technique for large midline tumors with anterior skull base invasion given the expansive working corridor that it allows for during tumor resection and cranial base reconstruction. First described by Dandy as a modification of Cushing's unilateral frontal craniotomy, the bifrontal craniotomy originally necessitated significant frontal lobe resection

until Tonnis reported his success with the same approach while preserving brain tissue.[10]

The patient is positioned in a neutral supine position with the head slightly extended to assist in gravitational retraction for access to the cranial base for olfactory groove, planum sphenoidale, and tuberculum meningiomas. A standard bicoronal incision is made ideally behind the hairline if possible, extending to the bilateral zygomas. A skin incision is made through the scalp with care to spare the pericranium. The skin flap is elevated anteriorly (to about 10 mm above the orbital rim) by carefully dissecting through the avascular loose areolar layer while allowing the temporalis and pericranium to remain attached to the skull. The superficial temporal arteries may be visualized here and should be spared. Electrocautery can be used to release the pericranium at the posterior edge of the skin incision to maximize the length of the flap; then the lateral portions of the pericranial flap can be elevated from the superior temporal lines. The pericranial flap is pulled anteriorly using a periosteal elevator until the orbital rims bilaterally and the nasion medially (**Fig. 2**A).[11,12] The supraorbital nerve is encountered coursing over the supraorbital notch.

The craniotomy should be modified to balance obtaining adequate access to the underlying pathology, limiting frontal lobe retraction, and maintaining cosmesis. A standard bifrontal craniotomy can be made by placing burr holes on either side of the anterior superior sagittal sinus, stripping the dura thoroughly, connecting these burr holes with a craniotome and its footplate, extending the width of the craniotomy to about the midpupillary line, and then turning the drill to extend the craniotomy as anterior as allowed by the margin of the periorbital flap. The craniotomy is connected horizontally at the anterior edge with a straight side-cutting burr to carefully release the anterior and posterior tables of the frontal sinus. If the underlying pathology requires an extended craniotomy to be made, then the temporalis muscles must be retracted downward just enough to expose the keyhole using careful subfascial dissection to protect the facial nerve. To include the orbital rim in the craniotomy, one would make an additional burr hole at one or both MacCarty keyholes to have adequate exposure to the periorbita.[13,14] The burr holes on either side of the superior sagittal sinus are connected to those at the keyholes, and the craniotome is taken as low as possible at the orbital rim. This extended bifrontal craniotomy has the advantage of minimizing frontal lobe retraction, but has cosmetic implications. The mucosa of the frontal sinus is removed thoroughly and coagulated, and then

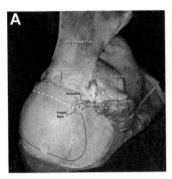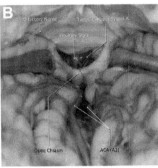

Fig. 2. Demonstration of a bicoronal craniotomy. (*A*) The pericranial flap is preserved for closure, the temporalis can be retracted inferiorly after a subfascial dissection if lower exposure is needed. A bicoronal craniotomy with orbit removal is demonstrated with the red line. The yellow dashed line indicates craniotomy without orbit removal. (*B*) Intradural exposure demonstrates bilateral anterior cerebral artery branches, optic chiasm and bilateral optic nerves, pituitary stalk, and bilateral olfactory nerves. A, artery; ACA, anterior cerebral artery; A2, second segment of the anterior cerebral artery; N, nerve.

filled with fat or muscle; autologous tissue is preferable.

The dura mater is incised using low transverse cuts on either side of the superior sagittal sinus at the posterior border of the craniotomy.[15] The sinus is then tied off at 2 spots using 0-silk sutures and is ligated. The falx is cut, and the dura mater is released and folded anteriorly. This approach permits wide exposure and control to the anterior fossa including the olfactory nerves, optic nerves and chiasm, pituitary stalk, and anterior cerebral artery branches (**Fig. 2**B). After resection of the tumor, the dura is closed in a watertight fashion and the previously harvested pericranial flap can be folded over the frontal sinus and tucked underneath the frontal lobes to cover any anterior skull base defect.[16]

TRANSPETROSAL APPROACH

The transpetrosal approach can provide access to the petroclival area and is commonly used in petroclival meningiomas. This approach can unlock the tentorium and connect the supratentorial and infratentorial spaces. The temporal lobe can be retracted significantly, which allows for a wider operative field. This approach was modernized, refined, and popularized by Graham,[17] Hakuba and colleagues,[18] and Al-Mefty and colleagues.[19,20] The posterior petrosectomy, ligation of the superior petrosal sinus, disconnection of the tentorium, and elevation of the temporal lobe is considered to be the foundational portion of this approach, while other skull base techniques can be used if certain additional regions need to be accessed. An anterior petrosectomy (or Kawase approach) can provide supplementary exposure if the petrous apex and the region inferior to the Meckel cave is involved by the pathologic condition at hand.[21,22]

The incision begins in the middle of the zygomatic arch and curves posteriorly and inferiorly to form a C-shape that includes the entire mastoid process (**Fig. 3**A). A cutaneous flap consisting of the subcutaneous layer and the galea is raised and reflected anteriorly. At the mastoid region, the pericranium consists of the temporalis fascia and the sternocleidomastoid (SCM) fascia, which are tightly fused together, and serves as an ideal vascularized flap that aids in obtaining a watertight closure. The vascular pedicle can be left attached to the temporalis fascia as advocated for by Fukushima and colleagues[23] or to the SCM fascia as described by Borba and colleagues.[24]

The mastoid process, suboccipital area, and temporal area are exposed after elevation of the cutaneous flap, fascia, and temporalis (**Fig. 3**B). Burr holes are placed on either side of the transverse sinus to avoid major sinus injury (see **Fig. 3**B). The "kidney bean"-shaped craniotomy is completed, exposing the dura of both the middle and posterior fossae. The junction of the sigmoid sinus and superior petrosal sinus forms an acute angle referred to as the *sinodural angle* (**Fig. 3**C), which is an important landmark in a mastoidectomy. A mastoidectomy begins with the removal of the superficial cortical bone and the antrum, which is a large cellular cavity located posterior to the external auditory canal. The antrum is usually the first cavity encountered and is easy to identify given its superficial location. The antrum is connected to the tympanic cavity anteriorly, and the incus is usually the next structure to be visualized when drilling the antrum. The facial nerve is immediately posterior to the incus, and the lateral semicircular canal is immediately posterior to the facial nerve (**Fig. 3**D).

Inferiorly, the jugular bulb is fully skeletonized as the inferior vertex of the Trautman triangle. The digastric ridge is a cortical bony ridge that signifies the inferior limit of the facial nerve. If needed, the prefacial recess can be removed carefully where the chorda tympani nerve resides. The posterior and superior semicircular canals are the limits of

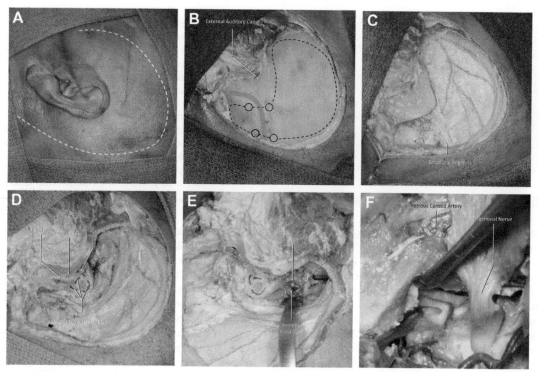

Fig. 3. Illustration of a transpetrosal approach. (*A*) The incision (*white dashed line*) starts anterior to the tragus and forms a U-shaped incision covering the entire mastoid process. (*B*) Four burr holes (*black circles*) are placed by the sinus (*blue transparent strip*) so that the sinus is not violated and can be carefully strapped; a kidney-bean shaped craniotomy is planned (black dashed *line*). (*C*) The sinodural angle is demonstrated, which is formed by the transverse sinus and superior petrosal sinus. (*D*) A mastoidectomy is performed; the incus, chorda tympani, facial nerve, and labyrinth are demonstrated. The presigmoid access can be established anterior to the sigmoid sinus. (*E*) An anterior petrosectomy is demonstrated, with boundaries of V3 anteriorly, GSPN laterally, and internal acoustic canal posteriorly; addition of the anterior petrosectomy can enlarge the exposure to the petroclival area, especially if the Meckel cave (*F*) and area inferior to it is involved. GSPN, greater superficial petrosal nerve; N, nerve; V3, vertebral artery, third segment.

the exposure in this presigmoid trajectory. Partial resection with careful sealing with bone wax may preserve hearing and has been referred to as the *transcrusal approach*.[25,26] The presigmoid and temporal dura is opened with ligation of the superior petrosal sinus. Care should be taken to preserve the vein of Labbe. A line connecting the sinodural angle and the lateral semicircular canal denotes the level of the internal acoustic canal (IAC). Section of the tentorial with protection of the trochlear nerve can unlock and free up temporal lobe elevation, which is the key maneuver in this approach that permits wide access to the petroclival area.

The anterior petrosectomy, or the Kawase approach, is an additional osteotomy that provides access to the petrous apex region, the Meckel cave, and the dorsum sellae. The boundary includes the mandibular nerve, the greater superficial petrosal nerve, and the IAC (**Fig. 3**E, F).

In petroclival meningiomas, the trigeminal nerve is usually displaced laterally by the tumor and the

trochlear nerve can commonly be encased by the meningioma. Wide access provided by tentorium section permits safe resection.

RETROSIGMOID CRANIOTOMY

Fedor Krause is commonly credited with performing the first retrosigmoid craniotomy in 1905.[27–29] Since then, the retrosigmoid approach has been a standard approach for pathology in the posterior fossa, specifically the cerebellopontine angle, petrous face, and petroclival regions.[30] The retrosigmoid approach remains the preferred approach for meningiomas in this region.[30–32]

The preference of the senior author (IFD) is to position the patient in the supine position. The trunk is positioned on the operative edge of the table so that the head is near the edge of the bed, which shortens the working distance to the microscope. A gel roll is placed under the ipsilateral shoulder to avoid excessive stretching of the neck veins and to facilitate the head turning 90°

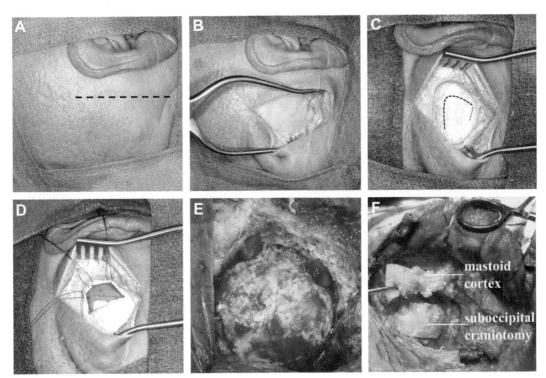

Fig. 4. Illustration of a retrosigmoid approach. (*A*) A retroauricular incision is planned. (*B*) The suboccipital bone is exposed including the digastric groove. (*C*) After a retrosigmoid craniotomy, the dura can be opened (*D*) close to and along the transverse and sigmoid sinus (*black dashed line*). An additional relaxation cut (*red dashed line*) can be performed if access to the cerebello-medullary cistern is needed. (*E*) A trans-temporal craniotomy (or expanded retrosigmoid approach) can be carried out to expose the entirety of the sigmoid sinus (*E*); the mastoid cortex can be harvested for cosmetics in closure (*F*).

with the contralateral zygoma parallel to the floor. The trunk of the bed is elevated approximately 25° to facilitate venous drainage. The Mayfield 3-pin fixation device is then applied, and the head is rotated to the contralateral side until the contralateral zygoma parallel to the floor. The head is mildly flexed while maintaining 2-finger breadth width between the jaw and clavicle. The course of the transverse sinus can be identified as a palpable groove through the scalp. This course is confirmed, and the craniocaudal extent of the transverse-sigmoid junction is approximated using the superior nuchal line.[33] This approximation is further confirmed using the neuronavigation system. A linear incision is planned approximately 2-finger breadths posterior to the external auditory canal with one-third of the incision lying above the transverse-sigmoid junction and two-thirds lying below it (**Fig. 4**A). Neuromonitoring is routinely used with monitoring motor evoked potentials, somatosensory evoked potentials, brainstem auditory evoked responses, and cranial nerve VII routinely performed. Depending on tumor location and size, cranial nerves IV and VI can also be monitored, as well as the lower cranial nerves.

The dissection is performed through the skin, subcutaneous tissues, and nuchal musculature, which are swept laterally to expose the mastoid and the digastric groove (**Fig. 4**B). A single burr hole is placed at the asterion, and a posterior craniotomy flap is turned to expose the transverse and sigmoid sinuses. The dural incision borders the transverse and sigmoid sinuses, leaving a narrow cuff of dura to facilitate tight closure. There is typically no need for lumbar drain placement, as an inferior dural incision parallel to the foramen magnum can be made, which facilitates access to the lateral part of cisterna magna to drain cerebrospinal fluid (**Fig. 4**C, D). This also obviates mannitol or furosemide in these cases. Following opening of the dura, microneurosurgical technique is used to resect the meningioma. Once resection of the tumor is completed, primary dural closure is typically performed. If unable to perform a tight dural closure, muscle can be used to supplement the closure or, rarely, a dural patch can be sewn in place. The mastoid air cells are usually occluded with bone wax or abdominal fat. The craniotomy flap is fit so that the anterior-superior portion is flush and covering the sinuses.

To expand the operative corridor, adjuncts can be performed to broaden the exposure. In patients with significant nuchal muscle bulk, a muscular flap is raised involving the temporalis, sternocleidomastoid, and the splenius capitis muscles. The scalp is exposed while preserving the musculature and reflected forward. Monopolar electrocautery is used to create a muscular flap starting at the mastoid base, arcing superiorly, and coursing back posteriorly and inferiorly. The sternocleidomastoid muscle is then reflected medially and inferiorly to expose the mastoid process and digastric groove. The remaining suboccipital musculature is then in a subperiosteal fashion and retracted inferiorly.

If there is a need to expand access to the cerebellopontine angle, a transmastoid approach (**Fig. 4**E, F) can be performed using a partial mastoidectomy[34]; this skeletonizes the sigmoid sinus in its entirety and allows for its mobilization during dural opening. This allows for easier access to the ventral brainstem and the medial aspects of the cerebellopontine angle cistern.[34]

The jugular bulb can also be skeletonized, and the infrajugular space drilled, allowing low-lying access in the posterior fossa. When opening dura, a low-lying incision in the posterior fossa can lead to accessing the cisterna magna and releasing cerebrospinal fluid; this facilitates brain relaxation, allowing us to work in the cerebellopontine angle in an easier fashion.

When looking to tackle meningiomas that may extend into the middle fossa, Kawase triangle can be drilled from the posterior aspect. This reverse Kawase approach can be used to drill the petrous apex posteriorly. The tentorium is cut in parallel to the petrous ridge, under visualization of the trochlear nerve, and the portions in Meckel cave, posterior cavernous sinus, and the middle fossa.[35]

TRANSCONDYLAR CRANIOTOMY

There have been various modifications since the initial transcondylar approach was described by Babu and colleagues[36], Bertalanffy and Seeger[37], and Heros.[38,39] The transcondylar approach is designed to access low clivus and ventral foramen magnum meningiomas. The key maneuver in this approach is to drill the occipital condyle so that the operating corridor is flattened from a lateral access viewpoint.

There are various versions of the incision, including the horseshoe, C-shaped, and "lazy-S" incision. The authors prefer the C-shaped incision based at the mastoid process (**Fig. 5**A). The cutaneous flap can be reflected anteriorly to the mastoid process, the suboccipital muscles can be dissected in a layer-by-layer fashion (**Fig. 5**B), a lateral to medial muscular dissection can optimize lateral access,[36] while the muscle bulk is avoided (**Fig. 5**C). This muscle dissection technique can expose the entire length of C1 while no muscle is attached to the lateral tubercle. To provide access to the ventral foramen magnum, the occipital condylar osteotomy is the key step following completion of a unilateral suboccipital craniotomy and C1 hemilaminectomy.

Depending on the extent of ventral access needed, there are 2 approaches offering different lateral approaching angles: far lateral and extreme lateral approaches. An extreme lateral approach is defined when the dura 1 cm or more ventral to the vertebral artery dural entry site can be accessed.[36] This approach provides a trajectory lateral to the spinal accessory nerve, which allows for better exposure to the ventral foramen magnum (**Fig. 5**D). When this approach is performed, it is imperative to position the patient in a manner in which the occipital condyle has not shifted in relation to the C1 articular surface. In other words, the patient's head should not be rotated in relation to the neck (**Fig. 5**E).

If needed, the C1 transverse foramen can be opened, and the vertebral artery can be transposed medially to provide even further lateral access and ventral exposure. The condyle can be drilled until the hypoglossal canal is opened. If more condyle needs to be removed, an occipital-cervical fusion can be considered to ensure postoperative stability. The jugular tubercle is the bony protrusion between the hypoglossal canal and jugular bulb over which the spinal accessory nerve travels. Removal of the jugular tubercle can expand and extend the exposure rostrally, which is referred to as "the ELITE approach" by Fukushima and colleagues.[23]

The dura can subsequently be opened using a C-shaped incision. The dentate ligament is usually the first to be incised after the arachnoid layer is released. Addressing posterior inferior cerebellar artery aneurysms may be possible via the vagoaccessory triangle, which is medial to the spinal accessory nerve.[40] However, ventral foramen magnum meningiomas require further access lateral to the spinal accessory nerve, for which reason an extensive condylar osteotomy that obtains maximum lateral access is critical in this case (**Fig. 5**F).

CRANIOTOMIES IN FALCOTENTORIAL MENINGIOMAS

The falcotentorial meningioma constitutes its own entity given the deep-seated location and important vascular relationships in near proximity. There

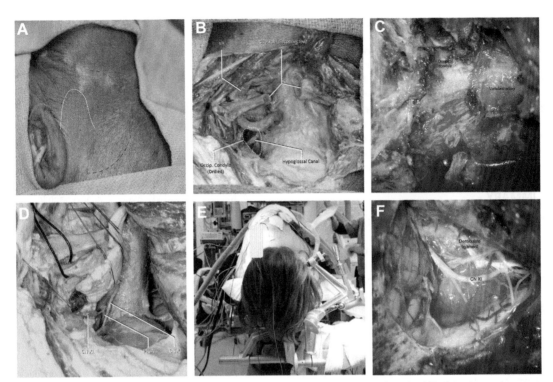

Fig. 5. Illustration of a transcondylar craniotomy. (*A*) A C-shaped incision (*red dashed line*) is planned to center the mastoid process (*yellow dashed line*). (*B*) A suboccipital craniotomy, hemilaminectomy of C1, and occipital condylar osteotomy are performed to complete the craniotomy. The occipital condyle is drilled until the hypoglossal canal is skeletonized. (*C*) Intraoperative image demonstrated similar exposure. (*D*) The dura is opened, and the dentate ligament is incised; the PICA is demonstrated branching off the vertebral artery. Sufficient access lateral to the spinal accessory nerve is obtained. (*E*) Patient positioning; relatively minimum rotation of the neck is used to avoid anatomic shift of the occipital-cervical joint. (*F*) Intraoperative image demonstrated a right sided transcondylar craniotomy in a foramen magnum meningioma; wide access lateral to the spinal accessory permits optimal dura base control and maneuverability. CN XI, glossopharyngeal nerve; CN XII, hypoglossal nerve; Occip, occipital; PICA, posterior inferior cerebellar artery; VA, vertebral artery.

are several eloquent and vulnerable neurovascular structures in this area, including the vein of Galenic group, the straight sinus, the pineal gland, the tectum, and the medial posterior choroidal arteries.[41] Management of falcotentorial meningiomas is also highly individualized because many craniotomies and approaches can provide access to this region. The occipital transtentorial approach and supercerebellar infratentorial approach are commonly used in falcotentorial meningiomas. Selection of the approach is performed by considering the origin of the meningioma, growth pattern, and directional displacement of the veins of Galenic group.[42]

The occipital transtentorial approach involves a craniotomy near the junction of the sagittal sinus and transverse sinus, and it used the interhemispheric trajectory given the lack of bridging veins in the occipital area. The patient can be positioned laterally with the approaching side down, so the ipsilateral occipital lobe can be retracted down with gravity, and the operating corridor can be maintained with no manual retraction. This technique minimizes retraction on the medial occipital lobe, which is the primary visual cortex. Both tentorium and falx can be incised open to provide exposure to the infratentorial space and contralateral supratentorial area.

The supracerebellar infratentorial approach uses a midline or paramedian craniotomy with the transverse sinus exposed. A sitting position can facilitate cerebellar retraction by gravity, but a preoperative echocardiogram is warranted due to the risk of air embolism. The free space is naturally larger in the infratentorial space than the supratentorial space without retraction on the cerebellum. The tentorium can be opened lateral to the straight sinus bilaterally to permit access if there is any supratentorial tumor extension. A steep tentorial slope angle is an unfavorable factor in a supracerebellar infratentorial approach due to the upward working angle.[41,43]

The anterior interhemispheric trans-splenial approach is another approach to the pineal area advocated by Spetzler,[44] which avoids medial occipital lobe and utilizes the anterior bridging vein-free zone. However, this approach is surgically challenging due to the long reaching distance. A torcular craniotomy, which combines bilateral occipital and supracerebellar trajectories and centers the torcular, provides maximum exposure to the falcotentorial junction but should be reserved for extreme cases given its degree of invasiveness.[45]

SUMMARY

Open craniotomy continues to be the primary surgical treatment in meningiomas, and Simpson grade 1 resection should always be the goal of meningioma surgery. Exposure is of paramount importance to obtain optimal maneuverability. Preoperative evaluation plays the most crucial role in approach selection, and planning should be carefully tailored in an individualized fashion. Every craniotomy should take advantage of the possible adjunctive osteotomies, given that every additional millimeter in exposure will be rewarded during surgical resection of meningioma.

CLINICS CARE POINTS

- Dispite multiple adjuvent therapy options available, open surgical resection remains as main treatment modality.
- Individulized approach selection is of paramount improtance in indivadual pathology.

DISCLOSURES

None.

FINANCIAL SUPPORT

None.

ACKNOWLEDGMENTS

None.

REFERENCES

1. Cushing H. Meningiomas: their classification, regional behavior, life history, and surgical end result111. Springfield: Charles C Thomas; 1938. p. 735.
2. Altay T, Couldwell WT. The frontotemporal (pterional) approach: an historical perspective. Neurosurgery 2012;71(2):481–92.
3. Coscarella E., Vishteh A.G., Spetzler R.F., et al., Subfascial and submuscular methods of temporal muscle dissection and their relationship to the frontalis branch of the facial nerve, J Neurosurg, 92 (5), 2000, 877–880.
4. MacCarty C, Kenefick T, McConahey W, Kearns T. Ophthalmopathy of Graves' disease treated by removal of roof lateral walls and lateral sphenoid ridge: review of 46 cases. Mayo Clin Proc 1970; 45(7):488–93.
5. Zabramski JM, Kiriş T, Sankhla SK, et al. Orbitozygomatic craniotomy. J Neurosurg 1998;89(2):336–41.
6. Al-Mefty O, Anand VK. Zygomatic approach to skull-base lesions. J Neurosurg 1990;73(5):668–73.
7. Hernesniemi J, Ishii K, Niemelä M, et al. Lateral supraorbital approach as an alternative to the classical pterional approach. In: New Trends of Surgery for Stroke and Its Perioperative Management. Vienna: Springer; 2005. p. 17–21.
8. Dolenc V. Direct microsurgical repair of intracavernous vascular lesions. J Neurosurg 1983;58(6):824–31.
9. Krisht AF. Transcavernous approach to diseases of the anterior upper third of the posterior fossa. Neurosurg Focus 2005;19(2):1–10.
10. Morales-Valero SF, Van Gompel JJ, Loumiotis I, Lanzino G. Craniotomy for anterior cranial fossa meningiomas: historical overview. Neurosurg Focus 2014;36(4):E14.
11. Chi J.H., Parsa A.T., Berger M.S., et al., Extended bifrontal craniotomy for midline anterior fossa meningiomas: minimization of retraction-related edema and surgical outcomes. Operative Neurosurgery. 2006, 59(suppl_4), ONS-426-ONS-434.
12. Dolci RLL, Todeschini AB, Santos ARLD, et al. Endoscopic endonasal double flap technique for reconstruction of large anterior skull base defects: technical note. Braz J Otorhinolaryngol 2019;85(4): 427–34.
13. Rhoton AL Jr. The anterior and middle cranial base. Neurosurgery 2002;51(suppl_4). S1-S273-S1-302.
14. Chandler JP, Silva FE. Extended transbasal approach to skull base tumors. Technical nuances and review of the literature. Oncology (Williston Park, NY) 2005;19(7):913–9 [discussion: 920, 923].
15. Dunn IF, Zhao X, Pelargos PE, et al. Anterior Fossa Pathology: Open Surgical Approaches. Contemporary Skull Base Surgery. Cham: Springer; 2022. p. 197–213.
16. Obeid F, Al-Mefty O. Recurrence of olfactory groove meningiomas. Neurosurgery 2003;53(3):534–43.
17. Graham MD. Surgical exposure of the facial nerve indications and techniques. J Laryngol Otol 1975; 89(6):557–75.
18. Hakuba A, Nishimura S, Jang BJ. A combined retroauricular and preauricular transpetrosal-transtentorial approach to clivus meningiomas. Surg Neurol 1988;30(2):108–16.

19. Al-Mefty O, Fox JL Sr, Smith RR. Petrosal approach for petroclival meningiomas. Neurosurgery 1988; 22(3):510–7.

20. Gross BA, Tavanaiepour D, Du R, et al. Evolution of the posterior petrosal approach. Neurosurg Focus 2012;33(2):E7.

21. Kawase T, Toya S, Shiobara R, et al. Transpetrosal approach for aneurysms of the lower basilar artery. J Neurosurg 1985;63(6):857–61.

22. Van Gompel JJ, Alikhani P, Youssef AS, et al. Anterior petrosectomy: consecutive series of 46 patients with attention to approach-related complications. J Neurol Surg B Skull Base 2015;76(05):379–84.

23. Fukushima T, Day J, Maroon J. Manual of skull base dissection. Pittsburgh: AF Neuro Video; 1996. p. 111–23.

24. Rassi M.S., Zamponi Jr J.O., Cândido D.N., et al., Combined presigmoid and retrosigmoid approach to petroclival meningiomas. J Neurol Surg B Skull Base. 2018;79(S 05):S402-S403.

25. Horgan MA, Delashaw JB, Schwartz MS, et al. Transcrusal approach to the petroclival region with hearing preservation: Technical note and illustrative cases. J Neurosurg 2001;94(4):660–6.

26. Tayebi Meybodi A, Liu JK. Endoscopic-assisted combined transcrusal anterior petrosal approach for resection of large petroclival meningioma: operative video and nuances of technique. Neurosurg Focus: Video 2022;6(2):V10.

27. Basma J, Anagnostopoulos C, Tudose A, et al. History, Variations, and Extensions of the Retrosigmoid Approach: Anatomical and Literature Review. J Neurol Surg B Skull Base 2022;83(Suppl 2):e324–35.

28. Elhammady MS, Telischi FF, Morcos JJ. Retrosigmoid Approach:: Indications, Techniques, and Results. Otolaryngol Clin 2012;45(2):375–97.

29. Fraenkel J, et al. I. Contribution to the surgery of neurofibroma of the acoustic nerve: with remarks on the surgical procedure. Ann Surg 1904;40(3): 293.

30. Samii M, Tatagiba M, Carvalho GA. Resection of large petroclival meningiomas by the simple retrosigmoid route. J Clin Neurosci 1999;6(1):27–30.

31. Bambakidis NC, Kakarla UK, Kim LJ, et al. Evolution of surgical approaches in the treatment of petroclival meningiomas: a retrospective review. Operative Neurosurg 2007;61:ONS202–11.

32. DeMonte F, McDermott MW, Al-Mefty O. Al-Mefty's meningiomas. Georg Thieme Verlag; 2011.

33. Day JD, Jordi XK, Manfred T, et al. Surface and superficial surgical anatomy of the posterolateral cranial base: significance for surgical planning and approach. Neurosurgery 1996;38(6):1079–84.

34. Abolfotoh M, Dunn IF, Al-Mefty O. Transmastoid retrosigmoid approach to the cerebellopontine angle: surgical technique. Operative Neurosurgery 2013; 73(suppl_1):ons16–23.

35. Tatagiba M, Rigante L, Mesquita Filho P, et al. Endoscopic-assisted posterior intradural petrous apicectomy in petroclival meningiomas: a clinical series and assessment of perioperative morbidity. World Neurosurg 2015;84(6):1708–18.

36. Babu RP, Sekhar LN, Wright DC. Extreme lateral transcondylar approach: technical improvements and lessons learned. J Neurosurg 1994;81(1): 49–59.

37. Bertalanffy H, Seeger W. The dorsolateral, suboccipital, transcondylar approach to the lower clivus and anterior portion of the craniocervical junction. Neurosurgery 1991;29(6):815–21.

38. Heros RC. Lateral suboccipital approach for vertebral and vertebrobasilar artery lesions. J Neurosurg 1986;64(4):559–62.

39. George B, Dematons C, Cophignon J. Lateral approach to the anterior portion of the foramen magnum: application to surgical removal of 14 benign tumors. Surg Neurol 1988;29(6):484–90.

40. Meybodi AT, Moreira LB, Zhao X, et al. Anatomical analysis of the vagoaccessory triangle and the triangles within: the suprahypoglossal, infrahypoglossal, and hypoglossal–hypoglossal triangles. World neurosurgery 2019;126:e463–72.

41. Zhao X, Belykh E, Przybylowski CJ, et al. Surgical treatment of falcotentorial meningiomas: a retrospective review of a single-institution experience. J Neurosurg 2019;133(3):630–41.

42. Bassiouni H, Asgari S, König H-J, et al. Meningiomas of the falcotentorial junction: selection of the surgical approach according to the tumor type. Surg Neurol 2008;69(4):339–49.

43. Syed HR, Jean WC. A novel method to measure the tentorial angle and the implications on surgeries of the pineal region. World Neurosurgery 2018;111: e213–20.

44. Yağmurlu K, Zaidi HA, Kalani MYS, et al. Anterior interhemispheric transsplenial approach to pineal region tumors: anatomical study and illustrative case. J Neurosurg 2017;128(1):182–92.

45. Quiñones-Hinojosa A, Chang EF, Chaichana KL, et al. Surgical considerations in the management of falcotentorial meningiomas: advantages of the bilateral occipital transtentorial/transfalcine craniotomy for large tumors. Operative Neurosurg 2009; 64:ons260–8.

Endoscopic Endonasal and Keyhole Surgery for Skull Base Meningiomas

Ilaria Bove, MD[a,b],*, Stephanie Cheok, MD[a], Jacob J. Ruzevick, MD[a], Gabriel Zada, MD, MS[a]

KEYWORDS

- Meningioma • Skull base • Keyhole • Endoscopic endonasal approach • Supraorbital approach

KEY POINTS

- Minimally invasive supraorbital and endonasal endoscopic approaches (EEAs) are safe and favorable approaches for selected anterior skull base (ASB) meningiomas.
- The supraorbital technique is ideal for unilateral or midline ASB meningiomas. Visualization and tumor resection can be supplemented with 0° and angled endoscopes.
- A supraorbital approach is more frequently selected if the meningiomas are larger than 3 cm or for lesions that extend laterally beyond one or both of the optic nerves, internal carotid arteries, or anterior clinoid processes.
- Advantages of EEA include a magnified view, direct midline exposure, early access to skull base, dura, and feeling vessels allowing for devascularization of the tumor and decompression of the optic apparatus.
- The superiorly oriented angle of approach allows the intervening arachnoid plane to protect the vascular supply of the optic apparatus to further improve visual outcomes in these patients.

INTRODUCTION

Meningiomas constitute 30% of all intracranial tumors, of which ASB meningiomas comprise approximately 10%.[1,2] These tumors can originate from the dura along the olfactory groove, planum sphenoidale (PS), and the tuberculum sellae (TS). Generally, symptoms are caused from mass effect against adjacent neurovascular structures, particularly to the olfactory nerves, optic nerves (ONs) and chiasm, cavernous sinus and its neurovascular contents, and/or the frontal lobes. For large, growing and symptomatic ASB meningiomas, the primary treatment is surgery, and the goal of meningioma surgery is to achieve gross total or maximal safe resection to minimize tumor recurrence. Historically, the resection of ASB meningioma has been achieved by transcranial approaches (TCAs).[3] Numerous TCAs are available to treat ASB meningiomas including the pterional, bifrontal, transbasal, and orbitozygomatic approaches. To access ASB meningiomas, TCAs often mandate some degree of brain retraction, sagittal sinus transection, or ON manipulation, and challenges related to edema, venous drainage, and wound healing represent the main potential complications. The last several decades have shown the evolution and implementation of minimally invasive approaches that benefit from the use of endoscope. These include the endoscopic endonasal approach (EEA) and the supraorbital keyhole minicraniotomy, performed via an eyebrow incision with or without endoscopic assistance. Decision-making and case selection

[a] Department of Neurological Surgery, The University of Southern California Keck, School of Medicine, Los Angeles, CA, USA; [b] Division of Neurosurgery, Department of Neurological Sciences, Università degli Studi di Napoli Federico II, Naples
* Corresponding author.
E-mail address: ilariabove90@gmail.com

Neurosurg Clin N Am 34 (2023) 393–402
https://doi.org/10.1016/j.nec.2023.02.003
1042-3680/23/© 2023 Elsevier Inc. All rights reserved.

depend on the anatomic and imaging features of the meningioma and its relationship to critical neurovascular structures. In this article, we describe the supraorbital keyhole and extended endoscopic endonasal approaches (EEEAs) for the resection of ASB meningiomas.

SUPRAORBITAL KEYHOLE APPROACH

The supraorbital keyhole craniotomy is a tailored approach for ASB pathology and was first described by Krause in the early 1900s and then popularized by Perneczky in the 1990s, primarily for anterior circulation aneurysm ligation.[4,5] The supraorbital approach represents a minimally invasive surgical approach to reach anterior cranial fossa floor and the parasellar region. Patient selection depends on the position of the tumor and its relationship to surrounding bony and neurovascular structures, which is determined using preoperative MR and CT imaging (eg, see **Fig. 1**). The goal of the approach is to provide adequate access to the ASB and to be able to excise the tumor, with minimal retraction of the gyrus rectus. This technique allows the surgeon to approach and work between both ONs, as well as both inferior and superior to the optic chiasm, using a very minimal eyebrow or traditional hairline incision and a well-placed 3 × 2 cm craniotomy immediately above the orbital roof. Visualization can be enhanced by the use of endoscope, in particular angled endoscopes, which provide better views and access to the sellar region, the circle of Willis, the anterior third ventricle, the anterior interhemispheric fissure, the upper third of the clivus, the interpeduncular cistern, and the medial aspect of the ipsilateral middle cranial fossa and temporal lobe.[6] A supraorbital approach is more frequently selected if the meningiomas are larger than 3 cm or for lesions that extend laterally beyond one or both of the ONs, internal carotid arteries, or anterior clinoid processes. These are anatomic areas that often require standard microsurgical instruments, and therefore inaccessible from an endonasal corridor. Compared with the pterional craniotomy, this approach requires less brain retraction during tumor dissection; compared with EEA, it has a minimal risk of postoperative cerebrospinal fluid (CSF) leakage or sinonasal morbidity.[7] Drawbacks include the possibility for damage to the frontalis branch of the facial nerve, and the risk of violating the frontal sinus during the bony opening.[8] Careful planning is required regarding the design of the bone flap to avoid frontal paranasal sinus violation, or repair in cases when the mucosa of the frontal sinus is breached. The supraorbital notch serves as a reliable landmark to indicate the lateral extension of the ipsilateral frontal sinus. If the decision is made to use intraoperative neuronavigation, this could also be used as an aid to maximize the medial craniotomy extension while preserving the frontal sinus cavity.

SURGICAL TECHNIQUE

The patient is positioned supine, with the head typically elevated 15°, extended 10° to 20°, and rotated to the contralateral side between 45° and 60° depending on the location of the tumor (anterior tumors such as olfactory groove meningiomas [OGMs] require more rotation). Stereotactic navigation guidance is often useful for plotting the approach trajectory and facilitating avoidance of the frontal sinus. In patients with large frontal sinuses, careful deliberation of the approach must be made and a plan to repair or cranialize the sinus using a pericranial flap or packing must be made before the operation. Each patient receives prophylactic intravenous antibiotics, and the eyebrows are scrubbed. Patients' eyes are covered with eye protector gels and tape. The supraorbital notch is located by palpation, and a skin incision lateral to the notch is planned. The incision is made within the eyebrow extending from the supraorbital notch to the lateral edge of the brow. The scalp then can be retracted superiorly, and the frontalis muscle cut in the line of the incision. A pericranial flap may be prepared at this point and retracted inferiorly along the supraorbital rim, especially in case of large frontal sinuses. The supraorbital nerve should be preserved to prevent permanent numbness of the forehead. Using blunt dissection, the temporalis muscle is dissected inferomedially from the superior temporal line only enough to expose McCarty's keyhole. A single burr hole is drilled with a standard drill bit, and the dura is dissected from the inner table of the skull. A craniotomy of approximately 2 × 3 cm in size situated immediately above the orbital rim is then performed (eg, see **Fig. 2**). Navigation is usually used to mark this border ahead of time, and all effort is made to avoid exposing the frontal sinus. In case of inadvertent exposure of the sinus, we first note whether the mucosa is disrupted. If not, the sinus breach can often be waxed off successfully. If so, the mucosa may stripped and gelfoam soaked in povidone iodine may use to obliterate the sinus. Next, a coarse diamond drill bit is used to drill the orbital rim as flat as possible so the dura can be tacked up without hindrance. The orbital rim is not usually removed, however the bony irregularities on the supraorbital ridge and the orbital roof are drilled to maximize the

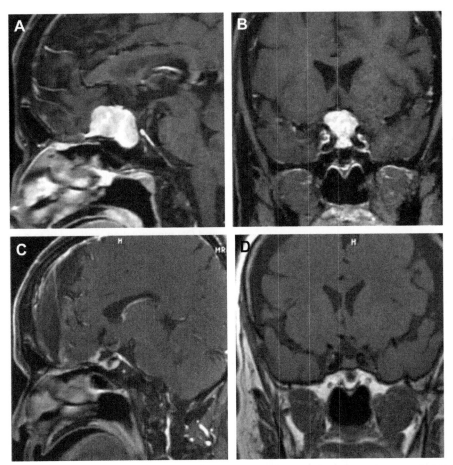

Fig. 1. Preoperative sagittal (*A*) and coronal (*B*) MRIs of a TSM approached through a supraorbital keyhole approach. Postoperative sagittal (*C*) and coronal (*D*) MRIs showed the GTR of the tumor.

surgical exposure and minimize the requirement for brain retraction. An extradural anterior clinoidectomy may be performed if needed. The dura is opened in a C-shape manner and reflected over the orbital rim [for example, see **Fig. 3**]. The operating microscope is typically used for this phase. The olfactory tract is identified and can be followed posteriorly to the ipsilateral ON and optico-carotid cistern. To expand the subfrontal surgical corridor, the proximal Sylvian fissure and

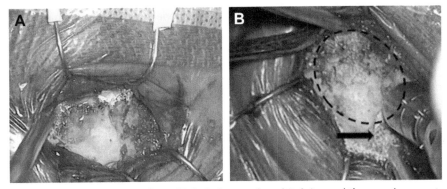

Fig. 2. (*A*) A pericranial flap has been reflected inferiorly over the orbital rim, and the superior aspect of the temporalis muscle has been dissected inferolaterally. (*B*) The craniotomy (*dashed black circle*) extends from the burr hole (*Black arrow*) laterally to the lateral edge of the frontal sinus medially.

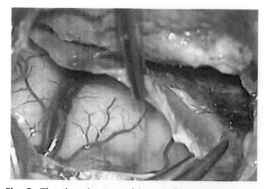

Fig. 3. The dura is opened in a C-shape manner and reflected over the orbital rim.

optico-chiasmatic cistern are opened, and CSF is drained to relax the frontal lobe. Microsurgical dissection is carried out to separate the tumor, preserving the arachnoid plane. The meningioma is identified, devascularized and debulked in piecemeal fashion, using a combination of an ultrasonic aspirator and bipolar coagulation [for example, see **Fig. 4**]. Once the tumor debulking is achieved, the surgical bed may be inspected for residual tumor with the aid of angled endoscopes. The dural attachment is coagulated and hemostasis is achieved. In cases of optic canal involvement, deroofing of the optic canal is carefully done using a diamond drill under constant irrigation to avoid thermal damage, and the falciform ligament is cut. The dura is closed in a multilayer watertight manner, and the cranial flap is fixed with miniplates and screws [for example, see **Fig. 5**]. The incision is closed in three layers, including subcuticular closure of the skin. Postoperative head elevation and cold compress application help minimize periorbital edema.

ENDOSCOPIC ENDONASAL APPROACH

After the introduction of EEEA, the indications of endoscopic endonasal surgery have been expanded from the posterior wall of frontal sinus to the odontoid process in a midline sagittal plane and from the midline to the middle fossa in a coronal plane.[9–13] For a transtuberculum approach to gain access to the suprasellar cistern, bony removal of the prechiasmatic sulcus, sella and limbus sphenoidale allow treatment of selected midline skull base lesions with a significant suprasellar component (ie, meningioma, craniopharyngioma, macroadenoma), which were historically approached from above. Generally, the most amenable lesions to be selected for endoscopic endonasal management are those that are predominantly midline, maintain their arachnoid plane

as evidenced by a lack of peritumoral edema, and those which do not encase neurovascular structures [for example, see **Fig. 6**]. On the other hand, major drawbacks of this approach include the requirement for skull base reconstruction, leading to an increased risk for CSF leak, possible loss of olfaction and other sinonasal complications.[14,15] The use of neuronavigation as well as the Doppler flow probe, with the refinement of reconstruction techniques (ie, 3F, the gasket seal, and nasoseptal flap [NSF]) have been critical in keeping the complication rate acceptably low. The endoscopic technique allows early devascularization of tumor prior to resection, early bilateral decompression of ONs and chiasm, less brain and ON manipulation, and owing to a perspective from below, allows the intervening diaphragm and arachnoid plane to protect the vascular supply of the optic apparatus. The configuration of the sphenoid sinus and the TS—the suprasellar notch - should be evaluated, especially in cases with an acute angle (type I, ie, angle < 118° is the most troublesome).[16] In cases of OGMs, the main advantage of EEA is that it provides a wide ventral corridor with the most direct access to the ASB, specifically the cribriform plate and PS, allowing early vascular control of the anterior and posterior ethmoidal arteries and early devascularization of the tumor without brain retraction. Additionally, EEA allows easier drilling of the hyperostotic bone and complete resection of the dural attachment, leading to more possible resection and lower rates of tumor recurrence.[17] The major limitations of EEA for OGMs include the inevitable risk of anosmia, especially in patients with preoperative preserved olfaction, and limited resection in cases of lateral extension of the lesion and/or its basal dural attachment beyond the medial orbital walls bilaterally.

SURGICAL TECHNIQUE

Under general anesthesia, the patient is positioned supine with the trunk raised 10°-15°, the head is extended 10° to 20°, and slightly turned toward the surgeon. A Mayfield (MAYFIELD Surgical Devices) head holder is placed and neuronavigation system is registered. A lumbar drain may be inserted before the operation, particularly for extended EEAs. For the reconstruction of the osteodural defect and fat harvest, the patient's abdomen or leg is prepared. The nasal phase starts with the insertion of the 0° endoscope into the right nostril to identify the main anatomic landmarks. The usual technique involved in the initial phase is holding the endoscope in the nondominant hand and one instrument in the dominant

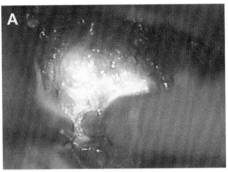
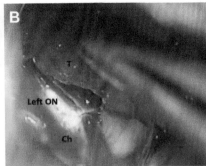

Fig. 4. (*A*) The meningioma is identified, devascularized, and debulked in piecemeal fashion, using a combination of an ultrasonic aspirator and bipolar coagulation. (*B*) Sharp dissection of the tumor from optic chiasm and left optic nerve. Ch, optic chiasm; Left ON, left optic nerve; T, tumor.

hand. During tumor dissection and intracranial manipulation, the technique involves the dual surgeon, binostril technique. The inferior and middle turbinates are gently dislocated laterally and a full turbinectomy is generally not performed unless needed to expand the working aperture. The endoscope is moved forward; the roof of the choana and the sphenoethmoid recess with the sphenoid ostium are identified. The mucosa that covers the anterior wall of the sphenoid sinus is dissected, preserving the septal branch of the sphenopalatine artery, which is important to maintain perfusion to the NSF. The NSF is harvested according to original description.[18] The anterior sphenoidotomy is performed starting 1,5 cm above the choana to identify and access the sphenoid ostium. The nasal septum is then detached from the vomer, and its posterior portion removed with the microdrill and/or Kerrison rongeur from the sphenoid bone and a wide sphenoidotomy is performed, with complete removal of the rostrum and flattening of the floor of the sphenoid. Bilateral posterior ethmoidectomies are performed for extended approaches to provide a view over the lateral aspects and at the anterior extent of the PS. After removal of the sphenoid mucosa, important landmarks of the posterior sphenoid wall, such as the clival recess, sella, ON protuberances, opticocarotid recesses, and internal carotid artery protuberances, must be identified to aid in intraoperative orientation. The location of these structures can be confirmed using stereotactic navigation. The amount of bony resection must be tailored to an individual's pathology. Additional bone removal of the TS, posterior portion of the PS and between the protuberances of the ONs is required to access the suprasellar region. The bony removal starts at the midline of the TS that can be thinned with a diamond drill bit [for example, see **Fig. 7**]. A Kerrison rongeur is used to complete the removal of the bone from the planum up to the falciform ligament, a useful landmark that usually represents the anterior limit of the bony and dural opening. The sellar floor and TS are removed to expose the superior intercavernous sinus (SIS). In cases of lesions compressing this sinus, the latter can be obstructed so that its transgression does not cause any bleeding.

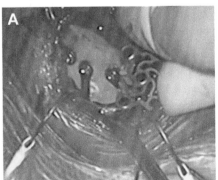
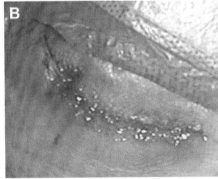

Fig. 5. (*A*, *B*) Following removal and hemostasis, the dura is closed in a multilayer watertight manner, and the cranial flap is fixed with miniplates and screws.

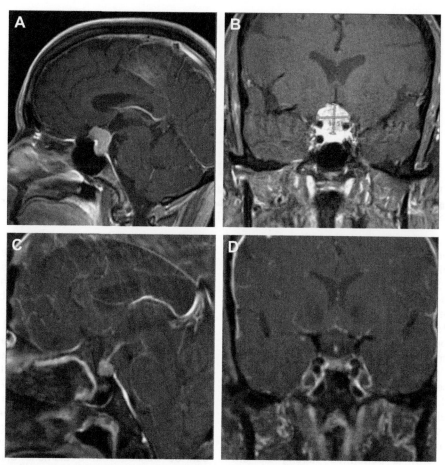

Fig. 6. Sagittal (*A*) and coronal (*B*) MRIs of typical TMS, approached through an endoscopic endonasal approach. Postoperative Sagittal (*C*) and coronal (*D*) MRIs showed the gross total removal of the tumor.

However, it is preferable to seal or ligate the SIS before accessing the tumor, and this structure can be cauterized and sharply divided prior to fully opening the dura. Laterally, just at the confluence of the internal carotid artery (ICA) and medial aspect of the optic canal, the medial opticocarotid recess represents a critical landmark (eg, see **Fig. 8**). Thus, the opening over the planum has a trapezoidal shape, with the short bases at the level of the TS. The posterior portion of the PS is removed paying attention to avoid damaging the posterior ethmoidal arteries that pass through a thin osseous channel at the level of junction with the ethmoid planum. The dura can then be opened sharply along the midline following localization with the neuronavigation instrument and a Doppler flow probe. Once the dura is opened in a French-door fashion, the arachnoid is opened sharply and tumor is visualized and removed according to the same paradigms of microsurgery: internal debulking, careful microdissection away from the optic chiasm, the pituitary stalk, and the superior

hypophyseal arteries. The AComA complex is located above the optic chiasm, which is usually protected by an arachnoid sheath. Internal debulking is performed with the aid of curved suctions, microscissors, and bipolar coagulation, and in case of firm tumor consistency, the ultrasonic surgical aspirator may be useful (eg, see **Fig. 9**). In case of OGMs, an extended transcribriform technique is used. Bilateral maxillary antrostomies are performed to prevent iatrogenic sinusitis and to expose the orbital floor. A wide bilateral sphenoidotomy is performed to expose the sella turcica, carotid protuberances, bilateral optic canals, TS, and PS. To expose the entire cribriform plate, particularly for large tumors that extend lateral to the middle turbinates, bilateral total ethmoidectomies are performed to expose the junction of the lamina papyracea with the fovea ethmoidalis. During the posterior ethmoidectomy, it is important to recognize an Onodi cell or spheno-ethmoidal air cell, which is a posterior ethmoid cell that is positioned superolateral to

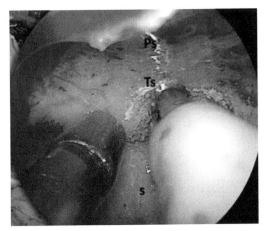

Fig. 7. The bony removal starts with the TS that can be thinned with a diamond drill bit. PS, planum sphenoidale; s, sella turcica; TS, *tuberculum sellae*.

the sphenoid sinus. This is an anatomic variant in which the ON and carotid artery may course through the lateral aspect of these Onodi cells.

Reconstruction often consists of a multilayer closure involving autologous fat grafting for dead space, dural reconstruction using fascia or a dural substitute, and placement of the NSF to provide broad bony coverage and apposition (eg, see **Fig. 10**).

DISCUSSION

In 1971, Donald Wilson was the first to describe the "keyhole" approach in cranial surgery as a method to minimize iatrogenic injury to normal brain during surgery.[19] Initial efforts on surgical management of large ASB meningiomas were limited to frontal lobectomy. With the advent of microscopes, many surgeons continued to use the bifrontal approach to spare significant frontal lobe resection. Unilateral pterional craniotomy and trans-sylvian approaches, popularized by

Yasargil and colleagues, were followed by the fronto-orbitozygomatic approach, which provided more basal exposure and less brain retraction.[20] The ideal approach for ASBs should provide adequate exposure of tumor, the surrounding structures, and the dural attachments. The selection of approach must be taken according to patient-related factors, tumor features (size, consistency, extension, location), its relationship to critical anatomic structures and surgeon experience. Both the supraorbital and endonasal endoscopic approaches usually provide adequate corridors for ASB pathologic condition. In carefully selected patients, these tailored minimally invasive approaches can provide direct access to the lesion and minimize brain retraction. Ottenhausen and colleagues[21] presented an algorithm, which incorporates the specific characteristics of supraorbital, EEA, and TCA approaches to aid in surgical decision-making. These algorithms include lateral extension beyond the internal carotid artery, ON, lamina papyracea, and involvement of cribriform plate and the presence or not of olfactory function. The supraorbital approach, through subfrontal corridor, is suitable for TS meningiomas with lateral extension up to the internal carotid arteries and anterior clinoid processes, or lateral extension beyond the lamina papyracea. In cases of OGMs, this route is usually used in cases of preserved olfaction or disrupted olfaction without cribriform plate invasion. Borghei-Razavi and colleagues[22] in a cadaveric study affirmed that the spheno-ethdmoidal suture represents a limit of the approach but also showed how the drilling of the superior two-thirds of the crista galli is possible with the aid of an endoscope.

During the last 2 decades, the improvements in endoscopic technique and refinements of instrumentations have allowed the endoscope to overcome some limits of the supraorbital approach. The endoscope allows for enhanced illumination

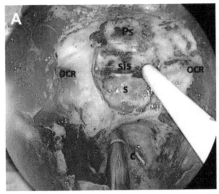

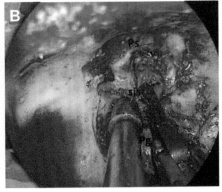

Fig. 8. (*A*) Identification of ICA using Doppler flow probe and (*B*) coagulation and cutting of superior intercavernous sinus (sis). c, clivus; OCR, optic carotid recess; Pg, pituitary gland; Ps, planum sphenoidale; s, sella turcica.

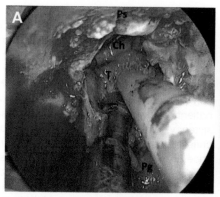
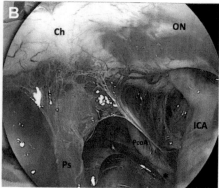

Fig. 9. (A) Internal debulking is performed in case of firm tumor with an ultrasonic surgical aspirator. (B) After careful dissection of the chiasm, the stalk, and the superior hypophyseal arteries, surgical cavity is examined to ensure the absence of any residual tumor. Pg, pituitary gland; ON, optic nerve; Ps, pituitary stalk; *, third cranial nerve; Ch, chiasm; PcoA, posterior communicating artery.

and improved visualization, especially of "hidden" areas beyond the anatomic corners of the surgical field that are not adequately visualized by the microscope. Compared with the subfrontal and pterional approaches, the supraorbital keyhole approach offers less brain retraction, avoids the need for splitting the Sylvian fissure and retraction of the frontal and/or temporal lobes. Further advantages include shorter operative time, reduced postoperative pain, and better cosmetic outcome. Iacoangeli and colleagues compared the traditional craniotomies to the supraorbital approach and did not find any significant difference in the extent of resection or complications while demonstrating improved cosmetic results.[23] However, the main drawbacks of this approach are the risk of lesioning the frontal sinus during the craniotomy and subsequent need for repair depending on extent of breach and injury to the frontotemporal branch of the facial nerve. The EEA provides another attractive minimally invasive approach to treat ABS meningiomas. The EEA tends to be selected in cases without significant lateral

extension or vascular encasement (internal carotid artery [ICA]/anterior cerebral artery [ACA]) for both TS meningiomas and for OGM. Advantages of EEA include close-up view, direct midline exposure, early devascularization and decompression of optic apparatus, with minimal or no neurovascular manipulation, owing to a superiorly oriented approach, which allows the intervening arachnoid plane to protect the vascular supply of the optic apparatus. This anatomic consideration may account for the fact that the incidence of postoperative visual deterioration is 2 to 5 times higher following a transcranial versus endonasal approach.[24] A recent metanalysis by Muskens and colleagues[25] showed that EEA afforded higher rates of postoperative visual improvement compared with TCA. Improvement or normalization of vision after the removal of meningioma via EEA can be achieved in approximately 85% of cases, particularly in case of TS meningiomas. According to Fahlbusch and Schott, Raco and colleagues,[26,27] and Magill and colleagues,[28] tumor size is another important characteristic in

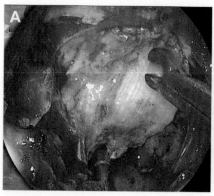
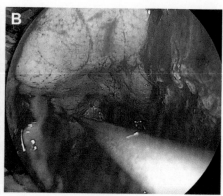

Fig. 10. A multilayer closure involving autologous fat grafting for dead space, dural reconstruction using fascia or a dural substitute (A), and apposition of the NSF (B).

the determination of visual outcome; patients harboring tumors smaller than 3 cm (or 17 mm according to USCF tumor score) having better visual outcomes. The vascular supply to the ONs and chiasm, which include small subchiasmatic perforating arteries, are especially vulnerable to compromise and can be difficult to visualize from a suprachiasmatic view provided by pterional, subfrontal, and transbasal approaches. TCAs are usually recommended for tumors larger than 3 cm because these tumors may extend laterally to areas inaccessible from an endonasal corridor and often encase critical neurovascular structures that require microsurgical dissection. The main disadvantages of this route include compromised olfaction and the risk of CSF. The reported risk of CSF rhinorrhea postoperatively in several clinal series ranging from 23% to 40%.[3,20] However, it is important to underlie how the introduction the vascularized NSF and the refinement of the reconstruction techniques have decreased the rate of CSF leak between 5% and 10%.[29,30]

CONFLICTS OF INTEREST

None.

PRIOR PRESENTATIONS

None.

CLINICS CARE POINTS

- Ideally, meningioma surgery requires a Simpson grade I resection, including the removal of the tumor, surrounding dura, and invaded bone. However, at the skull base, given the proximity of critical neurovascular structures, these goals must sometimes be modified.

- Some ABS meningiomas will remain unsuitable for minimally invasive routes and still require traditional transcranial surgery.

- During preoperative planning, the surgical team must determine the main goals of surgery keeping in mind both the tumor and patient characteristics. Only after an accurate history, physical examination, and radiological review will goals of surgery be determined, whether it is gross total resection, maximal safe resection, or vision preservation.

- Decision-making and case selection are the keys to successful surgery.

REFERENCES

1. Gardner PA, Kassam AB, Thomas A, et al. Endoscopic endonasal resection of anterior cranial base meningiomas. Neurosurgery 2008;63(1):36–52 [discussion: 52-4].
2. Abbassy M, Woodard TD, Sindwani R, et al. An Overview of Anterior Skull Base Meningiomas and the Endoscopic Endonasal Approach. Otolaryngol Clin North Am 2016;49(1):141–52.
3. Gadgil N, Thomas JG, Takashima M, et al. Endoscopic resection of tuberculum sellae meningiomas. J Neurol Surg B Skull Base 2013;74(4):201–10.
4. Mitchell P, Vindlacheruvu RR, Mahmood K, et al. Supraorbital eyebrow minicraniotomy for anterior circulation aneurysms. Surg Neurol 2005;63(1):47–51 [discussion: 51].
5. Reisch R, Perneczky A, Filippi R. Surgical technique of the supraorbital key-hole craniotomy. Surg Neurol 2003;59(3):223–7.
6. Gazzeri R, Nishiyama Y, Teo C. Endoscopic supraorbital eyebrow approach for the surgical treatment of extraaxialand intraaxial tumors. Neurosurg Focus 2014;37(4):E20.
7. Zada G. Editorial: The endoscopic keyhole supraorbital approach. Neurosurg Focus 2014;37(4): E21.
8. Fatemi N, Dusick JR, de Paiva Neto MA, et al. Endonasal versus supraorbital keyhole removal of craniopharyngiomas and tuberculum sellae meningiomas. Neurosurgery 2009;64(5 Suppl 2):269–84 [discussion: 264-6].
9. Kato T, Sawamura Y, Abe H, et al. Transsphenoidal-transtuberculum sellae approach for supradiaphragmatic tumours: technical note. Acta Neurochir 1998;140(7):715–8 [discussion: 719].
10. Cook SW, Smith Z, Kelly DF. Endonasal transsphenoidal removal of tuberculum sellae meningiomas: technical note. Neurosurgery 2004;55(1):239–44 [discussion: 244-6].
11. de Divitiis E, Cavallo LM, Cappabianca P, et al. Extended endoscopic endonasal transsphenoidal approach for the removal of suprasellar tumors: Part 2. Neurosurgery 2007;60(1):46–58 [discussion: 58-9].
12. Kassam A, Snyderman CH, Mintz A, et al. Expanded endonasal approach: the rostrocaudal axis. Part I. Crista galli to the sella turcica. Neurosurg Focus 2005;19(1):E3.
13. Couldwell WT, Weiss MH, Rabb C, et al. Variations on the standard transsphenoidal approach to the sellar region, with emphasis on the extended approaches and parasellar approaches: surgical experience in 105 cases. Neurosurgery 2004; 55(3):539–47 [discussion: 547-50].
14. Kassam AB, Prevedello DM, Carrau RL, et al. Endoscopic endonasal skull base surgery: analysis of

complications in the authors' initial 800 patients. J Neurosurg 2011;114(6):1544–68.

15. Cappabianca P, Cavallo LM, Colao A, et al. Surgical complications associated with the endoscopic endonasal transsphenoidal approach for pituitary adenomas. J Neurosurg 2002;97(2):293–8.

16. de Notaris M, Solari D, Cavallo LM, et al. The "suprasellar notch," or the tuberculum sellae as seen from below: definition, features, and clinical implications from an endoscopic endonasal perspective. J Neurosurg 2012;116(3):622–9.

17. Fernandez-Miranda JC, Gardner PA, Prevedello DM, et al. Expanded endonasal approach for olfactory groove meningioma. Acta Neurochir (Wien). Mar 2009;151(3):287–8 [author reply: 289-90].

18. Hadad G, Bassagasteguy L, Carrau RL, et al. A novel reconstructive technique after endoscopic expanded endonasal approaches: vascular pedicle nasoseptal flap. Laryngoscope 2006;116(10): 1882–6.

19. Wilson DH. Limited exposure in cerebral surgery. Technical note. J Neurosurg 1971;34(1):102–6.

20. Morales-Valero SF, Van Gompel JJ, Loumiotis I, et al. Craniotomy for anterior cranial fossa meningiomas: historical overview. Neurosurg Focus 2014;36(4): E14.

21. Ottenhausen M, Rumalla K, Alalade AF, et al. Decision-making algorithm for minimally invasive approaches to anterior skull base meningiomas. Neurosurg Focus 2018;44(4):E7.

22. Borghei-Razavi H, Truong HQ, Fernandes-Cabral DT, et al. Minimally Invasive Approaches for Anterior Skull Base Meningiomas: Supraorbital Eyebrow, Endoscopic Endonasal, or a Combination of Both? Anatomic Study, Limitations, and Surgical Application. World Neurosurg 2018;112:e666–74.

23. Iacoangeli M, Nocchi N, Nasi D, et al. Minimally Invasive Supraorbital Key-hole Approach for the Treatment of Anterior Cranial Fossa Meningiomas. Neurol Med -Chir 2016;56(4):180–5.

24. Koutourousiou M, Fernandez-Miranda JC, Stefko ST, et al. Endoscopic endonasal surgery for suprasellar meningiomas: experience with 75 patients. J Neurosurg 2014;120(6):1326–39.

25. Muskens IS, Briceno V, Ouwehand TL, et al. The endoscopic endonasal approach is not superior to the microscopic transcranial approach for anterior skull base meningiomas-a meta-analysis. Acta Neurochir 2018;160(1):59–75.

26. Fahlbusch R, Schott W. Pterional surgery of meningiomas of the tuberculum sellae and planum sphenoidale: surgical results with special consideration of ophthalmological and endocrinological outcomes. J Neurosurg 2002;96(2):235–43.

27. Raco A, Bristot R, Domenicucci M, et al. Meningiomas of the tuberculum sellae. Our experience in 69 cases surgically treated between 1973 and 1993. J Neurosurg Sci 1999;43(4):253–60 [discussion: 260-2].

28. Magill ST, Morshed RA, Lucas CG, et al. Tuberculum sellae meningiomas: grading scale to assess surgical outcomes using the transcranial versus transsphenoidal approach. Neurosurg Focus 2018; 44(4):E9.

29. Cavallo LM, Solari D, Somma T, et al. The 3F (Fat, Flap, and Flash) Technique For Skull Base Reconstruction After Endoscopic Endonasal Suprasellar Approach. World Neurosurg 2019;126:439–46.

30. Garcia-Navarro V, Anand VK, Schwartz TH. Gasket seal closure for extended endonasal endoscopic skull base surgery: efficacy in a large case series. World Neurosurg 2013;80(5):563–8.

Management of Intraventricular Meningiomas

Michael A. Bamimore, DO[a,b], Lina Marenco-Hillembrand, MD[a],
Krishnan Ravindran, MD[a], David Agyapong, BS[c], Elena Greco, MD[d],
Erik H. Middlebrooks, MD[a,d], Kaisorn L. Chaichana, MD[a,*]

KEYWORDS

- Meningiomas • Ventricles • Hydrocephalus • Cerebrospinal fluid • Neuro-oncology

KEY POINTS

- Several intracortical and intracallosal surgical approaches can be adopted for the safe, maximal resection of intraventricular meningiomas, depending on the anatomic placement of the tumor.
- Gross total tumor resection via piecemeal technique can alleviate neurologic symptoms stemming from tumor size.
- Main surgical limitations involve preserving surrounding tissue function.

INTRODUCTION

Meningiomas are among the most common primary brain tumors.[1–3] Intraventricular meningiomas (IVMs) comprise a small subset, 0.7% to 3% of all meningiomas, originating from collections of arachnoid cells within the choroid plexus.[4–6] These tumors represent a higher proportion of intracranial tumors in the pediatric population as compared with the adult population.[4,7] They are commonly observed in the lateral ventricles (80%), followed by the third (15%) and fourth (5%) ventricle, respectively.[4]

IVMs are often benign and asymptomatic; this allows them to grow to considerable sizes, up to 7.3 cm in diameter, before clinical presentation.[8,9] They are often discovered incidentally on computed tomography (CT) and MRI. On CT scans, tumors may seem as hyperdense or isodense, relative to the cerebrum, depending on the degree of calcification andcellularity.[2] The classic observation on MRI is a sharply defined, homogenous mass with a dural attachment.[2] IVMs have many similar imaging features as the extraventricular counterparts but more frequently show calcification. MRI is a poor predictor of the World Health Organization (WHO) grade in meningiomas.[8,10]

The WHO classifies IVMs as grades I, II, and III, representing benign, atypical, and malignant tumors, respectively.[2] Malignant lesions are usually the most aggressive.[4] Symptomatic intraventricular tumors often elicit generalized symptoms associated with signs of elevated intracranial pressure. Common symptoms at presentation include headache, nausea, and visual deficits.[11] Lesions in the third and fourth ventricles may present with obstructive hydrocephalus. Therapeutic options for intraventricular meningiomas include observation, microsurgical resection, and radiosurgery.[12] Ultimately, the decision on how to treat an intraventricular meningioma depends on several clinical factors including the perceived tumor grade,

[a] Department of Neurological Surgery, Mayo Clinic, 4500 San Pablo Road, Jacksonville, FL 32224, USA; [b] Department of Neurological Surgery, Cooper University Hospital, Camden, NJ, USA; [c] School of Medicine, Robert Wood Johnson Medical School, New Brunswick, NJ, USA; [d] Department of Radiology, Mayo Clinic, Jacksonville, FL, USA
* Corresponding author.
E-mail address: chaichana.kaisorn@mayo.edu

Neurosurg Clin N Am 34 (2023) 403–415
https://doi.org/10.1016/j.nec.2023.02.005
1042-3680/23/© 2023 Elsevier Inc. All rights reserved.

presence of peritumoral edema and intratumoral necrosis, hydrocephalus, tumor growth rate (if monitored), as well as the presence of symptoms.[13]

EPIDEMIOLOGY

Tumors of the meninges are the most common primary brain tumors, accounting for up to 37% of histologically determined brain tumors.[2] The overall incidence of meningiomas is estimated to be about 97.5 per 100,000 individuals in the United States, with intraventricular meningiomas accounting for 0.7% to 3%.[4,14] Several genetic factors have been linked to the occurrence of IVMs, a prime example being a type 2 neurofibromatosis disorder.[4] Environmental factors have also been implicated in the occurrence of meningiomas. Studies have shown that exposure to ionizing radiation, for example, through brain imaging modalities, leads to an increased likelihood of developing meningiomas.[2] The fact that most meningiomas express progesterone receptors and that women are affected significantly more often than men suggest a possible role of hormones in the manifestation of meningiomas.[2,4]

PATIENT EVALUATION AND PREOPERATIVE CONSIDERATIONS

Initial patient evaluation should comprise a thorough history, accompanying a complete neurologic examination of extremities and cranial nerves. Subsequent imaging assessment should be undertaken via MRI with and without contrast.[13,14] Surgical indications for resection include documented radiographic tumor growth and symptomatic presentation from either acute obstructive hydrocephalus or intratumoral hemorrhage. IVMs are usually 2 to 5 cm in diameter at time of discovery and present with symptoms secondary to mass effect.[13,15] Visual field deficits, headaches, nausea, and vomiting are common presenting symptoms.[14]

Important IVM preoperative considerations include anatomic location within the ventricular system, presence of obstructive hydrocephalus, and overview of the 3-dimensional relational anatomy. Lesions located in the third ventricle necessitate preoperative neuroophthalmological and endocrinological evaluations owing to resultant mass effect on the optic chiasm and pituitary gland/stalk, respectively.[15] Preoperative catheter angiography for assessment of candidate's feeding vessels for embolization is often of lower yield in intraventricular meningiomas, where most of the blood supply may arise from medial and lateral posterior choroidal vessels.[4] Functional or diffusion tensor imaging-MRI may provide valuable insight into white matter tracts when considering a transcortical approach.[16,17]

SURGICAL MANAGEMENT OF INTRAVENTRICULAR MENINGIOMAS

Surgical intervention for intraventricular meningiomas has been shown to produce a reduction in presurgical symptoms.[18,19] Generally, strategies involve either advancing via an incision made on the cortex, with transcortical (trans-gyral or trans-sulcal) approaches, or advancing via an interhemispheric incision, through the corpus callosum. The size and location of tumors are crucial in adopting a particular approach for resection.[1] Appropriate spatial access for complete tumor resection, often by piecemeal fashion, with minimal regional damage may also influence the choice of approach.[20]

Early identification and coagulation of vascular feeds to tumors is important to avoid intraoperative hemorrhagic events.[12] In certain cases, adopting a longer surgical route through less vital portions of the brain merits consideration.[4] In addition, the placement of the lesion in the dominant or nondominant hemisphere should influence the decision of approach.[13]

INTRAVENTRICULAR LOCATIONS

The lateral ventricles are the most common site of origin for intraventricular meningiomas, accounting for ~80% of cases. Tumors within the third and fourth ventricles account for ~15% and ~5%, respectively (**Fig. 1**).[1,4]

MENINGIOMAS OF THE LATERAL VENTRICLES

Most of the meningiomas within the lateral ventricle originate from the atrium (~80%).[11,21] Tumors from the inferior temporal horns are rare and ones from the frontal horns even more so.[4] Studies suggest a preponderance of left-sided tumors compared with right-sided ones.[1]

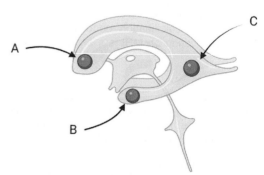

Fig. 1. Lateral ventricles.(*A*) lateral ventricle; (*B*) temporal horn; (*C*) atrium

Clinical Presentation and Imaging Characteristics

Meningiomas of the lateral ventricles usually remain asymptomatic until they are of considerable size.[1] Symptomatic presentation involves general neurologic symptoms associated with tumor mass effect and ventricular obstruction such as headaches, nausea, and vomiting.[4,5,12] Symptoms are often mild or sporadic, especially in the early stages, and may result in late hospital presentation.[4] Generalized or focal seizures, hemiparesis, and visual acuity defects have also been reported.[12,14] On MRI, tumors usually seem as smooth, homogeneously or heterogeneously enhancing intraventricular masses with sharp margins, sometimes accompanied by ventricular enlargement (**Fig. 2**).[22]

Surgical Anatomy

The ventricular region is well vascularized, with the internal carotid and basilar arteries arriving inferiorly and giving rise to several other arteries that span the region.[23] Arterial connections can be established from the anterior choroidal artery, posterior choroidal artery, or both.[4,20] These vascular

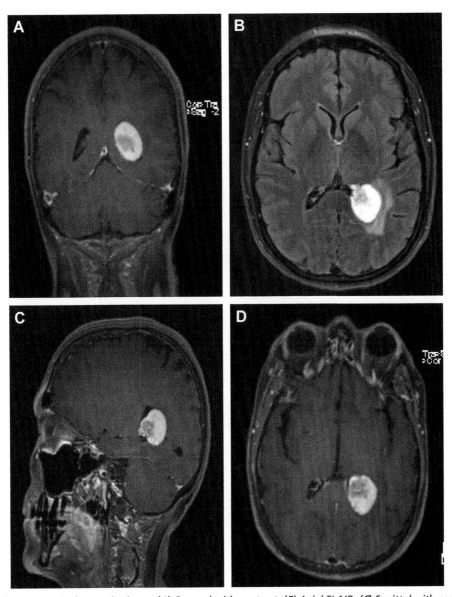

Fig. 2. Left intraventricular meningioma. (*A*) Coronal with contrast; (*B*) Axial FLAIR; (*C*) Sagittal with contrast; (*D*) Axial with contrast.

connections usually attach to the anterior or ante-roinferior tumor margin.

Subcortical white matter tracts such as the middle longitudinal fasciculus connect various cortical regions such as the precuneus (found in the posteromedial portion of the parietal lobe) and the cuneus (residing within the occipi-tal lobe between the parieto-occipital sulcus [POS] and the calcarine sulcus) to several intra- and interhemispheric regions of the brain **Fig. 3**.[24–28] Damage to these tracts during surgi-cal approach to IVMs may result in neurologic deficits and a reduced quality of life postsurgery (**Table 1**).[26,28–30]

Transcortical Approaches

Transcortical surgical approaches traverse the ce-rebral cortex directly to arrive at intraventricular meningiomas.[1] The point of dissection is usually within one of the cortical sulci, placed posteriorly, anteriorly, or temporally depending on the location of the tumor.[1,4] Frontal transcortical approaches

are usually reserved for lesions located within the frontal horn of the lateral ventricles.[4,15]

Parietal or Parieto-occipital Transcortical Approach

A parietal or parieto-occipital approach is partic-ularly helpful in extracting ventricular tumors reaching the superior aspect of the atrium.[12] Possible points of approach are the superior pa-rietal gyrus or the deep intraparietal sulcus.[4] Parietal approaches carry the risk of damaging white matter tracts such as the optic radiation, dorsal arcuate fasciculus, superior longitudinal fasciculus (SLF-I and -II), tapetum, middle longi-tudinal fasciculus, cingulum, vertical occipital fasciculus, and inferior fronto-occipital fasciculus (IFOF).[1,22,26,31] Monroy and colleagues, in addi-tion, highlighted the need to preserve the vertical rami, which is a network of fibers that connect the SLF-II and SLF-III to the borders of the intraparie-tal sulcus (**Fig. 4**).[31] These white matter tracts are thought to integrate and coordinate several

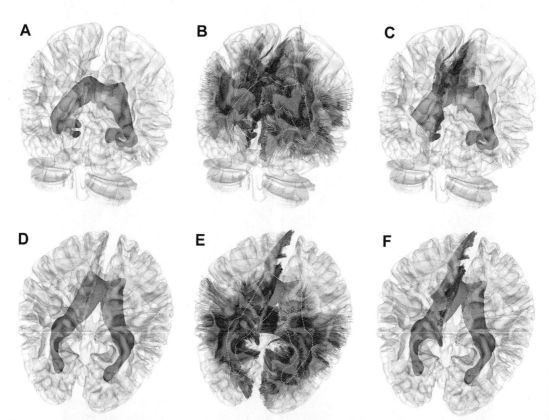

Fig. 3. Subcortical white matter tracts. (*A*) Posterior projection through cuneus; (*B*) Cuneal tracts (*dotted line:* outline of lateral ventricles); (*C*) Approach to atrium and posterior horn with splenium fibers of corpus callosum removed; (*D*) Posterior projection through precuneus; (*E*) Precuneal tracts (*dotted lines:* outline of lateral ventri-cles); (*F*) Approach to atrium and posterior horn with splenium fibers of corpus callosum removed. Cingulate = *red;* Corpus callosum = *blue;* Optic radiations = *yellow;* Superior longitudinal fasciculus I = *purple.*

Table 1
Anatomic connection, function, and deficits of white matter tracts

White Matter Tract	Anatomic Connection	Function	Deficit
Anterior commissure (AC)[28–30,32]	Connects olfactory bulb and cerebral regions between hemispheres	Olfactory, auditory, visual communication	Anosmia
Arcuate fasciculus (AF)[10,28–30]	Connects parts of the temporal gyrus to the midpart of the inferior and middle frontal gyri	Language processing, nonlinguistic communication	Impaired lexical, phonological, and semantic language processing
Cingulum[28,29,33]	Subcallosal gyrus to parahippocampal gyrus and uncus of temporal lobe	Coordinates emotional behavior, spatial processing, pain processing	Emotional behavioral changes; visuospatial, memory and attention deficits
Corpus callosum (CC)[29,33]	Connects left and right cerebral hemispheres	Facilitates coordination between left and right cerebral hemispheres	Motor, auditory, cognitive, and motor disconnection syndromes; impaired memory and problem-solving ability
Corticopontine fibers[29,30,34]	Projects from cerebral cortex to pontine nuclei	Coordination of voluntary motor function	Movement defects
Forceps major[29]	Interconnects parietal, occipital, and temporal lobes across hemispheres	Interhemispheric transfer of visual and language information	Disconnection syndromes
Forceps minor[29]	Connects prefrontal and occipital lobes across hemispheres	Facilitates coordination between left and right cerebral hemispheres	Disconnection syndromes
Fornix[29,32]	Main output of hippocampus	Memory processing	Memory loss
Inferior fronto-occipital fasciculus (IFOF)[28,30,35]	Connects the occipital cortex, temporo-basal areas, and superior parietal lobe to the frontal lobe	Lexical-semantic processing, visual spatial processing, attention	Spatial neglect, deficits in language development and processing
Inferior longitudinal fasciculus (ILF)[29,30]	Connects occipital and temporal lobes	Recognition and identification of visually perceived objects	Lexical and semantic language processing deficits
Lingular amygdaloid fasciculus (LAF)[26]	Connects the amygdala to the lingula	Social cognition	Unknown
Middle longitudinal fasciculus (MdLF)[26,30,31]	Interconnects superior temporal gyrus with parietal and occipital lobes	Processing acoustic information	Unknown
Sledge runner[29,30,36]	Interconnects the posterior part of the precuneus to the lingula	Visuospatial processing, recognition of places	Unknown

(continued on next page)

Table 1
(continued)

White Matter Tract	Anatomic Connection	Function	Deficit
Splenium[28–30,36]	Connects left and right cerebral hemispheres	Language, visuospatial information transfer and behavior	Visual and auditory disconnection syndromes
Superior longitudinal fasciculus (SLF) I[28–30]	Connecting the precuneus and superior frontal gyrus	Initiation of motor activity	Unknown
Superior longitudinal fasciculus (SLF) II[28–30]	Connects the angular gyrus and pars triangularis	Visual and oculomotor processes involved in spatial function	Dysfunction of spatial awareness
Superior longitudinal fasciculus (SLF) III[28–30]	Connects supramarginal gyrus to inferior frontal gyrus	Articulation, working memory, visuospatial attention	Dysfunction of spatial awareness
Thalamic radiations[28–30,37]	Connects thalamus to cerebral cortex	Relay sensory and motor information	Movement disorders, defect in arousal and consciousness
Tapetum[28–30]	Interconnects temporal lobes across hemispheres	Facilitates coordination between left and right cerebral hemispheres	Visual and auditory disconnection syndromes
Uncinate fasciculus (UF)[28–30,38]	Connects the middle, inferior frontal, and orbital gyri with the cortex of the anterior temporal lobe gyri, as well as the parahippocampal and hippocampal gyri	Episodic memory, language, and social emotional processing, making visual associations	Social/emotional defects, semantic memory retrieval deficits
Vertical occipital fasciculus (VOF)[28–30,39]	Connects dorsal and ventral visual cortices	Object recognition, reading	Reading impairment

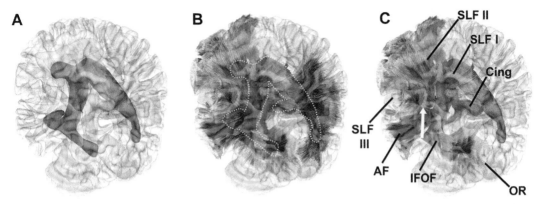

Fig. 4. Subcortical white matter tracts. Parietal or Parieto-occipital approach. *White arrow* designates ideal entry point. (*A*) Orientation of lateral ventricle; (*B*) White matter tracts through Kassam-Monroy Point (*dotted line* = outline of lateral ventricles); (*C*) Keyhole to atrium and posterior horn with splenium fibers of corpus callosum removed. AF = arcuate fasciculus (*cyan*), Cing = cingulate (*red*); IFOF = inferior fronto-occipital fasciculus (*pink*); OR = optic radiations (*yellow*); SLF = superior longitudinal fasciculus (SLF 1 = *purple*, SLF 2 = *orange*, SLF 3 = *teal*).

significant functions such as spatial awareness, visuospatial attention, gaze, numerical cognition, calculation, and grasping.

Monroy and colleagues recommend a surgical approach via the point of intersection between the posterior third of the intraparietal sulcus[32] and a lateral projection of the POS termed the IPS-POS (Kassam-Monroy [KM]) point.[31] An approach via the IPS-POS(KM) point using port-based techniques permits a safe parafascicular surgical trajectory to the atrium, reducing the risk of damage to the eloquent subcortical white matter tracts and the associated postsurgical complications (**Figs. 5 and 6**).[31]

Parietal or parieto-occipital approaches offer the opportunity for total resection of tumors, however, with an increased likelihood of intraoperative hemorrhagic events due to delayed access to choroidal arteries.[4,5]

Temporal Transcortical Approach

A temporal approach to resecting an intraventricular meningioma is best applied to more laterally placed lesions. A middle temporal gyrus approach affords the shortest and safest trajectory for lesions occupying the inferior aspect of the trigon (**Fig. 7**).[1,22] White matter tracts significantly endangered by temporal approaches include the optic radiation, anterior commissure, arcuate fasciculus, cingulum, uncinate fasciculus, IFOF, tapetum, and inferior longitudinal fasciculus. Extensive damage to the optic radiation can be avoided by keeping the dissection plane

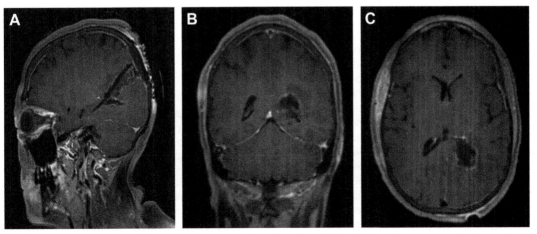

Fig. 5. IPS-POS (Kassam-Monroy) point, post-operative imaging. (*A*) Sagittal with contrast; (*B*) Coronal with contrast; (*C*) Axial with contrast.

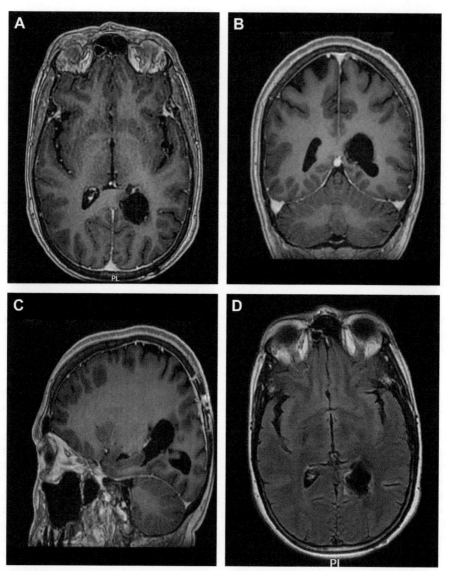

Fig. 6. IPS-POS (Kassam-Monroy) point, post-operative imaging. (*A*) Axial with contrast; (*B*) Coronal with contrast; (*C*) Sagittal with contrast; (*D*) Axial FLAIR.

parallel.[26,33] For lesions more on the superior aspect, the approach is usually situated closer to the parietal lobe to avoid the optic radiation.[22] A posterior-temporal approach is only recommended when there are preexisting visual field defects.[2] A pterional approach, going through the sylvian fissure, has also been found to be an appropriate approach for the rare lesions residing in the temporal horn.[4] Most temporal approaches allow early identification and coagulation of the tumor's blood supply and thus reduces the risk of intraoperative hemorrhagic events. Despite providing a shorter distance to certain tumors, other approaches may be favored over a temporal approach especially with dominant hemisphere

lesions, which pose a significantly high risk of postoperative hemianopia and speech disruption.[12]

PORT-BASED APPROACHES FOR INTRAVENTRICULAR MENINGIOMA? INDICATIONS?
Interhemispheric Approaches

Interhemispheric transcallosal approaches are favorable for the excision of lesions residing in the more superior aspects of the lateral ventricles.[15] This approach minimizes the risk of functional deficits following injury to subcortical tracts.[4,22] A unique risk of interhemispheric approaches is the

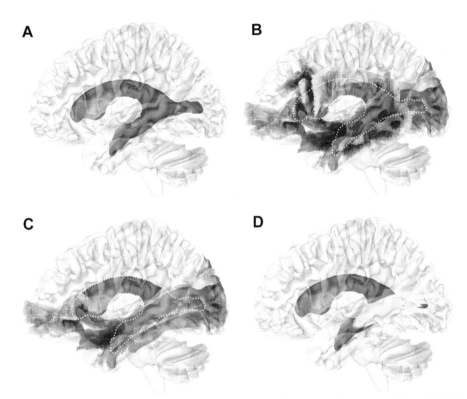

Fig. 7. Subcortical white matter tracts. Temporal approach. (*A*) Orientation of lateral ventricles; (*B*) White matter tracts through middle temporal gyrus (*dotted line* = outline of lateral ventricles); (*C*) arcuate fasciculus (AF) removed, inferior longitudinal fasciculus (ILF) and inferior fronto-occipital fasciculus (IFOF)visualized; (*D*) IFOF and ILF are removed, optic radiations (OR) is visualized overlying lower atrium and temporal horn. AF = *cyan*; ILF = *red*; IFOF = *pink*; OR = *yellow*.

chance of disconnection syndrome following damage to fibers such as SLF-I, cingulum, sledge runner, forceps major, and splenium.[17,33,34] This approach also carries an increased risk of hemorrhage due to late access to vasculature feeding the tumor.[23] A contralateral interhemispheric approach through the nondominant hemisphere can be adopted for the resection of tumors in the dominant hemisphere.[1] Such a technique requires electing an angle of approach that will grant adequate access to the tumor. Here, an increase in distance is endured in exchange for less contact with parenchyma of the dominant hemisphere.[1]

MENINGIOMAS OF THE THIRD VENTRICLE

Comprising 15% of ventricular meningiomas and only 0.1% to 0.18% of all intracranial meningiomas, third ventricle meningiomas are much rarer than their lateral ventricular counterparts.[4,35–38] As of 2015, there were only 90 documented cases of meningiomas in the third ventricle; however, despite this scarcity, most cases have been well researched and much is known about their features.[35,36]

Clinical Presentation and Imaging Characteristics

On CT imaging, third ventricle meningiomas typically seem hyperdense, with some showing calcification, obstructive hydrocephalus, and uniform enhancement.[5,35,39] MRI usually shows these meningiomas to be hypo- to isointense on T1-weighted images and iso- to hyperintense on T2.[5,35,39] In addition to imaging, clinical diagnostic symptoms resemble those of elevated intracranial pressure without any localized neurologic signs. Headache, vomiting, limb weakness, visual disturbances, and endocrine abnormalities are some of the most reported presentations associated with third ventricle meningiomas.[5,39]

Surgical Anatomy

Out of the various origins for third ventricle meningiomas—anterior, posterior, lateral, roof, and floor—tumors located posteriorly in the pineal region are the most common.[5,39] The most probable origin of third ventricle meningiomas is from arachnoid cells within the choroid plexus, resulting in a common blood supply for the tumors coming from the medial posterior choroidal artery; however, cases have been reported of the lateral posterior and anterior choroidal arteries being involved as well.[37]

Surgical Management and Approaches

When planning which surgical route to take, not only major deep venous structures but also the attachment of the tumor should be considered. Although third ventricle meningiomas are unique in that they have no dural attachment, surgical techniques have variable outcomes depending on the location of the tumor.[35] For posterior meningiomas, a posterior transcallosal route has been shown to have no major complications and is recommended if a surgeon feels comfortable with this technique.[35,37] An alternative is a supracerebellar infratentorial approach, which is predicated by the angle of the tentorium and the relationship of the deep draining veins to the tumor. For the anteriorly located tumors, an interhemispheric transcallosal transventricular transchoroidal approach is more suitable, as it allows for not only anterior access but also the ability to dissect the choroidal fissure in order to open the field of view.[40] Tumors occupying enough space to involve the floor or roof of the third ventricle are generally removed by one of the 3 anterior techniques: a transcortical transventricular transchoroidal approach, interhemispheric transcallosal interforniceal approach, or interhemispheric transcallosal transventricular transchoroidal approach.[5,35,40,41]

However, when considering a transcortical technique, the surgeon must consider the possibility of postoperative seizures or subdural fluid accumulation because of the cortical incision.[35] Finally, although research is scarce on third ventricle meningiomas, a recent review of the literature has found that a transcallosal interforniceal approach was the most successful in a patient population of 60.[37] However, more outcomes research is necessary to determine the optimal routes for each variation of third ventricle meningiomas.

MENINGIOMAS OF THE FOURTH VENTRICLE

Meningiomas of the fourth ventricle (MFV) are an extremely rare entity, representing 0.08% to 3% of all intracranial meningiomas and less than 0.1% to 6% of all intraventricular meningiomas.[42,43] These lesions originate from the arachnoid cap cells located in the stroma of the choroid plexus or tela choroidea in the roof of the fourth ventricle.[42,43] It is hypothesized that its rarity is due to the decreased bulk of the choroid plexus within the fourth ventricle versus the choroid plexus

found in the lateral ventricles. Histopathologically, greater than 80% of the meningiomas found in the fourth ventricle are benign (WHO grade I) and a small percentage are atypical (WHO grade II).[4]

Clinical Presentation and Imaging Characteristics

MFV are typically diagnosed between the third to the sixth decade of life and have a slight female predominance.[42–44] These tumors seem to be sporadic without significant association with other medical conditions, radiation therapy, or hormonal influences.[42] Clinically, patients with MFV most commonly present signs and symptoms associated with obstructive hydrocephalus caused by the tumor and increasing intracranial pressure secondary to the obstruction of cerebrospinal fluid (CSF) flow.[43] The most common presenting symptoms are headache (75%), ataxia (57.1%), vomiting (41.7%), dizziness (26.7%), and cranial nerve palsy (19.6%).[42,43]

On CT imaging, fourth ventricular meningiomas are typically hyperdense or isodense.[43] MRI of these lesions show tumors that are typically isointense or hypointense on T1-weighted imaging and usually show homogenous enhancement after contrast administration, although some can by heterogeneously enhancing. On T2-weighted imaging MFV are usually hyperintense.[43] Hydrocephalus is common on imaging, seen in about half of the patients (52.8%); however, it seems to be independent of maximum tumor diameter or tumor volume.[43]

Surgical Anatomy

The fourth ventricle is a tent-shaped midline cavity located between the cerebellum and the brainstem. It is ventral to the cerebellum, dorsal to the pons and medulla, and medial to the cerebellar peduncles. Rostrally it communicates with the third ventricle via the cerebral aqueduct, caudally it communicates with the cisterna magna via the foramen of Magendie, and laterally it communicates with the cerebellopontine angles via the lateral foramina of Luschka.

The fourth ventricle is grossly composed of a roof, floor, and 2 lateral recesses.

In the instance where the fourth ventricular meningioma originates from the inferior tela choroidea of the roof, invasion into the cerebellar parenchyma is highly likely, whereas tumors that originate from the choroid plexus tend to fill the ventricle without any signs of infiltration.[32] The blood supply of fourth ventricular meningioma usually arises from the posterior inferior cerebellar artery. In the absence of a posterior inferior cerebellar artery, the main feeder is the superior cerebellar artery.[42,43,45]

Surgical Management and Approaches

Generally, gross total resection is the primary treatment modality for MFV.[43] Usually, these tumors are resected using a median suboccipital craniotomy and telovelar approach, which provides access to the fourth ventricle by using the cerebello-medullary fissure and minimizes neural tissue damage.[46,47] If the tumor extends to the cerebellopontine angle, then a larger retrosigmoid suboccipital craniotomy extending to the posterior edge of the sigmoid sinus is preferred.[43] A telovelar approach is recommended versus the transvermian to access lesions in the fourth ventricle, as splitting the vermis can result in cerebellar mutism, manifesting with nystagmus, gait disturbance, oscillation of the head and neck, truncal ataxia, and disturbance in equilibrium.

In the largest series reported including 11 patients with MFV, postoperative complications occurred in 15.3% of cases. These included postoperative hematoma and transient neurologic symptoms after surgery (including urinary retention, oropharyngeal paralysis, bilateral abducens paralysis, mild vertigo, mild dysphasia, nystagmus, and nausea), most of which recovered on follow-up.[42] Recurrence rates for fourth ventricular meningiomas tend to be slightly higher than intraventricular meningiomas (6.8 vs 5.3%). Thus, follow-up is required to identify the optimal opportunity for potential intervention and prevent the new onset of neurologic deficits.

FUNCTIONAL AND NEUROLOGIC OUTCOMES

Intraventricular meningiomas can be resected with low morbidity and mortality. Visual field deficit remains a common postoperative neurologic deficit experienced following resection of lateral ventricular lesions, experienced in up to 5% to 20% of patients postoperatively.[11,48–50] Following transcortical approaches, postoperative seizures may be increased following resection.[51] Permanent motor deficits following resection of atrial meningiomas is reported to occur in up to 14% of patients.[52]

Recent years have seen more attention drawn to functional outcomes, although few studies report detailed neuropsychological outcomes. Following resection of lateral ventricle meningiomas, the proportion of patients with preserved or improved cognitive function is reported to be within 59% to 86%.[51–53] A 2019 systematic review by Schartz and colleagues analyzing 60 literature reported 65.6% of patients experienced a good outcome following third ventricular meningiomas resection.

In their analysis, hypothalamic dysfunction was noted in 4 patients.[37]

Future directions may include use of tubular retraction systems for minimally invasive tumor resection, of which early experience with intraventricular meningiomas has been reported with success.[54]

TUMOR RECURRENCE

Tumor recurrence following resection of intraventricular meningioma remains rare. Recent series have highlighted recurrence rates of approximately 5%.[55] Unsurprisingly, subtotal tumor resection has been identified as an important prognostic indicator for tumor recurrence.[56] Indeed, gross total resection can be typically achieved in nearly 95% of tumors with most recurrences arising from atypical or malignant lesions. Accordingly, few series report resection of recurrent lesions. Given the indolent nature of these lesions, residual tumor may have minimal clinical consequence and, if present, may be considered for either stereotactic radiosurgery or reoperation.

SUMMARY

To facilitate safe and efficacious resection of intraventricular meningiomas, a thorough understanding of patient preoperative imaging and ventricular neurovascular anatomy is crucial; this allows safe gross total resection to be achieved in most cases with minimal surgical morbidity.

CLINICS CARE POINTS

- The optimal surgical approach for intraventricular meningioma resection should minimize retraction of normal brain and minimize involvement of nonaffected cortical and subcortical regions.
- General principles of resection include obtaining proximal vascular control and tumor debulking in piecemeal fashion.
- Meningiomas in the lateral ventricles may be approached either transcortically (parietal, parieto-occipital or temporal) or interhemispheric transcallosal, ipsilaterally or contralaterally.
- Meningiomas in the third ventricle are best approached as pineal region tumors, either infratentorial supracerebellar, occipital transtentorial, or anterior/posterior transcallosal, depending on relationship to the velum interpositum and displacement of the internal cerebral veins

- Meningiomas of the fourth ventricle are best approached through a midline suboccipital telovelar approach.
- Preoperative and postoperative obstructive hydrocephalus may necessitate temporary or permanent CSF diversion.

DISCLOSURE

We have no conflict of interests or funding to disclose.

REFERENCES

1. Nayar VV, DeMonte F, Yoshor D, et al. Surgical approaches to meningiomas of the lateral ventricles. Clin Neurol Neurosurg 2010;112(5):400–5.
2. Moliterno J, Omuro A. *Meningiomas: comprehensive stratgies for management.* Springer; 2020.
3. Raguž M, Rotim A, Sajko T, et al. Microsurgical management of a rare incidental intraventricular meningioma: a case report and relevant literature review. Acta Clin Croat 2021;60(1):156–60.
4. Engelbert Knosp AB. Chapter 32: Meningiomas of the lateral and fourth ventricles. In: Franco DeMonte MWM, Ossama Al-Mefty. Al-Mefty's Meningiomas. Thieme; 2011.
5. Bhatoe HS, Singh P, Dutta V. Intraventricular meningiomas: a clinicopathological study and review. Neurosurg Focus 2006;20(3):E9.
6. Ma J, Cheng L, Wang G, et al. Surgical management of meningioma of the trigone area of the lateral ventricle. World Neurosurg 2014;82(5):757–69.
7. Muley KD, Shaikh ST, Deopujari CE, et al. Primary intraventricular meningiomas in children-experience of two cases with review of literature. Childs Nerv Syst 2017;33(9):1589–94.
8. Kim EY, Kim ST, Kim HJ, et al. Intraventricular meningiomas: radiological findings and clinical features in 12 patients. Clin Imaging 2009;33(3):175–80.
9. Lyngdoh BT, Giri PJ, Behari S, et al. Intraventricular meningiomas: a surgical challenge. J Clin Neurosci 2007;14(5):442–8.
10. Demaerel P, Wilms G, Lammens M, et al. Intracranial meningiomas: correlation between MR imaging and histology in fifty patients. J Comput Assist Tomogr 1991;15(1):45–51.
11. Liu M, Wei Y, Liu Y, et al. Intraventricular meninigiomas: a report of 25 cases. Neurosurg Rev 2006; 29(1):36–40.
12. Nanda A, Bir SC, Maiti T, et al. Intraventricular Meningioma: Technical Nuances in Surgical Management. World Neurosurg 2016;88:526–37.
13. Chen C, Lv L, Hu Y, et al. Clinical features, surgical management, and long-term prognosis of intraventricular meningiomas: A large series of 89 patients

at a single institution. Medicine (Baltim) 2019; 98(16):e15334.
14. Pereira BJA, de Almeida AN, Paiva WS, et al. Natural history of intraventricular meningiomas: systematic review. Neurosurg Rev 2020;43(2):513–23.
15. Fusco DJ, Spetzler RF. Surgical considerations for intraventricular meningiomas. World Neurosurg 2015;83(4):460–1.
16. Budu A, Mezei G, Choudhari KA. Minimally invasive tubular corticotomy using "Dandy cannula-glove technique" for trans-cortical approaches to the ventricular lesions. Technical note. Interdisciplinary neurosurgery : Advanced techniques and case management 2022;27:100946.
17. Fornari M, Savoiardo M, Morello G, et al. Meningiomas of the lateral ventricles. Neuroradiological and surgical considerations in 18 cases. J Neurosurg 1981;54(1):64–74.
18. Kashiwazaki D, Takaiwa A, Nagai S, et al. Reversal of cognitive dysfunction by total removal of a large lateral ventricle meningioma: a case report with neuropsychological assessments. Case Rep Neurol 2014;6(1):44–9.
19. Jiang Y, Lv L, Li J, et al. Clinical features, radiological findings, and treatment outcomes of high-grade lateral ventricular meningiomas: a report of 26 cases. Neurosurg Rev 2020;43(2):565–73.
20. Sumi K, Suma T, Yoshida R, et al. Massive intracranial hemorrhage caused by intraventricular meningioma: case report. BMC Neurol 2021;21(1):25.
21. Giulioni M, Martinoni M. Giant intraventricular meningioma. World Neurosurg 2014;82(5):e657–8.
22. Nayar VV, Foroozan R, Weinberg JS, et al. Preservation of visual fields with the inferior temporal gyrus approach to the atrium. J Neurosurg 2009;110(4): 740–3.
23. Dumitrescu AM, Costea CF, Furnică C, et al. Morphological aspects of the vasculogenesis and angiogenesis during prenatal edification of the circle of Willis: a review. Rom J Morphol Embryol 2021; 62(3):679–87.
24. Tanglay O, Young IM, Dadario NB, et al. Anatomy and white-matter connections of the precuneus. Brain Imaging Behav 2022;16(2):574–86.
25. Cavanna AE. The precuneus and consciousness. CNS Spectr 2007;12(7):545–52.
26. Bruni JE, Montemurro D. Human Neuroanatomy : a Text, brain Atlas and Laboratory dissection Guide. Oxford University Press, Incorporated; 2009.
27. Güngör A, Baydin S, Middlebrooks EH, et al. The white matter tracts of the cerebrum in ventricular surgery and hydrocephalus. J Neurosurg 2017;126(3): 945–71.
28. Muftah Lahirish IA, Middlebrooks EH, Holanda VM, et al. Comparison Between Transcortical and Interhemispheric Approaches to the Atrium of Lateral Ventricle Using Combined White Matter Fiber

Dissections and Magnetic Resonance Tractography. World Neurosurg 2020;138:e478–85.

29. Watson C, Kirkcaldie M, Paxinos G. The brain : an introduction to functional Neuroanatomy. Elsevier Science & Technology; 2010.

30. Latini F, Trevisi G, Fahlström M, et al. New Insights Into the Anatomy, Connectivity and Clinical Implications of the Middle Longitudinal Fasciculus. Front Neuroanat 2020;14:610324.

31. Monroy-Sosa A, Jennings J, Chakravarthi S, et al. Microsurgical Anatomy of the Vertical Rami of the Superior Longitudinal Fasciculus: An Intraparietal Sulcus Dissection Study. Oper Neurosurg (Hagerstown) 2019;16(2):226–38.

32. Groen RJ, du Toit DF, Phillips FM, et al. Anatomical and pathological considerations in percutaneous vertebroplasty and kyphoplasty: a reappraisal of the vertebral venous system. Spine 2004;29(13): 1465–71.

33. Botez-Marquard T, Botez MI. Visual Memory Deficits After Damage to the Anterior Commissure and Right Fornix. Arch Neurol 1992;49(3):321–4.

34. Koutsarnakis C, Kalyvas AV, Skandalakis GP, et al. Sledge runner fasciculus: anatomic architecture and tractographic morphology. Brain Struct Funct 2019;224(3):1051–66.

35. Li P, Diao X, Bi Z, et al. Third ventricular meningiomas. J Clin Neurosci 2015;22(11):1776–84.

36. Karki P, Yonezawa H, Bohara M, et al. Third ventricular atypical meningioma which recurred with further malignant progression. Brain Tumor Pathol 2015; 32(1):56–60.

37. Schartz D, D'Agostino E, Makler V, et al. Third ventricle World Health Organization Grade II meningioma presenting with intraventricular hemorrhage and obstructive hydrocephalus: A case report and literature review. Surg Neurol Int 2019;10:73.

38. Hanieh A. Meningioma of the third ventricle. Childs Nerv Syst 1989;5(1):41–2.

39. Uygur ER, Deniz B, Zafer K. Anterior third ventricle meningiomas. Report of two cases. Neurocirugia (Astur) 2008;19(4):356–60.

40. Mizowaki T, Nagashima T, Yamamoto K, et al. Optimized surgical approach to third ventricular choroid plexus papillomas of young children based on anatomical variations. World Neurosurg 2014;82(5): 912.e15–9.

41. Wajima D, Iida J, Nishi N. Third ventricular meningioma–case report. Neurol Med -Chir 2011;51(1): 75–8.

42. Pichierri A, Ruggeri A, Morselli C, et al. Fourth ventricle meningiomas: a rare entity. Br J Neurosurg 2011;25(4):454–8.

43. Luo W, Xu Y, Yang J, et al. Fourth Ventricular Meningiomas. World Neurosurg 2019;127:e1201–9.

44. Sadashiva N, Rao S, Srinivas D, et al. Primary intrafourth ventricular meningioma: Report two cases. J Neurosci Rural Pract 2016;7(2):276–8.

45. Zhang J, Shrestha R, PeiZhi Z, et al. Meningioma of the fourth ventricle with exceptional growth pattern. Clin Neurol Neurosurg 2013;115(8):1567–9.

46. Cohen-Gadol A. Telovelar Approach: A Practical Guide for Its Expansion to the Fourth Ventricle. World Neurosurg 2021;148:239–50.

47. Tomasello F, Conti A, Cardali S, et al. Telovelar Approach to Fourth Ventricle Tumors: Highlights and Limitations. World Neurosurg 2015;83(6): 1141–7.

48. Ødegaard KM, Helseth E, Meling TR. Intraventricular meningiomas: a consecutive series of 22 patients and literature review. Neurosurg Rev 2013; 36(1):57–64 [discussion: 64].

49. Nakamura M, Roser F, Bundschuh O, et al. Intraventricular meningiomas: a review of 16 cases with reference to the literature. Surg Neurol 2003;59(6): 491–503 [discussion: 503-4].

50. McDermott MW. Intraventricular meningiomas. Neurosurg Clin N Am 2003;14(4):559–69.

51. D'Angelo VA, Galarza M, Catapano D, et al. Lateral ventricle tumors: surgical strategies according to tumor origin and development–a series of 72 cases. Neurosurgery 2005;56(1 Suppl):36–45 [discussion: 38-45].

52. Schwartz C, Jahromi BR, Lönnrot K, et al. Clinical outcome after microsurgical resection of intraventricular trigone meningiomas: a single-centre analysis of 20 years and literature overview. Acta Neurochir 2021;163(3):677–87.

53. Grujicic D, Cavallo LM, Somma T, et al. Intraventricular Meningiomas: A Series of 42 Patients at a Single Institution and Literature Review. World Neurosurg 2017;97:178–88.

54. Jamshidi AO, Beer-Furlan A, Hardesty DA, et al. Management of large intraventricular meningiomas with minimally invasive port technique: a threecase series. Neurosurg Rev 2021;44(4):2369–77.

55. Teng H, Liu Z, Yan O, et al. Lateral Ventricular Meningiomas: Clinical Features, Radiological Findings and Long-Term Outcomes. Cancer Manag Res 2021;13:6089–99.

56. Wang X, Cai BW, You C, et al. Microsurgical management of lateral ventricular meningiomas: a report of 51 cases. Minim Invasive Neurosurg 2007;50(6): 346–9.

Spheno-Orbital Meningiomas

Cameron A. Rawanduzy, MD, Karol P. Budohoski, MD, PhD, Robert C. Rennert, MD, Alexander Winkler-Schwartz, MD, PhD, William T. Couldwell, MD, PhD*

KEYWORDS

- Spheno-orbital meningioma • En plaque meningioma • Frontotemporal • Orbital apex
- Hyperostosis

KEY POINTS

- Spheno-orbital meningiomas originate from the dura of the sphenoid wing and can locally invade the clinoid, cavernous sinus, orbital apex, rectus muscles, and periorbita.
- Evolution of imaging technology led to a greater understanding of growth characteristics; these tumors are defined by their soft tissue and hyperostotic components.
- The classic symptomatic triad is proptosis, visual deficit, and ocular paresis.
- Surgery is the definitive treatment for spheno-orbital meningiomas.
- Extent of resection should be tailored to the individual patient.

INTRODUCTION

Meningiomas are dural-based tumors arising from the arachnoid cap cells, otherwise known as meningothelial cells. Approximately 13% to 19% of intracranial tumors are meningiomas, and they are the most common primary brain tumor in adults. Most meningiomas are benign World Health Organization (WHO) grade I lesions, and they frequently present in the sixth and seventh decades of life.[1–3]

Genetic predispositions, radiation exposure, and female sex are associated risk factors for the development of meningiomas. The female predominance may be explained by the role of sex hormones—primarily estrogen, progesterone, and androgen receptors—that are present in meningiomas.[2]

Spheno-orbital meningiomas (SOMs) are an uncommon, but important subtype of intracranial meningiomas. SOMs arise from the sphenoid wing and extend into the orbit.[4] These menigiomas comprise up to 20% of all intracranial meningiomas, and although they tend to have a benign histopathology, their location and growth pattern invading the cranial nerve foramina and the intraorbital compartment present unique surgical challenges.[5–7] This review provides an overview of spheno-orbital tumors, their presentation, and an introduction to management strategies.

Historical Background

SOMs originate from the dura of the sphenoid wing and secondarily infiltrate the orbital compartment. SOMs represent approximately 4% of space-occupying orbital lesions, and they are the sixth most frequent orbital tumor, with a peak incidence in the sixth and seventh decade of life.[8,9]

Studies have found that female predominance is greater in SOMs than in meningiomas of other locations.[9] There is a suggested female-to-male distribution of 2:1, although there are consistent reports of a much greater female sex predilection of between 5:1 and 11:1 female to male.[5,10]

These tumors are complex and slow growing,[5] and they are characteristically distinct from sphenoid wing meningiomas in part because they have both an intraosseous and an orbital/periorbital component.[7] SOMs were first described by

Department of Neurosurgery, Clinical Neurosciences Center, University of Utah, 175 North Medical Drive East, Salt Lake City, UT 84132, USA
* Corresponding author.
E-mail address: neuropub@hsc.utah.edu

Neurosurg Clin N Am 34 (2023) 417–423
https://doi.org/10.1016/j.nec.2023.02.006
1042-3680/23/© 2023 Elsevier Inc. All rights reserved.

Cushing and Eisenhardt in 1938[3,10,11] as "hyperostosing meningioma of ala magna," and in the computed tomography (CT) era the term was modernized and SOM was adopted. Magnetic resonance imaging (MRI) has since led to greater understanding of the tumor characteristics such as the prominent soft tissue components that invade surrounding structures.[12] Cushing defined the sphenoidal ridge as having 3 separate components: the deep inner/clinoidal segment; the middle/alar segment; and the outer/pterional segment. The clinoidal and alar segments compose the margin of the lesser sphenoid wing, and the pterional segment is the margin of the greater wing.[13] Cushing characterized these sphenoidal ridge tumors as either globoid/nodular-shaped or flat "meningioma en plaque" tumors that originate from the dura of the sphenoid ridge and spread along the sphenoid wing.[3,10] The globoid tumors are space-occupying lesions whose location can be medial, middle, or lateral, whereas en plaque meningiomas are flat and expansive, infiltrate the dura, and comprise a thin, diffuse, sheetlike layer over the contours of the inner table of the skull.[3,6,14]

Hyperostosis is present in many of these tumors, but especially in the en plaque subtype.[4,11,15,16] Because of the presence of intraosseous growth, a thin carpetlike soft tissue mass forms at the dura, and the bony tumor growth invades the sphenoid bone and spreads throughout the orbit.[17] The lesser sphenoid wing, orbital roof, lateral orbital wall, and the floor of the middle fossa, as well as the anterior clinoid process (ACP), superior orbital fissure (SOF), and optic canal (OC), are commonly involved.[18]

Compressive symptoms can become apparent as the tumors increase in size[2] and there is invasion of neurovascular structures of the orbital apex (OA) and the optic nerve; the SOF and the nerves supplying extraocular muscles and the cavernous sinus (CS) with its content can pose challenges to surgical resection.[4]

Symptoms

The symptoms and prognosis are mostly influenced by the extent of the bony invasion, rather than dural involvement.[10] When symptomatic, patients often present with one or all of the classic triad of proptosis, visual impairment, and ocular paresis.[7,11,16,19,20] Proptosis is the most common clinical sign, reportedly affecting between 33% and 86% of patients.[9] Proptosis can be a consequence of hyperostosis of the orbital walls, intraorbital growth of the tumor, or reduction of venous drainage from dural infiltration at the SOF causing

venous stasis.[17] The intraorbital space is usually reduced because of hyperostosis and tumor invasion, and compression can rapidly cause visual symptoms and lead to irreversible visual loss.[12] Visual deterioration can be related to optic nerve compression of the tumor itself, either in the area of the OA or OC, or hyperostosis in the OC walls. The rate of visual impairment in SOMs ranges from 43.8% to 80%, and the rate of OC invasion has been reported to be 5.8% to 68.6%.[21]

Characteristic Features

SOMs originate at the sphenoid wing, involve the orbit, and consistently affect the orbital roof and the lateral orbital wall. The roof is made up of the frontal bone and lesser wing of the sphenoid and contains the trochlear fossa and supraorbital foramen. The lateral orbital wall is made up by the zygomatic bone and greater wing of the sphenoid.[22]

Extension into the OA, OC, and SOF is common.[23] The OA is the narrowest part of the orbit connecting the intracranial cavity to the orbit. The OA houses the OC, SOF, and inferior orbital fissure. The ACP is the projection formed by the medial and posterior ends of the lesser wing of the sphenoid bone,[24] and its removal is often necessary to fully decompress the optic nerve when resecting the SOM.[24] The OA is surrounded by the greater and lesser wings, the ethmoidal sinus, the palatine bone, and the annulus of Zinn,[24] a fibrous ring surrounding the OC and part of the SOF at the OA. Within the boundaries of the annulus of Zinn are the optic nerve, OA, oculomotor nerve, abducens nerve, and the nasociliary nerve. The annulus attaches to the optic strut, which functions to stabilize the extraocular muscles in the OA. Diplopia can occur if damage to this structure is sustained.[25]

Morphologically, SOMs have 2 components, intraosseous growth with associated hyperostosis and an intradural soft tissue component.[5] Some consider intraosseous meningioma and en plaque meningioma as separate entities; however, there is rarely singular bony or soft tissue involvement and they are usually associated with one another.[18] The distinction between intraosseous and en plaque meningioma is likely a result of their initial identification in the era before regular use of MRI. CT would not reveal the soft tissue component, whereas today, MRI can detect tumor invading surrounding soft tissue structures and the intraorbital space.[5]

The hallmark feature of these tumors is hyperostosis of the sphenoid wing, orbital wall, SOF, and OC.[9,26] Extensive tumors can reach the frontal and temporal bones.[19] Because of their inherent invasiveness, SOMs can display features of malignancy upon imaging, but these tumors tend to be WHO grade I.[4] The hyperostotic tumor causes destruction of the orbital wall and roof and can affect the ACP, CS, and middle or posterior cranial fossae.[20,23] Large tumors can compress the optic nerve and supraclinoid carotid artery.[14]

Natural History

SOMs are known to recur at greater rates than other meningiomas.[4,17] Reported recurrence rates vary from 0% to 71% in the literature, and recurrence time is usually delayed; recurrences appear after a mean of 6 years.[4] A study by Ho and colleagues[27] found tumors with a higher number of 1p and 6q deletions progressed more frequently after subtotal resection. Although genetic factors may play a role, at least in part recurrences are related to the inability of achieving gross total resection (GTR).

As expected, the extent of resection is in part correlated with the recurrence rate. Recurrence rates may be higher after grade III/IV resection when compared with grade I resection.[15,17,23] The multicompartmental nature of the tumor makes GTR challenging. Involvement of the SOF, OC, and OA can pose the greatest restriction to the extent of resection.[4,17,28] OA and diffuse type meningiomas have significantly higher rates of recurrence than tumors located in the lateral and medial sphenoid compartments because of the involvement of critical neurovascular structures more medially.[23] SOF involvement, extension to the infratemporal fossa and sphenoidal ethmoidal sinuses, and WHO grade II lesions are also implicated in higher rates of recurrence.[23] Reoperation is the treatment of choice for recurrent tumors, and radiosurgery is generally the choice for patients with WHO grade II tumors.[23]

SOMs can encase vasculature, and attempts to dissect tumor adherent to these vessels has resulted in rates of vascular injury upward of 20%. Leaving behind residual tumor and following up with fractionated stereotactic radiosurgery or radiosurgery may be more favorable. Near-total resection of low-grade meningiomas often leads to remnants that may not recur.[3]

Operative Technique

Optimal treatment strategy, including the preferred approach, the target extent of resection, and the necessity of orbital wall reconstruction are subjects of debate. Often, surgical planning and execution are guided by the surgeon's preference, experience, and level of comfort.[29]

Numerous approaches, both orbitocranial and cranioorbital, are available for resecting tumors affecting the skull base and orbit, and the lesion location influences the chosen surgical approach. Nonetheless, a frontotemporal craniotomy is often the preferred approach to SOM because of its versatility and the ability to visualize intracranial and intraorbital portions of the tumor from this approach. Although the orbital compartment may be unfamiliar territory, a frontotemporal craniotomy is well within the skull base neurosurgeon's armamentarium, and it provides a very suitable corridor to remove hyperostotic bone and decompress the optic nerve, foramen magnum, foramen ovale, and CS.[26] Furthermore, the frontotemporal craniotomy provides easy access into the lateral and superior orbit, where most of the SOMs are located.

The senior author (W.T.C.) has pursued more aggressive resection through the past three decades of practice, while achieving improvement in outcomes. Early on, more conservative resections yielded less satisfactory reductions in proptosis, whereas aggressive resections resulted in measurable improvements. These findings have been reported in a separate series,[26,29] and the preferred operative technique is detailed in the following discussion.

A standard frontotemporal craniotomy can be performed. Hyperostotic bone is often encountered after the myocutaneous flap is elevated and drilled, and any tumor invading the temporalis muscle will prompt resection of the muscle. The hyperostotic sphenoid wing is drilled down to the meningo-orbital band, which is cauterized and sharply cut. Dura of the frontal lobe is peeled from the orbital roof, and the dura of the temporal lobe is peeled from the middle fossa floor to expose the SOF, foramen rotundum, foramen ovale, and foramen spinosum. The dura is stripped from the lateral CS without entering the sinus. The middle meningeal artery is commonly a feeder artery to the tumor, and it is coagulated and cut. Once the dural portion of the tumor has been adequately resected, the lateral orbital wall of the orbit is drilled to completely expose the periorbita. The hyperostotic portion of the tumor can increase the probability of recurrence if not extensively resected, so drilling the roof of the orbit until normal bone is encountered is standard practice. The SOF is decompressed by drilling bone posteriorly. The second branch of the fifth cranial nerve is decompressed as it enters the foramen rotundum and pterygopalatine fossa. If the middle fossa floor is affected by tumor, the dura is stripped away from V3 and the foramen ovale is decompressed. The orbital roof is drilled if it is infiltrated by tumor,

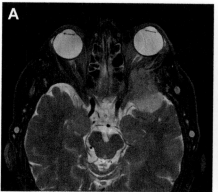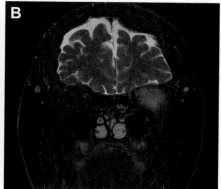

Fig. 1. The soft tissue component of the spheno-orbital tumor can be seen on (*A*) axial and (*B*) coronal magnetic resonance imaging. Extension commonly affects the frontal and temporal dura and infiltrates the orbital compartment affecting the orbital apex, periorbita, and extraocular muscles.

with care to avoid entering the nasal sinuses. Resection is extended posteriorly to the OC and ACP. A clinoidectomy is regularly performed to unroof the OC and decompress the optic nerve. When the periorbita is invaded by tumor, it is sharply opened, and tumor is dissected along a plane from the periorbital fat. In young patients, extraocular muscle tumor involvement is spared unless removing the tumor is likely to prevent recurrence. In older patients, the extraocular muscles are resected if invaded by tumor. These patients follow up with oculoplastic surgeons for normal globe repositioning. Finally, once satisfactory resection of the tumor of the orbital compartment is achieved, the dura is dissected down to the middle fossa, and any tumor-involved dura is removed.[26]

The decision to reconstruct the orbit after surgery is based on surgeon preferences. Reconstruction is theorized to prevent pulsatile exophthalmos, as well as to minimize cerebrospinal fluid leakage and infection risk and establish normal, symmetric eye position. There are multiple reports of similar outcomes without reconstruction.[11,15]

Treatment Nuances

Historically, patients with these tumors were not recommended as operative candidates because of the high mortality and morbidity.[18,29] Today, improved microsurgical techniques have solidified surgical resection as the standard management to alleviate symptoms such as proptosis and visual deficits.[29]

Recently, surgically treated SOMs are becoming increasingly complex, in part because of the period of observation before surgery and the greater adoption of radiosurgery for simpler tumors.[3]

Radiographic imaging is necessary to differentiate sphenoid wing meningioma from SOM. The combination of hyperostosis and orbital extension is the distinguishing characteristic. CT should be used as first-line imaging to identify bony involvement and hyperostosis. MRI in conjunction with CT will identify soft tissue components, dural involvement, and total extension (**Fig. 1**; **Fig. 2**).[1,10,11] MRI can also reveal increased vascularity in these tumors from external carotid artery supply.[7] In patients with known SOMs, large and/or fast-growing tumors, those growing >1 cm^3 per year, should undergo more regular serial imaging, potentially every 6 months, to guide treatment.[9]

It was previously thought that curative treatment of SOMs required the entirety of the intradural, periorbital, and hyperostotic tumor to be resected, and intracranial and facial sinuses needed to be opened in select cases.[23] Surgical goals and management have progressed, yet the invasion of critical neurovascular structures continues to make treatment challenging.[3,5,17] Simpson grade I resection is the gold standard, but it is often impossible, and GTR rates vary between 0% and 70% across treatment centers.[7] Extent of resection is determined by the tumor anatomy and what soft tissue structures are involved. If the CS, SOF, and Zinn fibrous ring are affected, GTR is unlikely. The intraconal orbit, pterygopalatine fossa, and encased vasculature can also limit GTR.[15] Therefore, the goals of surgery are to maximize the extent of resection into the dura, bone, and orbital compartments; minimize morbidity; and treat symptoms, that is, the triad of proptosis, visual deficits, and ocular paresis.[15]

Visual function deficits are directly related to the degree of bone hyperostosis, so it is imperative to remove all hyperostotic bone and decompress the optic nerve to ensure recovery.[11]

Complex surgical approaches to expose the intracranial and intraorbital structures are required,

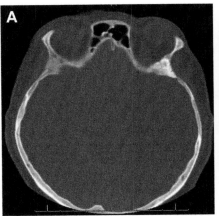
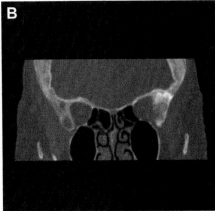

Fig. 2. Computed tomography should be obtained along with magnetic resonance imaging to understand the full scope of tumor involvement of the soft tissues as well as hyperostotic bone (*A, B*).

and close collaboration between neurosurgeons, maxillofacial, and oculoplastic surgeons is essential.[30] Approaches include transzygomatic, pterional, frontotemporal, combined transcranial-transmalar, or cranio-orbital.[18] Involvement of neurovascular structures must be considered to establish a realistic surgical goal while planning preoperatively.[26] Maximal safe resection involves periorbital resection (**Fig. 3**A and B) and decompressing the optic nerve (**Fig. 3**C). Some studies support periorbital resection to improve proptosis. Other investigators prefer to leave the periorbita.[4] In the authors' experience, periorbital tumor resection yields adequate visual and cosmetic results, and tumor control in the long-term is reasonable.[26] CS involvement generally should be left alone because good tumor control with adjuvant therapy has been demonstrated.[3] Unroofing of the OC is important for improvement in visual deterioration.[21] Visual acuity improves in 16.6% to 85% of patients,

and decompression of the optic nerve is advocated to improve visual acuity.[17]

There are some advocates for postoperative radiotherapy for long-term tumor control in managing patients with subtotal resections; this is debatable because meningiomas are inherently slow-growing tumors.[30] Tumor location in relation to the optic apparatus must be considered when opting for adjuvant radiation.[11]

Complications

The classic triad of proptosis, visual deterioration, and ocular paresis is the most common patient presentation, although there are other less common symptoms associated with these tumors. Acute intracranial hemorrhage is a rare but devastating complication.[31] In addition, there are reports of patients with SOMs presenting as mimicking idiopathic orbital inflammation.[8]

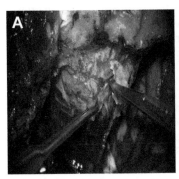
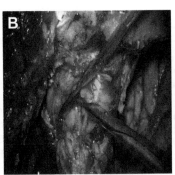
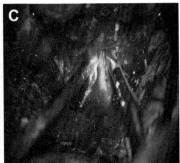

Fig. 3. Perioperative imaging demonstrating intraorbital resection technique. Drilling of the posterolateral wall and opening of the periorbita is essential to achieve near-total resection of the tumor (*A*). Tumor that has invaded the periorbita can be safely resected by identifying the plane between the periorbital fat and the tumor and dissecting in an anterior-to-posterior direction (*B*). Decompressing the optic nerve can ensure greater probability of improving visual acuity deficits (*C*).

The most common complications after resection are cranial nerve injuries including ophthalmoplegia from injury to the oculomotor, trochlear and abducens nerves, as well as facial numbness from injury to the trigeminal nerve.[15,17] Complications can result in transient or permanent neurological deficits. Extraocular muscle damage and rarely cerebral infarction due to damage to the internal carotid artery can occur postoperatively.[4] Other, often difficult-to-treat complications result from opening the paranasal sinuses. Typically, medial extension of the tumor can lead to opening of the sphenoid and/or ethmoidal sinuses, which may be difficult to identify intraoperatively and difficult to treat because of the lack of available vascularized tissue, which can be used for reconstruction of the skull base.

To avoid pulsating exophthalmos, reconstructing the orbital wall can be beneficial; however, this is mostly individual surgeon preference.[18]

SUMMARY

SOMs are complex skull base tumors that characteristically affect the intracranial and orbital compartments. Their natural history is not well elucidated; however, they display histopathologic properties and an epidemiologic profile similar to convexity meningiomas. Differentiating them from sphenoid wing meningiomas is the amalgamation of extensive intraosseous and soft tissue components, which can involve critical neurovascular structures and complicate surgery. Ultimately, lesions presenting symptomatically necessitate treatment, and near-total resection is feasible in select cases. Individualized operative planning is essential to establishing goals and managing expectations.

CLINICS CARE POINTS

- Spheno-orbital meningiomas are challenging to treat, and there is an elevated risk of recurrence due to involvement of critical structures limiting gross total resection.
- Innovative, minimally invasive surgical techniques are being developed, including orbitocranial approaches, to achieve targeted dissections and relief of symptoms in line with surgical goals.
- More aggressive resection can achieve improved outcomes as measured by proptosis and the need for future treatment including radiation or reoperation.

AUTHORS' CONTRIBUTIONS

C.A. Rawanduzy: methodology, writing – original draft, visualization; K.P. Budohoski: methodology, writing – original draft, visualization; R.C. Rennert: methodology, writing – original draft, visualization; A. Winkler-Schwartz: methodology, writing – original draft, visualization; W.T. Couldwell: conceptualization, resources, supervision, project administration, writing – review and editing.

FUNDING

No funding was received for this research.

CONFLICTS OF INTEREST/COMPETING INTERESTS

The authors report no conflicts of interest.

DATA AVAILABILITY

Not applicable.

CODE AVAILABILITY

Not applicable.

ETHICAL APPROVAL

Not applicable.

CONSENT TO PARTICIPATE

Not applicable.

CONSENT FOR PUBLICATION

The patient consented to the publication of any relevant imaging in this article.

ACKNOWLEDGMENTS

We thank Vance Mortimer for assistance in preparing the operative images and Kristin Kraus for editorial assistance.

REFERENCES

1. Muhsen B.A., Aljariri A.I., Hashem H., et al., En-plaque sphenoid wing grade II meningioma: Case report and review of literature, Ann Med Surg (Lond), 74, 2022,103322.
2. Kaiser A.E., Reddy S.V., Von Zimmerman M.A., et al., Gross and histological examination of a large spheno-orbital meningioma, Cureus, 12 (9), 2020, e10256.
3. Sughrue ME, Rutkowski MJ, Chen CJ, et al. Modern surgical outcomes following surgery for sphenoid wing meningiomas. J Neurosurg 2013;119(1):86–93.

4. Nagahama A, Goto T, Nagm A, et al. Spheno-orbital meningioma: surgical outcomes and management of recurrence. World Neurosurg 2019;126:e679–87.

5. Young J., Mdanat F., Dharmasena A., et al., Combined neurosurgical and orbital intervention for spheno-orbital meningiomas - the Manchester experience, Orbit, 39 (4), 2020, 251–257.

6. Güdük M, Özduman K, Pamir MN. Sphenoid Wing Meningiomas: Surgical Outcomes in a Series of 141 Cases and Proposal of a Scoring System Predicting Extent of Resection. World Neurosurg 2019; 125:e48–59.

7. Menon S., Sandesh O., Anand D., et al., Sphenoorbital meningiomas: optimizing visual outcome, J Neurosci Rural Pract, 11 (3), 2020, 385–394.

8. Rodríguez-Colón G., Bratton E.M., Serracino H.,et al., Sphenoid wing meningioma with extraocular muscle involvement mimicking idiopathic orbital inflammation, Ophthalmic Plast Reconstr Surg, 33 (3S Suppl 1), 2017, S97–S99.

9. Saeed P, van Furth WR, Tanck M, et al. Natural history of spheno-orbital meningiomas. Acta Neurochir 2011;153(2):395–402.

10. Simas NM, Farias JP. Sphenoid wing en plaque meningiomas: Surgical results and recurrence rates. Surg Neurol Int 2013;4:86.

11. Shrivastava R.K., Sen C., Costantino P.D., et al., Sphenoorbital meningiomas: surgical limitations and lessons learned in their long-term management, J Neurosurg, 103 (3), 2005, 491–497.

12. Talacchi A., De Carlo A., D'Agostino A., et al., Surgical management of ocular symptoms in sphenoorbital meningiomas. Is orbital reconstruction really necessary?, Neurosurg Rev, 37 (2), 2014, 301–309, [discussion: 309-10].

13. MacCarty CS. Meningiomas of the sphenoidal ridge. J Neurosurg 1972;36(1):114–20.

14. Magill S.T., Vagefi M.R., Ehsan M.U., et al., Sphenoid wing meningiomas, Handb Clin Neurol, 170, 2020, 37–43.

15. Dalle Ore C.L., Magill S.T., Rodriguez Rubio R., et al., Hyperostosing sphenoid wing meningiomas: surgical outcomes and strategy for bone resection and multidisciplinary orbital reconstruction, J Neurosurg, 134 (3), 2020, 711–720.

16. Leroy HA, Leroy-Ciocanea CI, Baroncini M, et al. Internal and external spheno-orbital meningioma varieties: different outcomes and prognoses. Acta Neurochir 2016;158(8):1587–96.

17. Terrier LM, Bernard F, Fournier HD, et al. Sphenoorbital meningiomas surgery: multicenter management study for complex extensive tumors. World Neurosurg 2018;112(0):e145–e156.

18. Ringel F, Cedzich C, Schramm J. Microsurgical technique and results of a series of 63 spheno-orbital meningiomas. Neurosurgery 2007;60(4 Suppl 2):214–21 [discussion: 221-2].

19. Kiyofuji S., Casabella A.M., Graffeo C.S., et al., Sphenoorbital meningioma: a unique skull base tumor. Surgical technique and results, J Neurosurg, 133 (4), 2020, 1044–1051.

20. Shapey J., Jung J., Barkas K., et al., A single centre's experience of managing spheno-orbital meningiomas: lessons for recurrent tumour surgery, Acta Neurochir, 161 (8), 2019, 1657–1667.

21. Mariniello G., de Divitiis O., Bonavolontà G., et al., Surgical unroofing of the optic canal and visual outcome in basal meningiomas, Acta Neurochir, 155 (1), 2013, 77–84.

22. Murdock N, Mahan M, Chou E. Benign Orbital Tumors. In: StatPearls [Internet]. FL: StatPearls Publishing, Treasure Island; 2022.

23. Mariniello G., de Divitiis O., Corvino S., et al., Recurrences of Spheno-Orbital Meningiomas: Risk Factors and Management, World Neurosurg, 161 (0), 2022, e514–e522.

24. Engin Ö, Adriaensen G.F.J.P., Hoefnagels F.W.A., et al., A systematic review of the surgical anatomy of the orbital apex, Surg Radiol Anat, 43 (2), 2021, 169–178.

25. Ma C., Zhu X., Chu X., et al., Formation and fixation of the annulus of Zinn and relation with extraocular muscles: a plastinated histologic study and its clinical significance, Invest Ophthalmol Vis Sci, 63 (12), 2022, 16.

26. Kim R.B., Fredrickson V.L. and Couldwell W.T., Visual outcomes in spheno-orbital meningioma: a 10-year experience, World Neurosurg, 158, (0), 2022, e726–e734.

27. Ho C-Y, Mosier S, Safneck J, et al. Genetic profiling of orbital meningioma. Brain Pathol 2015;25(2): 193–201.

28. Yang J, Ma SC, Liu YH, et al. Large and giant medial sphenoid wing meningiomas involving vascular structures: clinical features and management experience in 53 patients. Chin Med J (Engl) 2013; 126(23):4470–6.

29. Bowers CA, Sorour M, Patel BC, et al. Outcomes after surgical treatment of meningioma-associated proptosis. J Neurosurg 2016;125(3):544–50.

30. Sandalcioglu I.E., Gasser T., Mohr C., et al., Sphenoorbital meningiomas: interdisciplinary surgical approach, resectability and long-term results, J Cranio-Maxillo-Fac Surg, 33 (4), 2005, 260–266.

31. Frič R., Hald J.K. and Antal E.A., Benign sphenoid wing meningioma presenting with an acute intracerebral hemorrhage - a case report, J Cent Nerv Syst Dis, 8 (0),2016, 1–4.

Spinal Meningiomas
Diagnosis, Surgical Management, and Adjuvant Therapies

Vijay M. Ravindra, MD, MSPH[a,b,c], Meic H. Schmidt, MD, MBA[d,*]

KEYWORDS

- Spinal meningioma • Atypical • Myelopathy • Intraoperative monitoring

KEY POINTS

- Spinal meniniomga is the most common intradural tumor.
- Spinal meningiomas are typically benign.
- Surgical resection is the prefered treatment.

INTRODUCTION

Spinal meningiomas are the most common intradural tumor of the spine (**Tables 1–3**). They are mostly managed with operative resection, with the goal of achieving gross total resection while minimizing neurological dysfunction. Advances in surgical techniques and adjuvant treatment modalities have further improved the opportunities to achieve a cure. In this article, we review the current management of spinal meningiomas including diagnosis, surgical treatment, and adjuvant therapies.

Epidemiology

Meningiomas arise from meningothelial arachnoid cap cells and accounted for 36.8%–37.6% of the Central Brain Tumor Registry of the United States[1]; spinal meningiomas are much less frequent and represent 5%–10% of all meningiomas.[2,3] Intradural spinal tumors have an incidence of 64 per 100,000 person-years and account for 3% of primary central nervous system (CNS) tumors[4]; spinal meningiomas are the most common intradural spinal tumors. Spinal meningiomas are described anatomically as intradural, extramedullary lesions (**Fig. 1**). The differential diagnosis for intradural, extramedullary lesions, which account for two-third of all intraspinal neoplasms overall,[5] includes

- Meningioma
- Schwannoma
- Neurofibroma

Spinal meningiomas mostly occur between 40 and 70 years of age[6] and are most commonly found in middle-aged women, with a female-male ratio as high as 4:1,[7] a greater disparity of women to men than what is seen with cranial meningiomas. As theorized with intracranial meningiomas, the higher incidence and prevalence in women may be a result of tumor/tissue response to sex hormones.[6,8] Although the relationship of sex hormones and meningioma growth and development is suspected, other receptor types may contribute to pathogenesis:[8]

- Steroid receptors
- Peptidergic receptors
- Growth factor receptors
- Aminergic receptors

a Department of Neurosurgery, Clinical Neurosciences Center, University of Utah, 175 North Medical Drive East, Salt Lake City, UT 84132, USA; b Department of Neurosurgery, University of California San Diego, 9500 Gilman Drive, La Jolla, CA 92093, USA; c Department of Neurosurgery, Naval Medical Center San Diego, 34800 Bob Wilson Drive, San Diego, CA 92134, USA; d Department of Neurosurgery, University of New Mexico, 1155 University Bldvd. Southeast, Albuquerque, NM 87131, USA
* Corresponding author. UNMH, Bldg 235, Room Neurosurgery North, 2 ACC, MSC 10 5615, Albuquerque, NM 87131-0001.
E-mail address: mhschmidt@salud.unm.edu

Neurosurg Clin N Am 34 (2023) 425–435
https://doi.org/10.1016/j.nec.2023.02.007

Table 1
McCormick scale for grading spinal meningioma

Grade	Definition
0	No symptoms or neurological deficits
I	Neurologically normal, mild focal deficit not significantly affecting function of involved limbs; mild spasticity or reflex abnormality; normal gait
II	Presence of sensorimotor deficit affecting function of involved limb; mild to moderate gait difficulty; severe pain or dysesthetic syndrome impairing patient's quality of life; patient still functions and ambulates independently
III	More severe neurological deficit; requires cane/brace for ambulation of significant bilateral upper extremity impairment; may or may not function independently
IV	Severe deficit; requires wheelchair or cane/brace with bilateral upper extremity impairment; usually not independent

From McCormick PC, Torres R, Post KD, Stein BM. Intramedullary ependymoma of the spinal cord. J Neurosurg. 1990;72(4):523-532. https://doi.org/10.3171/jns.1990.72.4.0523.

Most spinal meningiomas are histologically benign or World Health Organization (WHO) grade I; however, lesions may be atypical (WHO grade II) or anaplastic (WHO grade III),[9–11] requiring further

Table 2
Simpson classification for grading extent of resection in spinal meningiomas

Grade	Definition
1	Macroscopically complete removal of tumor with excision of its dural attachment
2	Macroscopically complete removal of tumor with coagulation of its dural attachment
3	Macroscopically complete removal of tumor, without resection or coagulation of its dural attachment
4	Partial removal, leaving tumor in situ

Donald Simpson, The Recurrence Of Intracranial Meningiomas After Surgical Treatment, J Neurol Neurosurg Psychiatry, Simpson et al. 20:22-39, 1957.

Table 3
Frankel scale for grading spinal injury and disability

Frankel Grade	Definition
A	No motor or sensory function below the level of injury
B	Some preserved sensory function
C	Some preserved motor function, unable to walk
D	Preserved useful motor function, able to walk
E	Normal motor and sensory function

(*Adapted from* Frankel, H., Hancock, D., Hyslop, G. et al. The value of postural reduction in the initial management of closed injuries of the spine with paraplegia and tetraplegia. Spinal Cord 7, 179–192 (1969). https://doi.org/10.1038/sc.1969.30)

treatment. The histological subtypes mirror those of cranial meningiomas; psammomatous (WHO grade I), meningothelial (WHO grade I), and transitional (WHO grade I) subtypes are the most commonly seen ones among spinal meningiomas.

In contrast to intracranial meningiomas, spinal meningiomas have a lower recurrence rate,[9,10,12] which may suggest less-aggressive histopathology, although patients found to have lesions with psammomatous pathological characteristics have worse neurological outcomes.[12] The rate of malignant transformation of spinal meningiomas is low at 3%.[10]

The presentation of spinal meningiomas varies from asymptomatic to severe paraplegia or quadriparesis. The resulting neurological morbidity and symptoms are caused by spinal cord compression, either acute or chronic. Because spinal meningiomas grow slowly, even mild neurological deficits may be the result of significant spinal cord compression. Patients most commonly present with

- Generalized back pain, radicular pain, or mechanical pain
- Sensory loss, dermatomal and nondermatomal, may be reflective of the location of spinal cord compression
- Weakness
- Sphincter disturbances, including urinary dysfunction (incontinence, incomplete emptying, retention)

Despite significant neurological deficit in some cases, surgical treatment can be curative, with few complications and rapid functional recovery.[6,13–16]

Patients with a spinal meningioma can be assessed and graded on neurological dysfunction using the McCormick scale.[17]

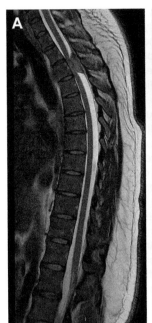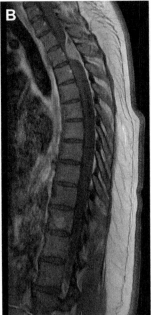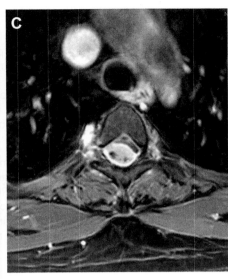

Fig. 1. Sagittal (*A*) T2-weighted image demonstrating isointense signal of the dorsally situated lesion in the mid-thoracic spine. Sagittal (*B*) and axial (*C*) T1-weighted post–contrast-enhanced images demonstrating homogeneous contrast enhancement with a distinct dural attachment.

Although the diagnosis of spinal meningioma may be made based on imaging characteristics, tissue diagnosis and confirmation dictate the need for further treatment.

Management Principles

Although most spinal meningiomas are detected because of symptoms explained by the lesion, a subset of lesions are detected incidentally. For these lesions or other small, noncompressive lesions, management options typically involve surveillance imaging. For symptomatic lesions, treatment may involve symptom control (medication for pain, neuropathic pain, and so forth), surgical excision, external beam radiation therapy, and, on rare occasions, chemotherapy.[18] For patients with symptomatic spinal meningiomas, the primary treatment is maximal surgical resection. Further adjuvant treatment for incompletely resected lesions and more aggressive histopathological subtypes is a subject of study and controversy.[19–21]

The outcomes of surgical treatment for spinal meningiomas are favorable overall[6,7,13–16,22–24]; however, individual outcomes depend on tumor size and location and, most importantly, the premorbid state of the patient. Although derived for intracranial meningiomas, the Simpson classification[25] is used in defining the extent of resection for spinal meningiomas.

Genetic and Molecular Markers

Spinal meningiomas can harbor a deletion of chromosome 22q and the associated gene NF2.[26,27] DNA microarray analysis demonstrated that spinal meningiomas had greater likelihood of chromosome 22 deletion than intracranial meningiomas.[27] In fact, complete or partial loss of chromosome 22 has been demonstrated in more than 50% of patients with spinal meningiomas.[26,28] Ketter and colleagues[28] demonstrated that each of 23 patients with spinal meningiomas had a normal chromosomal set or a monosomy of chromosome 22, and this genotype was not associated with disease recurrence.

Spinal meningiomas can have either complete or partial loss of chromosome 22, along with loss of 1p, 9p, and 10q with the gain of 5p and 17q.[26] These chromosomal aberrations are encountered in the atypical and anaplastic subtypes. Additionally, spinal meningiomas likely originate from a single-cell clone versus a collection of cells; 35 of 1555 genes were more highly expressed in spinal meningiomas than intracranial meningiomas,[27] including those involved in

- Transcription: *Hox* genes, *NR4* family of genes, *KLF4*, *FOSL2*, and *TCF 8*
- Intracellular signaling: *RGS16*, *DUSP5*, *DUSP1*, *SOCS3*, and *CMKOR*
- Extracellular signaling: *L6*, *TGFB1I4*, *CYR61*, and *CDH2*

Additional genes that have been implicated in spinal meningioma development include

- Matrix metalloproteinase-9: functions in protein upregulation with respect to cell growth and invasion[29]
- SMARCE1: involved in regulation of secondary DNA structure within chromosomes and is associated with multiple spinal meningioma formation[30]

Intracranial meningiomas have been more extensively sequenced, with multiple mutations (DAL1, TIMP, p16, p15, p14ARF, NDRG2, ADTB1, DLC1, c-myc, bcl-2, and STAT3) discovered that have yet to be defined in spinal meningiomas.[31] Further studies of the genetics and molecular targets will undoubtedly improve the management of spinal meningiomas.[32]

Tumor Locations

Spinal meningiomas can occur anywhere along the dura of the spinal column, but their most commonly reported location is the thoracic spine (67%–84%), followed by the cervical (14%–27%) and lumbar (2%–14%) spine.[6,7,13–16,22]

Patients aged 50 yeaes or younger had a higher frequency of spinal meningiomas in the cervical spine (39%), most commonly in the upper cervical spine.[32] Levy[16] reported location varied by sex, with thoracic spine meningiomas being more common in females. In addition to location along the spinal column, the relationship within the spinal canal and specifically the spinal cord is a common method of classifying spinal meningiomas. Most occur lateral to the spinal cord neural structures (68%), followed by posterior (18%), and then anterior (15%). Careful study of preoperative imaging aids in understanding the anatomy and surgical challenges with resection and reconstruction. Spinal meningiomas are primarily intradural, extramedullary lesions although 5%–14% may have an extradural component,[6,13–16,22] and a rare lesion may be entirely extradural.[6,14,15] Multiple spinal meningiomas can occur as well, but this is uncommon.

PATIENT EVALUATION

Patients commonly present with delayed onset of neurological symptoms. Upon evaluation with a detailed history, patients will often report symptom duration lasting 1–2 years prior to the initial presentation[14–16,22]; however, some patients may have protracted symptoms (>2 years) including chronic pain, radiculopathy, sensory disturbance, or weakness. Back pain or radiculopathy occurs

before weakness and sensory changes; sphincter dysfunction is typically a late finding.[7]

Magnetic resonance imaging (MRI) is the preferred imaging modality for evaluation of suspected spinal cord lesions based on symptoms and neurological findings. If MRI cannot be performed, then computed tomography myelography can be used for evaluating spinal pathology. The widespread availability and use of MRI has improved detection on average by 6 months earlier,[22] which subsequently leads to improved neurological function on presentation for surgery. Intraspinal meningiomas demonstrate classic MRI characteristics, including isointense signal on T1- and T2-weighted images with homogenous contrast enhancement with gadolinium administration (see **Fig. 1**). An algorithmic approach can aid in evaluating patients with intraspinal meningiomas (**Fig. 2**). The differential diagnosis for intradural lesions includes

- Metastatic lesion
- Dropped metastatic lesion from intracranial disease
- Primary CNS tumor (glioma, astrocytoma)
- Schwannoma
- Neurofibroma
- Meningioma
- Lipoma
- Malignant peripheral nerve sheath tumor

The degree of spinal cord compression is often associated with the onset and severity of the patient's symptoms. Because of better diagnostic techniques, the incidence of lesions, including spinal meningiomas, is growing, leading to a potential management dilemma about when to intervene.[33] Corell and colleagues[34] found that patients with intradural tumor occupying >65% of the cross-sectional area of the spinal canal were more likely to have preoperative symptoms and deficit; the authors concluded that patients with >65% canal occupancy should be considered for surgery because of the risk of growth causing neurological deficits.

SURGICAL APPROACH

The goals of surgical treatment of intraspinal meningiomas include excision to confirm histological diagnosis and decompression of the neural elements. The approach is dependent on location along the spinal column, size of the lesion, and relationship to the spinal cord. For lesions posterior and lateral to the spinal cord, a laminectomy is typically used. Multilevel approaches with or without fusion adjunct and laminoplasty are also used (**Fig. 3**). Minimally invasive resection of

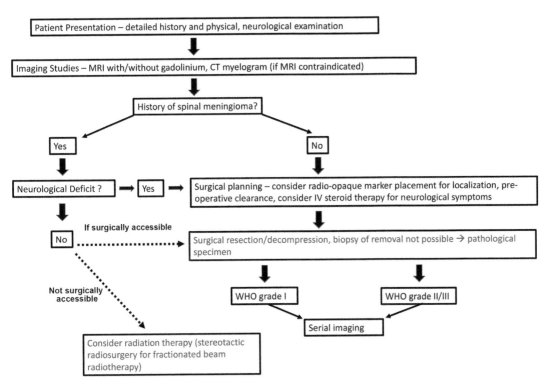

Fig. 2. Treatment algorithm for evaluating patients with suspected spinal cord meningioma. CT, computed tomography; IV, intravenous.

intradural-extramedullary spinal tumors has been described.[35] For thoracic lesions, the use of a radio-opaque marker can help with localization and limit the extent of bony opening.[36] For meningiomas anterior to the neural elements, more lateral bone removal from the facet joint and articular surface may be necessary; the decision to place instrumentation and stabilize the spine should be based on the extent of bone removal and risk of instability.

Ventral meningiomas in the cervical spine may be best approached anteriorly via a corpectomy to provide an adequate window for tumor removal; spinal reconstruction is necessary, and dural repair can often be difficult in this setting. For lesions lateral or anterior to the spinal cord located at T3-L2, a lateral extracavitary approach[37] or costotransversectomy[38] can be used to allow for circumferential neural decompression. A lateral extracavitary approach may require posterior fixation because of extensive pedicle removal and disruption of the ipsilateral facet joint. Costotransversectomy requires partial laminectomy and facetectomy, and arthrodesis may not be needed unless the anterior column is violated. With these 2 techniques, attention should be paid to the great vessels and radicular arteries, which must be carefully studied.[37,38]

Factors associated with the need for spinal instrumentation and arthrodesis[38] include multi-level exposure, disruption of the facet joints, and corpectomy.[39–41] Intraspinal meningiomas at biomechanical junctional locations, including the occipitocervical, cervicothoracic, and thoracolumbar junctions, are at risk of instability.[41–43] Stabilization should be considered for lesions in this location.[44] A classification scheme for intra-spinal meningiomas and the surgical approach and need for fusion has been reported,[38] but this decision should be made on a case-by-case basis based on bone removal, ligamentous disruption, and biomechanics. Most patients do not require fusion, but surveillance after surgery for the development of spinal deformity is necessary.

The use of microsurgical technique, ultrasonic aspiration, and neurophysiologic monitoring has made surgery more feasible, but removal of intraspinal meningiomas remains a challenge to neurosurgeons. The obvious risk is worsened neurological functioning, which can manifest as motor or sensory disturbances or autonomic dysfunction. Intraoperative ultrasound can be used to provide real-time information about the size, shape, and morphology of the spinal cord.[45] This can also be useful in tailoring bone removal

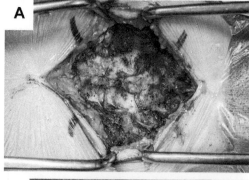

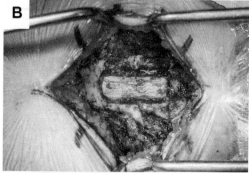

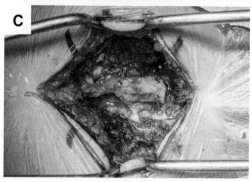

Fig. 3. (*A*) Intraoperative photograph demonstrating the bony exposure needed to perform a single- or multi-level laminectomy for resection. (*B*) Photograph showing laminectomy and exposure of the dural surface. (*C*) Intraoperative photograph demonstrating 2-level laminoplasty after spinal meningioma resection.

by clearly identifying the cranial and caudal extent of the tumor.

The surgical technique chosen should avoid or minimize displacement and manipulation of the spinal cord while ensuring tumor exposure, specifically the dural attachment. Several measures can be taken to achieve this goal, including sectioning of the dentate ligament. Removal can be carefully performed once the exposure has been completed, dura opened, and arachnoid plane identified.

Grossly intraspinal meningiomas are firm lesions with a distinct fibrous capsule which regularly have

a distinct dural attachment (**Fig. 4**). Once the capsule is identified and opened sharply, internal debulking is performed with bipolar electrocautery, suction, ultrasonic surgical aspirator, microscissors, or a laser.[6] As the tumor is reduced in size, it is gently mobilized away from the neural elements toward the dural attachment. This step is difficult in lesions with ventral extension or a ventral attachment. Once the dural attachment is addressed, the decision must be made to resect any remaining dura that appears diseased or is involving tumor. In some meningiomas, the attachment may be quite diffuse, and complete removal is not achievable.

As noted above, the Simpson classification is used to describe and define the extent of resection for spinal meningiomas,[25] even though it was initially validated in intracranial lesions. For intraspinal meningiomas, especially those in the anterior and lateral corridors, the dural attachment of spinal meningiomas is often cauterized rather than removed because of the difficulty in repairing dural defects in these corridors. An alternative strategy is to separate the dura into its inner and outer leaflets to allow resection of the tumor from the inner leaflet and closure of the outer leaflet primarily. In any case, Simpson grade I–III resection can achieve symptom resolution and is associated with low recurrence rates in atypical spinal meningiomas.[46] After tumor removal, the dural opening is closed in a watertight fashion, either by using a dural patch or primarily (**Fig. 5**).

Although surgery is the primary treatment for intraspinal meningiomas, lesions in the anterior corridor, en plaque meningiomas, recurrent tumors with scarring, and meningiomas with calcification are encumbered by potential barriers to complete resection.[6,14–16,22] Surgical resection of tumors with these characteristics requires careful planning and counseling. Considerations include cerebrospinal fluid (CSF) diversion, postoperative adjuvant therapy, and close imaging surveillance.

Neurophysiologic Monitoring

Neurophysiologic monitoring is a surgical adjunct that aims to minimize the potential of neurological deficits during surgery. These modalities can provide the surgical team with information with respect to extent of tissue manipulation and resection and the potential of functional preservation.[14]

The two most frequently used techniques—transcranial motor evoked potential (Tc-MEP) and somatosensory evoked potentials (SSEPs) monitoring—have both been approved for use by the US Food and Drug Administration.[47] Depending on the location of the meningioma, additional

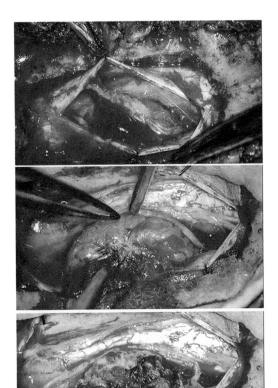

Fig. 4. Intraoperative photographs after dural opening identifying the spinal meningioma, which grossly appears purple in appearance with evidence of a firm capsule and definitive plane between the dura and tumor.

methods of monitoring as an adjunct include spontaneous and stimulated electromyography, direct spinal cord stimulation, and reflex monitoring.[48]

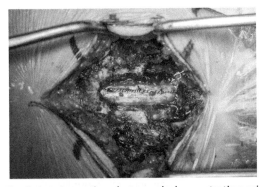

Fig. 5. Intraoperative photograph demonstrating primary dural closure following spinal meningioma resection with a running 4-0 Nurolon suture. Closure should be performed in a watertight fashion to prevent cerebrospinal fluid leak.

Tc-MEPs are widely available.[49,50] The modality works by the application of a high-voltage stimulus to electrodes on the scalp, which in turn activates the motor pathways to elicit a motor contraction (muscle MEP) or nerve action potential (D-wave) that is recorded and can provide information about the integrity of the motor tracts during resection.[48] Tc-MEP is most helpful for tumors situated anteriorly or anterolaterally and those compressing the corticospinal tract,[14] but it is commonly used in conjunction with SSEP for spinal tumors, regardless of location.

SSEP functions by providing a stimulus to peripheral nerves. In the upper extremity, the stimulus travels from the median or ulnar nerve to the spinal cord and brachial plexus, where the Erb's point potential is generated, which then travels to the dorsal column nuclei, yielding the N13 potential. The fibers then pass via the medial lemniscus to reach the thalamus, where a part of the N20 potential is generated. Then after arriving at the primary sensory cortex, the N20 and P22 potentials are generated.[48] In the lower extremity from the posterior tibial nerve at the foot is the most typical site used, but alternate sites include the peroneal nerve at the fibular head or the tibial nerve in the popliteal fossa. In the lower extremity, the SSEP travels past the popliteal fossa, generating a popliteal potential, before reaching the lumbosacral plexus. As the impulses enter the cauda equina, N21, a lumbar potential, is generated. SSEP monitoring is most useful for lesions situated posteriorly or posterolaterally and those that are compressing the dorsal columns,[14] but SSEP and MEP are often used in conjunction for intraspinal neoplasms, regardless of location.

Surgical Complications

Complications related to surgical resection of intraspinal meningiomas are also related to the extent of neural compression present on presentation and the resultant manipulation of these structures during resection. The mortality rate for surgical treatment of spinal meningiomas ranges from 0% to 3%[51]; most commonly, the cause of death is unrelated to the intraspinal meningioma. With the need for a large dural opening and subsequent repair, there is a 0%–4% risk of CSF leak.[7] Additional perioperative complications can include

- Pulmonary embolism
- Hematoma (either subdural or epidural)
- Pneumonia—hospital or community acquired
- Myocardial infarction
- Deep venous thrombosis
- Urinary tract infection
- Surgical site infection

Patients should be monitored for delayed spinal deformity, specifically postlaminectomy kyphosis.

FUNCTIONAL AND NEUROLOGICAL OUTCOME

Overall, patients who undergo surgery for intraspinal meningiomas have good functional and neurological outcomes. The Frankel scale is used to provide common language[52] for grading spinal injury and disability in this setting.

Sandalcioglu and colleagues[9] demonstrated that 96% of patients who underwent surgery for intraspinal meningiomas reported an improvement or at least unchanged neurological function. Functional improvement can occur in up to 95% of cases, with neurological decline occurring in fewer than 10%.[6,13–16,22] Even patients who present with significant neurological dysfunction can experience a full recovery.[16,22] Transient worsening may occur and can be a result of surgical manipulation or edema within the neural structures.[6,15,22] Sandalcioglu and colleagues[9] demonstrated that patient age in the range of 76–80 years and tumors that were completely calcified were risk factors for deterioration; in the same study, there was no association between dural attachment, tumor extension, or resection grade and neurological deterioration.

Health-Related Quality-of-Life Outcomes

Health-related quality-of-life (HRQoL) characteristics are globally defined as the aspects of the quality of life that are most affected by ill health; assessment of these is frequently used to quantify the self-perceived health status. In a study of 84 patients treated surgically for spinal meningiomas, Pettersson-Segerlind and colleagues[53] found no difference in HRQoL over a mean follow-up of 8.7 years after surgery when compared with a control population; furthermore, all patients who were working before the surgery returned to work after the surgery, with the majority doing so within 3 months.

SPINAL MENINGIOMA RECURRENCE

Intraspinal meningiomas are deemed less aggressive than their intracranial counterparts in light of demonstrating a significantly lower proliferative activity, a decreased density of macrophage infiltrates, and an increased time to tumor progression.[54] As with any neoplasm, recurrence is a concern; however, the rate of recurrence for intraspinal meningiomas is low, ranging from 1.3% to 6.4%.[6,13–16] The slow rate of growth and presentation in the later years are also factors that

contribute to the low rate of recurrence.[7] Patients with recurrence tend to have en plaque lesions with some infiltration or have undergone partial resection.[22]

Unlike intracranial meningiomas, excision of the dural attachment for intraspinal meningiomas is not associated with recurrence.[6,13,14,22] Cohen-Gadol and colleagues[32] reported higher recurrence rates in patients older than 50 years because of a higher number of cervical spine lesions, extension of tumors into the extradural space, and en plaque growth, all of which have been associated with challenging initial resection and presenting barriers to complete removal.

PHARMACOLOGIC TREATMENT OPTIONS

Medical management has been reported for meningiomas. Hydroxyurea, interferon-alpha 2B, and octreotide have all been used to treat refractory, high-grade intracranial meningiomas.[55] For intracranial meningiomas, cytotoxic agents, hormonal agents, immunomodulators, and growth factor–specific targets are theorized to play roles moving forward for management.[56] Such information about potential medical management is lacking for intraspinal meningiomas, but it is hoped that the growing molecular biomarker and genetic evidence will provide information for targeted therapy. Nevertheless, for patients with neurological symptoms caused by spinal meningiomas, it is likely that surgical removal will remain the most effective method of treatment to improve neurological function.

ADJUVANT RADIOTHERAPY AND RADIOSURGERY

Radiotherapy can be used in the settings of subtotal resection or recurrent lesions,[47] but its role has not been fully identified.[13,15] Radiotherapy can be considered for grade III spinal meningiomas or grade II spinal meningiomas after recurrence or subtotal resection.[45,57] Conversely, there is evidence that WHO grade II histology intraspinal meningiomas may not require adjuvant radiotherapy after surgery, and instead gross-total resection without adjuvant radiotherapy may provide adequate short-term tumor control.[46]

Radiotherapy can also be considered as an alternative primary treatment when surgery is too risky because of the lesion location or patient-level comorbid conditions,[13,15,16] but treatment in these settings is based on radiologic findings rather than histopathology. Gerszten and colleagues[58] demonstrated this in 10 intraspinal meningiomas and other benign spinal tumors;

however, this is not a common management strategy.[59] Management with initial radiation may ultimately result in the need for surgery if there is neurological decline. This treatment method should be reserved for patients who cannot tolerate surgery or present with recurrent tumors without neural element compression that are not surgical candidates.

SUMMARY

Meningiomas are the most common spinal tumors encountered in adults and can often be treated successfully with surgical resection alone. Pathological evaluation is necessary, however, because higher-grade lesions may require adjuvant therapy. Radiation therapy may be used as an adjuvant for subtotal resections of higher-grade lesions (WHO grade II or III). In the future, individualized molecular and genetic information may help tailor treatments and provide potential medical targets for nonsurgical care.

CLINICS CARE POINTS

- Spinal meningiomas are benign tumors that account for about 8% of all meningiomas and 25%–30% of all spinal canal tumors.
- Patient presentation can be variable and is highly dependent on lesion location and the degree of spinal cord compression.
- The main treatment is surgical excision, including the dural attachment when possible, while minimizing neurological dysfunction.
- Radiation therapy can be used for more aggressive pathological lesions (WHO grade II or III) or those that are unresectable because of unacceptable neurological morbidity.
- Emerging molecular and genetic targets may represent adjuvant treatment options for both surgical and nonsurgical treatment.

DISCLOSURE

The authors have nothing to disclose.

Video 1. Case example of a 65-year-old woman who presented with 6 months of progressive weakness with associated bowel and bladder incontinence. Imaging demonstrated a T1-T2 intradural, extramedullary lesion consistent with a spinal cord meningioma. She underwent a T1-T2 laminoplasty for resection. Note the meningioma

is located ventrolateral to the spinal cord. Once the dura was opened, sharp dissection was used to develop a plane between the tumor and normal spinal cord structures. The tumor was then systematically coagulated using bipolar electrocautery, microscissors, and the surgical ultrasonic aspirator. Once the meningioma was freed from its attachment to the spinal cord, it was rolled toward its dural attachment and removed. The dura was coagulated to remove additional tumor cells. At the conclusion of the resection, the dura was primarily repaired using a running 4-0 Nurolon suture.

REFERENCES

1. Ostrom QT, Patil N, Cioffi G, et al. CBTRUS statistical report: primary brain and other central nervous system tumors diagnosed in the United States in 2013-2017. Neuro Oncol 2020;22(12 Suppl 2):iv1–96.
2. Champeaux C, Weller J, Katsahian S. Epidemiology of meningiomas. A nationwide study of surgically treated tumours on French medico-administrative data. Cancer Epidemiol 2019;58:63–70.
3. Westwick HJ, Shamji MF. Effects of sex on the incidence and prognosis of spinal meningiomas: a surveillance, epidemiology, and end results study. J Neurosurg Spine 2015;23(3):368–73.
4. Ostrom QT, Gittleman H, Liao P, et al. CBTRUS statistical report: primary brain and central nervous system tumors diagnosed in the United States in 2007-2011. Neuro Oncol 2014;16(Suppl 4):iv1–63.
5. Albanese V, Platania N. Spinal intradural extramedullary tumors. Personal experience. J Neurosurg Sci 2002;46(1):18–24. Available at: https://www.ncbi.nlm.nih.gov/pubmed/12118219. Published 2002/07/16.
6. Solero CL, Fornari M, Giombini S, et al. Spinal meningiomas: review of 174 operated cases. Neurosurgery 1989;25(2):153–60. Available at: https://www.ncbi.nlm.nih.gov/pubmed/2671779. Published 1989/08/01.
7. Gottfried ON, Gluf W, Quinones-Hinojosa A, et al. Spinal meningiomas: surgical management and outcome. Neurosurg Focus 2003;14(6):e2.
8. Parisi J, Mena H. Nonglial tumors. In: Nelson J, Parisi J, Schochet S Jr, editors. Principles and practice of neuropathology. St Louis: Mosby; 1993. p. 203–66.
9. Sandalcioglu IE, Hunold A, Muller O, et al. Spinal meningiomas: critical review of 131 surgically treated patients. Eur Spine J 2008;17(8):1035–41.
10. Setzer M, Vatter H, Marquardt G, et al. Management of spinal meningiomas: surgical results and a review of the literature. Neurosurg Focus 2007;23(4):E14.

11. Maiuri F, De Caro ML, de Divitiis O, et al. Spinal meningiomas: age-related features. Clin Neurol Neurosurg 2011;113(1):34–8.

12. Schaller B. Spinal meningioma: relationship between histological subtypes and surgical outcome? J Neuro Oncol 2005;75(2):157–61.

13. Gezen F, Kahraman S, Canakci Z, et al. Review of 36 cases of spinal cord meningioma. Spine (Phila Pa 1976) 2000;25(6):727–31.

14. King AT, Sharr MM, Gullan RW, et al. Spinal meningiomas: a 20-year review. Br J Neurosurg 1998;12(6): 521–6.

15. Roux FX, Nataf F, Pinaudeau M, et al. Intraspinal meningiomas: review of 54 cases with discussion of poor prognosis factors and modern therapeutic management. Surg Neurol 1996;46(5):458–63 [discussion: 463-464].

16. Levy WJ Jr. Bay J, Dohn D. Spinal cord meningioma. J Neurosurg 1982;57(6):804–12.

17. McCormick PC, Torres R, Post KD, et al. Intramedullary ependymoma of the spinal cord. J Neurosurg 1990;72(4):523–32.

18. Jecko V, Weller J, Houston D, et al. Epidemiology and survival after spinal meningioma surgery: a nationwide population-based study. Asian Spine J 2022. https://doi.org/10.31616/asj.2021.0213.

19. Champeaux C, Wilson E, Brandner S, et al. World Health Organization grade III meningiomas. A retrospective study for outcome and prognostic factors assessment. Br J Neurosurg 2015;29(5): 693–8.

20. Champeaux C, Houston D, Dunn L. Atypical meningioma. A study on recurrence and disease-specific survival. Neurochirurgie 2017;63(4):273–81.

21. Champeaux C, Dunn L. World Health Organization Grade II Meningioma: A 10-year retrospective study for recurrence and prognostic factor assessment. World Neurosurg 2016;89:180–6.

22. Klekamp J, Samii M. Surgical results for spinal meningiomas. Surg Neurol 1999;52(6):552–62.

23. Namer IJ, Pamir MN, Benli K, et al. Spinal meningiomas. Neurochirurgia 1987;30(1):11–5.

24. Peker S, Cerci A, Ozgen S, et al. Spinal meningiomas: evaluation of 41 patients. J Neurosurg Sci 2005;49(1):7–11. Available at: https://www.ncbi.nlm.nih.gov/pubmed/15990713. Published 2005/07/02.

25. Simpson D. The recurrence of intracranial meningiomas after surgical treatment. J Neurol Neurosurg Psychiatr 1957;20(1):22–39.

26. Arslantas A, Artan S, Oner U, et al. Detection of chromosomal imbalances in spinal meningiomas by comparative genomic hybridization. Neurol Med -Chir 2003;43(1):12–8 [discussion: 19].

27. Sayagues JM, Tabernero MD, Maillo A, et al. Microarray-based analysis of spinal versus intracranial meningiomas: different clinical, biological, and genetic characteristics associated with distinct patterns of gene expression. J Neuropathol Exp Neurol 2006;65(5):445–54.

28. Ketter R, Henn W, Niedermayer I, et al. Predictive value of progression-associated chromosomal aberrations for the prognosis of meningiomas: a retrospective study of 198 cases. J Neurosurg 2001; 95(4):601–7.

29. Barresi V, Alafaci C, Caffo M, et al. Clinicopathological characteristics, hormone receptor status and matrix metallo-proteinase-9 (MMP-9) immunohistochemical expression in spinal meningiomas. Pathol Res Pract 2012;208(6):350–5.

30. Smith MJ, O'Sullivan J, Bhaskar SS, et al. Loss-of-function mutations in SMARCE1 cause an inherited disorder of multiple spinal meningiomas. Nat Genet 2013;45(3):295–8.

31. Pham MH, Zada G, Mosich GM, et al. Molecular genetics of meningiomas: a systematic review of the current literature and potential basis for future treatment paradigms. Neurosurg Focus 2011;30(5):E7.

32. Cohen-Gadol AA, Zikel OM, Koch CA, et al. Spinal meningiomas in patients younger than 50 years of age: a 21-year experience. J Neurosurg 2003;98(3 Suppl):258–63.

33. Weber C, Gulati S, Jakola AS, et al. Incidence rates and surgery of primary intraspinal tumors in the era of modern neuroimaging: a national population-based study. Spine (Phila Pa 1976) 2014;39(16): E967–73.

34. Corell A, Cerbach C, Hoefling N, et al. Spinal cord compression in relation to clinical symptoms in patients with spinal meningiomas. Clin Neurol Neurosurg 2021;211:107018.

35. Tredway TL, Santiago P, Hrubes MR, et al. Minimally invasive resection of intradural-extramedullary spinal neoplasms. Neurosurgery 2006;58(1 Suppl): ONS52–8.

36. Binning MJ, Schmidt MH. Percutaneous placement of radiopaque markers at the pedicle of interest for preoperative localization of thoracic spine level. Spine (Phila Pa 1976) 2010;35(19):1821–5.

37. Amin B, Abdulhak M. Lateral extracavitary approach. In: Baaj A, Mummaneni P, Uribe J A, et al, editors. Handbook of spine surgery. New York: Thieme; 2012. p. 290–5.

38. Misra SN, Morgan HW. Avoidance of structural pitfalls in spinal meningioma resection. Neurosurg Focus 2003;14(6):e1.

39. Herman JM, Sonntag VK. Cervical corpectomy and plate fixation for postlaminectomy kyphosis. J Neurosurg 1994;80(6):963–70.

40. Inoue A, Ikata T, Katoh S. Spinal deformity following surgery for spinal cord tumors and tumorous lesions: analysis based on an assessment of the spinal functional curve. Spinal Cord 1996;34(9):536–42.

41. Papagelopoulos PJ, Peterson HA, Ebersold MJ, et al. Spinal column deformity and instability after

lumbar or thoracolumbar laminectomy for intraspinal tumors in children and young adults. Spine (Phila Pa 1976) 1997;22(4):442–51.

42. Oxland TR, Lin RM, Panjabi MM. Three-dimensional mechanical properties of the thoracolumbar junction. J Orthop Res 1992;10(4):573–80.

43. Schlenk RP, Kowalski RJ, Benzel EC. Biomechanics of spinal deformity. Neurosurg Focus 2003;14(1):e2.

44. Wiggins GC, Mirza S, Bellabarba C, et al. Perioperative complications with costotransversectomy and anterior approaches to thoracic and thoracolumbar tumors. Neurosurg Focus 2001;11(6):e4.

45. Mimatsu K, Kawakami N, Kato F, et al. Intraoperative ultrasonography of extramedullary spinal tumours. Neuroradiology 1992;34(5):440–3.

46. Sun SQ, Cai C, Ravindra VM, et al. Simpson Grade I-III resection of spinal atypical (World Health Organization Grade II) Meningiomas is associated with symptom resolution and low recurrence. Neurosurgery 2015;76(6):739–46.

47. Ravindra VM, Schmidt MH. Management of spinal meningiomas. Neurosurg Clin N Am 2016;27(2): 195–205.

48. Stecker MM. A review of intraoperative monitoring for spinal surgery. Surg Neurol Int 2012;3(Suppl 3): S174–87.

49. Burke D, Hicks R, Stephen J, et al. Assessment of corticospinal and somatosensory conduction simultaneously during scoliosis surgery. Electroencephalogr Clin Neurophysiol 1992;85(6):388–96.

50. Kalkman CJ, Drummond JC, Kennelly NA, et al. Intraoperative monitoring of tibialis anterior muscle motor evoked responses to transcranial electrical stimulation during partial neuromuscular blockade. Anesth Analg 1992;75(4):584–9.

51. Kwee LE, Harhangi BS, Ponne GA, et al. Spinal meningiomas: Treatment outcome and long-term follow-up. Clin Neurol Neurosurg 2020;198:106238.

52. Frankel HL, Hancock DO, Hyslop G, et al. The value of postural reduction in the initial management of closed injuries of the spine with paraplegia and tetraplegia. I. Paraplegia 1969;7(3):179–92.

53. Pettersson-Segerlind J, von Vogelsang AC, Fletcher-Sandersjoo A, et al. Health-related quality of life and return to work after surgery for spinal meningioma: a population-based cohort study. Cancers 2021; 13(24):6371.

54. Wach J, Lampmann T, Guresir A, et al. Proliferative potential, and inflammatory tumor microenvironment in meningioma correlate with neurological function at presentation and anatomical location-from convexity to skull base and spine. Cancers 2022;14(4):1033.

55. Sherman WJ, Raizer JJ. Medical management of meningiomas. CNS Oncol 2013;2(2):161–70.

56. Moazzam AA, Wagle N, Zada G. Recent developments in chemotherapy for meningiomas: a review. Neurosurg Focus 2013;35(6):E18.

57. Sun SQ, Cai C, Murphy RK, et al. Management of atypical cranial meningiomas, part 2: predictors of progression and the role of adjuvant radiation after subtotal resection. Neurosurgery 2014;75(4): 356–63 [discussion: 363].

58. Gerszten PC, Chen S, Quader M, et al. Radiosurgery for benign tumors of the spine using the Synergy S with cone-beam computed tomography image guidance. J Neurosurg 2012;117(Suppl): 197–202.

59. Gerszten PC, Quader M, Novotny J Jr, et al. Radiosurgery for benign tumors of the spine: clinical experience and current trends. Technol Cancer Res Treat 2012;11(2):133–9.

Management of Atypical and Anaplastic Meningiomas

Dominique Higgins, MD, PhD[a], Ashish H. Shah, MD[b], Ricardo J. Komotar, MD[b],*, Michael E. Ivan, MD, MBS[b]

KEYWORDS

- Malignant meningioma • Atypical meningioma • Anaplastic meningioma • Radiation therapy
- Chemotherapy • Recurrence

KEY POINTS

- The overall incidence of atypical and anaplastic meningiomas is low; however, these tumors remain aggressive and difficult to control.
- Despite aggressive treatment of malignant meningiomas the average reported 5-year survival rates are in the range of 30%–60%.
- Obtaining a gross total resection via surgery remains the best first-line treatment for overall survival; however, in most patients adjuvant radiotherapy is also recommended.
- Predictors of overall survival are tumor size, age, location, histopathologic findings, and more recently methylation and mutation status.
- New insights into the biologic basis of meningioma growth have identified several exciting targeted therapeutic interventions that have shown promise to improving the current pharmacologic treatment options.

INTRODUCTION

Although meningiomas are generally thought of as benign lesions, a small proportion displays more aggressive behavior. Although difficult to assess their incidence, recent data support that 1.5% of all meningiomas are not benign.[1] These aggressive meningiomas can arise either de novo or progress from lower grade tumors as evident by recurrence.[2] In fact, approximately 20% to 35% of benign meningiomas tumors recur as atypical (World Health Organization [WHO] grade II), and 1% to 3% as anaplastic (WHO grade III). Although benign meningiomas have a low risk of recurrence of approximately 10%, atypical and anaplastic meningiomas are characteristically more aggressive in nature, and are associated with higher recurrence risks of 29% to 52% and 50% to 94%, respectively.[3,4] Unlike benign meningiomas, which seem to be linked to estrogen levels and are more common in women, atypical and anaplastic meningiomas are more common among men. They also seem to have a greater predilection for the cerebral convexities. With each update to the WHO grading, the definition of atypical and anaplastic meningiomas has evolved, and with it the percentage of tumors meeting diagnostic criteria has increased.[5]

Surgery remains a mainstay of treatment of meningiomas that have either grown from prior imaging or those that produce symptoms. Typically, neurosurgeons aim for Simpson grade 1 resection (gross total resection [GTR] with excision of the dural tail and overlying invaded cranium). If a GTR is not attainable, clinicians may opt for a subtotal resection (STR) and adjuvant radiotherapy (RT). The decision to use adjuvant RT is based on the extent of resection and the histopathologic tumor characteristics, and is generally added in cases of atypical and anaplastic meningiomas.[3,6] Unfortunately, when patients fail to respond to this standard initial therapy, current treatment

[a] Department of Neurosurgery, University of North Carolina; [b] Department of Neurosurgery, University of Miami, University of Miami Brain Tumor Initiative
* Corresponding author. 1095 Northwest 14th Terrrace, Miami, FL 33136, USA.
E-mail address: RKomotar@med.miami.edu

Neurosurg Clin N Am 34 (2023) 437–446
https://doi.org/10.1016/j.nec.2023.02.011

options are extremely limited and the morbidity and mortality among these patients increase significantly because of neurologic deterioration secondary to aggressive growth, compression of neural structures by the tumor, and peritumoral edema.

Aided by rapid advances in biotechnology, understanding of meningiomas at the molecular level has grown vastly in recent years, in particular with regard to the tumor genetic alterations and methylation changes. With this, interest in targeted therapies has emerged in an effort to treat aggressive meningiomas, which have failed traditional therapy. Results of many of these studies have been sobering, but drugs, such as everolimus and bevacizumab, have shown some promise. Several clinical trials are ongoing, and it is hoped will soon add to the armamentarium against this resilient disease.

PATIENT EVALUATION OVERVIEW

Atypical and anaplastic meningiomas present clinically similarly to their benign counterparts, and there are few clues to their more aggressive nature before tissue is obtained. Common symptoms include headaches, seizures, and focal neurologic deficits related to the location of the tumor. Paralleling the increasing use of diagnostic imaging, many tumors are also diagnosed incidentally.

Estrogen does not seem to play a role in the pathogenesis of high-grade meningiomas as it does in benign meningiomas. In fact, opposite to benign meningiomas, which have a much high incidence in females, atypical and anaplastic meningiomas have a two-fold increase in males.[7] The one factor consistently associated with atypical and anaplastic meningiomas is ionizing radiation, especially in younger patients. There are several reports of patients who received cranial irradiation for various tumors and later went on to develop high-grade radiation-induced meningiomas.[8]

To date, there are no reliable radiologic indicators of malignancy in meningiomas. Several features on MRI, including increased peritumoral edema, heterogeneous appearance, hyperintensity on diffusion weighted imaging, and characteristic fluid-attenuated inversion recovery appearance of the brain-meningioma interface have been found to have some predictive value, but all these features also are seen in benign meningiomas (**Fig. 1**).[8,9] Magnetic resonance spectroscopy has been used in small studies, showing increased lipid and lactate peaks in nonbenign meningiomas, but more work is needed to validate this and to assess what the role of this method might be in clinical practice.[10] PET imaging, and in particular DOTATE-PET, which is based on somatostatin analogues, has also been

shown to have utility in diagnosing recurrent meningiomas and is increasingly being used as a therapeutic guide.[11]

Location of the tumor has been shown to correlate to a patient's chance of recurrence and atypia. One group has identified that a non–skull base location increased the risk for grade II/III pathology by two-fold.[7] Additionally, skull base locations were associated with longer progression-free survival in atypical meningiomas. However, many of the transcriptional markers found associated with the various meningioma subtypes have correlated with location without negative prognostication.[12]

Although Cushing recognized the malignant potential of meningiomas in the 1930s, no uniform grading system gained widespread acceptance until the year 2000. In the 1990s, the Mayo Clinic group proposed a set of criteria for atypical and anaplastic meningiomas based on analysis of their large series, which demonstrated that in the absence of frank anaplasia, brain invasion was a highly significant predictor of recurrence risk, even in otherwise histologically benign-appearing tumors.[13] This prompted the inclusion of brain invasion as one of the criteria for atypical meningiomas, and significantly increased the number of tumors now classified as such. Based on these findings, WHO adopted the 2007 uniform grading criteria for atypical and anaplastic meningiomas, summarized in **Table 1**.[14] Analysis of our series of patients between 2000 and 2007 with this criteria showed that histochemical profiles of atypical and anaplastic meningiomas were similar to WHO grade I meningiomas. These markers included EMA and vimentin positivity and negative or weak staining for S-100 protein. Histologically, anaplasia seemed to be the most significant risk factor for early mortality. In the previously mentioned Mayo Clinic series, median survival for frankly anaplastic meningiomas was only 1.5 years. Among tumors with brain invasion but without anaplasia, median survival was 14.9 years with otherwise benign morphology and 10.4 years with atypical morphology. This difference did not reach statistical significance. Several reports have also found high MIB-1 labeling index to correlate with recurrence,[15] although the Mayo group initially concluded that MIB-1 labeling was mainly useful for grading in borderline cases. Also helpful in predicting tumor recurrence and overall survival in patients with atypical and anaplastic meningiomas is the Ki-67 proliferative index.[16]

Another predictor of survival and recurrence for patients with aggressive meningiomas is age. The CTBRUS data suggest that age has one of the

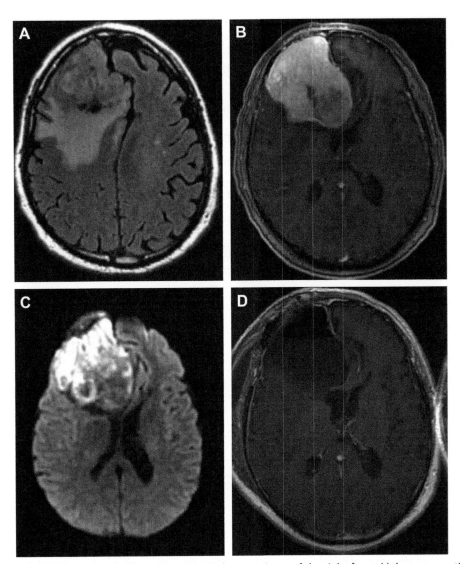

Fig. 1. Axial MRI findings of a patient with an atypical meningioma of the right frontal lobe preoperatively and postoperatively. (*A*) MRI T2 fast spin echo fluid-attenuated inversion recovery demonstrating significant peritumoral edema. (*B*) Diffusion sequence with significant hyperintensity commonly seen in higher grade meningiomas. (*C*) T1 fast spoiled gradient echo with contrast demonstrating the irregular outline of the meningioma and heterogeneous enhancement, consistent with higher grade meningioma. (*D*) Postoperative MRI, T1 sequence with contrast after gross total resection.

biggest effects on survival after diagnosis with malignant meningiomas with a 10-year survival of 84.4% for age 24 to 44 and 33.5% if greater than 75.[1] Larger tumor size on presentation also predicts poor survival mostly because of the tumor ability to encompass neurovascular structures.[17] Overall treatment of anaplastic meningiomas remains poor, with the average reported 5-year survival rates in the range of 30% to 60%.[18]

The WHO CNS5 grading criteria released in 2021 has continued to build on these findings, with an emphasis on molecular markers associated with atypical and anaplastic.[12] The criteria

for atypical meningiomas have remained largely unchanged with histologic subtypes of chordoid and clear cell being associated with grade 2, in addition to the presence of brain invasion (see **Table 1**). Clear cell subtypes were found to be highly associated with *SMARCE1* mutations as determined by loss of nuclear expression on immunostaining, and decreased transcriptional expression.[5,12,19] Anaplastic meningiomas, however, are no longer classified based on histology alone (papillary and rhabdoid). Meningiomas with mutations in the *TERT* promoter or homozygous deletions in *CDKN2A/B* are automatically

Table 1
WHO CNS5 classification for atypical and anaplastic meningiomas

Atypical meningioma	• 4–19 mitotic figures/10 high power fields OR
	• Brain invasion OR
	• Predominant choroid or clear cell morphology
	• Three of the following histologic features:
	  ○ Increased cellularity
	  ○ Small cells with high nuclear/cytoplasmic ratio
	  ○ Large and prominent nucleoli
	  ○ Patternless or sheetlike growth
	  ○ Foci of "spontaneous" or geographic necrosis

Anaplastic meningioma	• Excessive mitotic activity (>20 mitoses per 10 high power fields) OR • Focal or diffuse loss of meningothelial differentiation at the light microscopic level resulting in sarcoma, carcinoma, or melanoma-like appearance OR • TERT promoter mutation or CDKN2A/B deletion • Papillary or rhabdoid morphology no longer required

classified as grade 3, even in the absence of histologic criteria. Mutations in BAP1 is associated with rhabdoid subtype but does not automatically trigger an anaplastic subtype diagnosis. Future iterations of meningioma classification will likely take into account more broad molecular changes, such as methylation and chromosomal loss. Integrated grading systems have been proposed that take into account these factors.[20] For example, Nassiri and colleagues[20] have defined four molecular subtypes (immunogenic, benign NF2 wildtype, hypermetabolic, and proliferative) based on DNA, RNA, and methylome analyses that correlated with clinical outcomes.

SURGICAL TREATMENT OPTIONS

Surgery is the main treatment of all types of meningiomas, allowing definitive histopathologic diagnosis and possible cure. The goals and technique of surgery in atypical and anaplastic meningiomas are essentially the same as for benign meningiomas. Whenever safely possible, the lesion is completely excised with a margin of healthy dura around it, or a Simpson grade I excision. Any involved bone should be drilled out. Atypical and anaplastic meningiomas often adhere to underlying cortex, making complete resection more challenging. Extent of resection seems to be the most important modifiable predictor of long-term outcome, with several studies showing clear benefit to GTR.[21]

Meningiomas in general are often highly vascular. Resection of large tumors with evidence of hypervascularity on preoperative imaging can therefore sometimes be facilitated with embolization, especially when it is believed that the tumor's blood supply cannot be controlled early in surgery. This is usually accomplished using liquid embolic agents, such as Onyx, but other methods and agents have been used. However, embolization carries its own set of risks, from endovascular manipulation of the cerebral vasculature, and from inadvertent occlusion of healthy branches by stray embolic agent. It is therefore important to keep in mind that embolization is only worthwhile if it is believed that the combined risk of embolization and resection of the embolization is less than up-front resection of the tumor.[22]

Like benign meningiomas, atypical and anaplastic meningiomas can usually be resected with low risk of serious complications.[23] However, the morbidity and mortality are significantly lower when meningioma surgery is performed in a high-volume center while maintaining a maximal safe resection philosophy.[24] In a recent series of 45 atypical meningiomas, operated on a total of 62 times including reoperations, postoperative complications were reported in eight cases.[15] Only one of those complications was related to a reoperation. There were a total of five wound infections, one postoperative hematoma, one deep venous thrombosis, and one case of cerebrospinal fluid rhinorrhea.[15] The specific risk of venous thromboembolic complications was studied in a recent large series of meningiomas, 20% of which were either atypical or anaplastic. They reported venous thromboembolic events in 7% of patients, and identified weight and postoperative immobilization as the main risk factors. Histologic grade did not have an effect on the incidence of thromboembolic complications.[25]

Perioperative anticonvulsants are routinely used at many centers because of the potentially devastating effects that seizures can have in the postoperative period. However, in a meta-analysis comprising 19 studies and 698 patients with meningiomas (most of which were benign), routine use of anticonvulsants in meningioma did not prove beneficial for prevention of early and late postoperative seizures.[26] However, in patients who present with seizures preoperatively or develop seizures during the follow-up period, long-term antiepileptic treatment is usually required. At our institution, we use levetiracetam as the first-line treatment, and arrange for follow-up with an epileptologist for long-term care.

BRACHYTHERAPY

Implantation of radioactive seeds has been attempted in patients with recurrent atypical and anaplastic meningiomas. In one study, median survival of 8 years after implantation was achieved.[27] However, 27% of patients developed wound breakdown necessitating surgical intervention, and another 27% developed radiation necrosis, requiring reoperation in half. Despite this, brachytherapy offers a treatment option in tumors when radiosurgery is not an option.

RADIOTHERAPY TREATMENT OPTIONS

The decision to use radiation for atypical meningiomas remains controversial, because clear guidelines on the use of adjuvant treatments do not exist. Primarily, the decision to radiate these patients is largely governed by the extent of resection of the tumor. For patients who have STR or biopsy, adjuvant radiation treatment provides an improved progression-free survival as indicated by several studies.[28–34] Generally, the use of adjuvant fractionated external bean radiation or stereotactic radiosurgery after STR for atypical and anaplastic meningiomas is accepted in the neurosurgical community because of the high recurrence rate after surgery alone (grade IC recommendation).[14] Current guidelines of the National Comprehensive Cancer Network recommend GTR alone for accessible tumors with adjuvant RT reserved for incomplete resections or recurrences for atypical and WHO grade I meningiomas.[35] However, because of the increased risk for disease relapse in atypical meningiomas in up to 30% of cases even after GTR, the management paradigm for these lesions recently has been contented.[32]

Treatment with RT after GTR for atypical meningiomas has been associated with improved local control at 5 years. In a recent systematic review by our group, 5-year local control was improved 11% for patients in the GTR plus RT group compared with the GTR group ($P = 0.057$).[36]

Additionally, the recurrence rates were also significantly improved from 34% to 15% with the use of adjuvant RT ($P = 0.005$). Nevertheless, there was no improvement in overall survival for patients who received adjuvant RT and salvage RT after recurrence. **Table 2** demonstrates local recurrence rates for atypical meningiomas treated with GTR and GTR plus RT.[36] Typically, radiation treatment for external beam RT is dosed at 54 to 60 Gy fractionated over 6 weeks, albeit, stereotactic radiosurgery can also be efficacious depending on the size and location of the lesion.

A recent study evaluating RT in anaplastic meningiomas recommended RT after all surgical resections.[37] In this group 63 patients underwent surgery and then radiation. The 2-, 5-, and 10-year overall survival was 82%, 61%, and 40%, respectively, and the progression-free survival was 80%, 57%, and 40%. Of the nearly 50% of patients that recurred, there was a significant survival benefit to repeat surgery. These data must be re-examined in the context of updated grading criteria.

PHARMACOLOGIC TREATMENT OPTIONS

For treatment of refractory atypical and anaplastic meningiomas with aggressive pathologic features, occasionally pharmacologic treatment is necessary. Several clinical trials investigating the benefit of immunotherapeutic and hormonal agents have been performed with minimal benefit.[3] As a result of failed previous chemotherapeutic agents including hydroxyurea, a search for targeted therapies has ensued.[38–40] Several types of meningiomas have been found to have a high expression for certain molecular targets including platelet-derived growth factor, epidermal growth factor, vascular endothelial growth factor, insulin-like growth factor, and transforming growth factor-β.[3,41] Although clinical trials investigating epidermal growth factor receptor and platelet-

Table 2 Recurrence rates for atypical meningiomas treated initially with GTR or GTR plus RT			
	GTR (%)	**GTR plus RT (%)**	***P* Value**
Recurrence	33.7	15.0	0.005
1-y local control	90.1	97	0.09
5-y local control	55.1	67.7	0.057
Overall survival	89.7	89.4	0.95

derived growth factor receptor have been unfruitful, other targets, such as vascular endothelial growth factor, have demonstrated some early promise.[42–45] In a recent review by our group, the use of bevacizumab for treatment-refractory meningiomas resulted in a progression-free survival of 18 months (n = 44) based on a systematic review of three separate patient groups. Dosing for bevacizumab varies between 5 and 10 mg/kg intravenous/treatment.

Hormone influences on meningioma growth have been well documented during periods of hormonal excess.[46,47] The correlation between immunohistochemistry for endocrine markers (progesterone and estrogen) and tumor progression has resulted in a search for hormonal pharmacotherapy. Estrogen modulators have had little efficacy for meningiomas, however, secondary to their low expression rate. In a recent study of treatment-refractory meningiomas, tamoxifen only demonstrated minimal responses in 3 of 19 patients.[48] Progesterone receptors, however, seems to be more abundant on cell surfaces of meningiomas; therefore, a search for potential inhibitors ensued. Early studies using mifepristone (RU486), an antiprogesterone agent, has demonstrated some early promising results with radiographic regression in approximately 30% of patients.[49,50] Nevertheless, larger studies by the Southwest Oncology Group failed to demonstrate any significant benefit of RU486 for treatment-refractory meningiomas with nearly 90% disease progression despite treatment.[51] Growth hormone receptors also are nearly universal in meningiomas; therefore, potential growth hormone antagonists may be able to inhibit tumor growth through insulinlike growth factor-1 modulation. Some partial treatment effects have been demonstrated after treatment with somatostatin or similar hormonal therapeutics.[51]

TREATMENT RESISTANCE/COMPLICATIONS

For patients with disease progression or residual disease that receive radiation, clinicians must monitor for treatment effect by evaluating for potential pseudoprogression or radiation necrosis. Posttreatment changes after radiation may occur for meningiomas depending on treatment type and time after radiation. Tumor swelling and suspected pseudoprogression in radiated meningiomas typically responds to corticosteroids within the first 6 months. Lesional progression 6 months after RT raises suspicion for radiation necrosis or true tumor progression. Patients with lesions suspicious for tumor progression or radiation necrosis should be serially monitored for radiographic changes or worsening symptoms. Patients who

develop surgery- and radiation-refractory meningiomas continue to be difficult to treat. For recurrence WHO II/III meningiomas the progression-free survival at 6 month is only 29% and the treatment algorithm becomes more complex.[52] Repeat surgery for resection remains as the best option in patients who can tolerate such an intervention. An improved benefit was noted if the patient underwent a near total resection after tumor recurrence followed by RT versus a GTR followed by RT.[37] This suggests that attempts to achieve a GTR in these recurrent invasive meningiomas may sometimes be associated with increased risk. Therefore the best philosophy is maximal safe resection on the first and second surgery. **Fig. 2** provides suggested treatment/management protocols for atypical/anaplastic meningiomas.

EXPERIMENTAL THERAPIES

Certain patients with treatment-refractory meningiomas may be candidates for experimental therapies. Laser interstitial therapy relies on stereotactic navigation-based catheter systems to induce thermal ablation of the target lesion. For patients with multiple meningiomas, poor surgical candidates, or surgically inaccessible lesions, laser interstitial therapy may be an alternative option to cytoreductive surgery. Additional nonpharmacologic options including alternating electrical fields may also be a theoretical option for highly aggressive meningiomas. Alternating electric fields helps interfere with cellular mitoses during anaphase through an external device that is calibrated to the tumor location. Another potential treatment of recurrent aggressive meningiomas with a high proliferative index is tumor treating fields and was recently investigated as a clinical trial with results pending (NCT01892397). Finally, additional tumor markers continue to be isolated, such as increased PD-L1, which have been shown to increase expression on aggressive meningiomas and could lead to the use of checkpoint inhibitors.[53] These molecular targets are currently being investigated as potential targets for clinical trials.

EVALUATION OF OUTCOME AND LONG-TERM RECOMMENDATIONS

After treatment of atypical/anaplastic meningiomas, patients must be monitored closely for disease progression. The RANO criteria helps monitor treatment response by measuring maximal cross-sectional area and clinical outcome after treatment. Responses are categorized as complete (disappearance of lesion), partial (>50% radiographic change), stable (<50% radiographic response), or

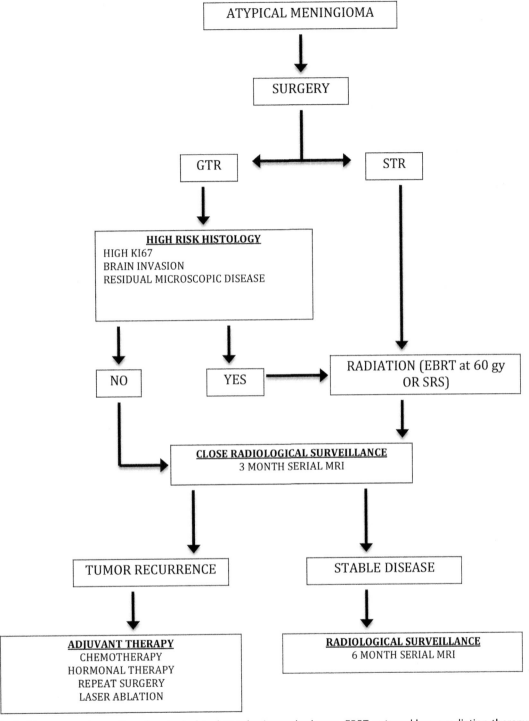

Fig. 2. Management paradigm for atypical and anaplastic meningiomas. EBRT, external beam radiation therapy; SRS, stereotactic radiosurgery. (*Data from* Ref.[14])

progression (increase in size by 25%). Although the RANO criteria applies definitely to gliomas, using the RANO criteria for meningioma response may also help guide management protocols. Careful monitoring every 3 to 6 months with serial contrast-enhanced MRIs may be necessary depending on pathology, proliferative index, extent of resection, and symptomatology.

SUMMARY

Atypical and anaplastic meningiomas represent a small percentage of meningiomas, with evolving classification criteria. These higher grade tumors, however, remain aggressive and difficult to treat. Surgery remains the initial treatment option for atypical and anaplastic meningiomas but recurrences remain more complex and difficult to treat. Advances in surgical, radiation, and medical therapies over the past few decades have resulted in a modest improvement in overall survival yet more prospective data are needed. Increasing numbers and variety of promising clinical trials have resulted from development of new minimally invasive techniques and innovative-targeted therapeutic interventions based on continuous research of these aggressive meningiomas.

CLINICS CARE POINTS

- Gross Total Resection of atypical and malignant meningiomas is highly recommended for first line management of these tumors when feasible and safe.
- Adjuvant Radiotherapy or Radiosurgery is recommended for all subtotally resected Grade II and all Grade III meningiomas.
- Adjuvant Radiotherapy for atypical meningiomas after Gross Total Resection is under investigation in multicenter clinical trials.

FUNDING

A.H. Shah's research is funded by the Florida Center for Brain Tumor Research and the Neurosurgery Research Education Fund.

REFERENCES

1. Ostrom QT, Gittleman H, Liao P, et al. CBTRUS statistical report: primary brain and central nervous system tumors diagnosed in the United States in 2007-2011. Neuro Oncol 2014;16(Suppl 4):1–63.
2. Moliterno J, Cope WP, Vartanian ED, et al. Survival in patients treated for anaplastic meningioma. J Neurosurg 2015;123(1):23–30.
3. Wen PY, Quant E, Drappatz J, et al. Medical therapies for meningiomas. J Neurooncol 2010;99(3):365–78.
4. Louis DN, Ohgaki H, Wiestler OD, et al. The 2007 WHO classification of tumours of the central nervous system. Acta Neuropathol 2007;114(2):97–109.
5. Chen WC, Perlow HK, Choudhury A, et al. Radiotherapy for meningiomas. J Neuro Oncol 2022;160(2):505–15.
6. Alexiou GA, Gogou P, Markoula S, et al. Management of meningiomas. Clin Neurol Neurosurg 2010;112(3):177–82.
7. Kane AJ, Sughrue ME, Rutkowski MJ, et al. Anatomic location is a risk factor for atypical and malignant meningiomas. Cancer 2011;117(6):1272–8.
8. Modha A, Gutin PH. Diagnosis and treatment of atypical and anaplastic meningiomas: a review. Neurosurgery 2005;57(3):538–50 [discussion: 38-50].
9. Enokizono M, Morikawa M, Matsuo T, et al. The rim pattern of meningioma on 3D FLAIR imaging: correlation with tumor-brain adhesion and histological grading. Magn Reson Med Sci 2014;13(4):251–60.
10. Yue Q, Isobe T, Shibata Y, et al. New observations concerning the interpretation of magnetic resonance spectroscopy of meningioma. Eur Radiol 2008;18(12):2901–11.
11. Prasad RN, Perlow HK, Bovi J, et al. 68)Ga-DOTATATE PET: the future of meningioma treatment. Int J Radiat Oncol Biol Phys 2022;113(4):868–71.
12. Horbinski C, Berger T, Packer RJ, et al. Clinical implications of the 2021 edition of the WHO classification of central nervous system tumours. Nat Rev Neurol 2022;18(9):515–29.
13. Perry A, Scheithauer BW, Stafford SL, et al. "Malignancy" in meningiomas: a clinicopathologic study of 116 patients, with grading implications. Cancer 1999;85(9):2046–56.
14. Sun SQ, Hawasli AH, Huang J, et al. An evidence-based treatment algorithm for the management of WHO grade II and III meningiomas. Neurosurg Focus 2015;38(3):E3.
15. Klinger DR, Flores BC, Lewis JJ, et al. Atypical meningiomas: recurrence, reoperation, and radiotherapy. World Neurosurgery 2015;84(3):839–45.
16. Bruna J, Brell M, Ferrer I, et al. Ki-67 proliferative index predicts clinical outcome in patients with atypical or anaplastic meningioma. Neuropathology 2007;27(2):114–20.
17. Ferraro DJ, Funk RK, Blackett JW, et al. A retrospective analysis of survival and prognostic factors after stereotactic radiosurgery for aggressive meningiomas. Radiat Oncol 2014;9:38.
18. Hanft S, Canoll P, Bruce JN. A review of malignant meningiomas: diagnosis, characteristics, and treatment. J Neuroncol 2010;99(3):433–43.
19. St Pierre R, Collings CK, Same Guerra DD, et al. SMARCE1 deficiency generates a targetable mSWI/SNF dependency in clear cell meningioma. Nat Genet 2022;54(6):861–73.

20. Nassiri F, Liu J, Patil V, et al. A clinically applicable integrative molecular classification of meningiomas. Nature 2021;597(7874):119–25.

21. Zhu H, Xie Q, Zhou Y, et al. Analysis of prognostic factors and treatment of anaplastic meningioma in China. J Clin Neurosci 2015;22(4):690–5.

22. Ashour R, Aziz-Sultan A. Preoperative tumor embolization. Neurosurg Clin N Am 2014;25(3):607–17.

23. Sughrue ME, Rutkowski MJ, Shangari G, et al. Risk factors for the development of serious medical complications after resection of meningiomas. Clinical article. J Neurosurg 2011;114(3):697–704.

24. Curry WT, McDermott MW, Carter BS, et al. Craniotomy for meningioma in the United States between 1988 and 2000: decreasing rate of mortality and the effect of provider caseload. J Neurosurg 2005;102(6):977–86.

25. Hoefnagel D, Kwee LE, van Putten EH, et al. The incidence of postoperative thromboembolic complications following surgical resection of intracranial meningioma. A retrospective study of a large single center patient cohort. Clin Neurol Neurosurg 2014;123:150–4.

26. Komotar RJ, Raper DM, Starke RM, et al. Prophylactic antiepileptic drug therapy in patients undergoing supratentorial meningioma resection: a systematic analysis of efficacy. J Neurosurg 2011;115(3):483–90.

27. Ware ML, Larson DA, Sneed PK, et al. Surgical resection and permanent brachytherapy for recurrent atypical and malignant meningioma. Neurosurgery 2004;54(1):55–63 [discussion: 63-4].

28. Aizer AA, Arvold ND, Catalano P, et al. Adjuvant radiation therapy, local recurrence, and the need for salvage therapy in atypical meningioma. Neuro Oncol 2014;16(11):1547–53.

29. Lee KD, DePowell JJ, Air EL, et al. Atypical meningiomas: is postoperative radiotherapy indicated? Neurosurg Focus 2013;35(6):E15.

30. Hammouche S, Clark S, Wong AH, et al. Long-term survival analysis of atypical meningiomas: survival rates, prognostic factors, operative and radiotherapy treatment. Acta neurochirurgica 2014;156(8):1475–81.

31. Sun SQ, Cai C, Murphy RK, et al. Management of atypical cranial meningiomas, part 2: predictors of progression and the role of adjuvant radiation after subtotal resection. Neurosurgery 2014;75(4):356–63 [discussion: 63].

32. Mair R, Morris K, Scott I, et al. Radiotherapy for atypical meningiomas. J Neurosurg 2011;115(4):811–9.

33. Park HJ, Kang HC, Kim IH, et al. The role of adjuvant radiotherapy in atypical meningioma. J Neurooncol 2013;115(2):241–7.

34. Jo K, Park HJ, Nam DH, et al. Treatment of atypical meningioma. J Clin Neurosci 2010;17(11):1362–6.

35. Nabors LB, Ammirati M, Bierman PJ, et al. National Comprehensive Cancer Network. Central nervous system cancers. J Natl Compr Canc Netw 2013;11(9):1114–51.

36. Hasan S, Young M, Albert T, et al. The role of adjuvant radiotherapy after gross total resection of atypical meningiomas. World Neurosurgery 2015;83(5):808–15.

37. Sughrue ME, Sanai N, Shangari G, et al. Outcome and survival following primary and repeat surgery for World Health Organization grade III meningiomas. J Neurosurg 2010;113(2):202–9.

38. Schrell UM, Rittig MG, Anders M, et al. Hydroxyurea for treatment of unresectable and recurrent meningiomas. I. Inhibition of primary human meningioma cells in culture and in meningioma transplants by induction of the apoptotic pathway. J Neurosurg 1997;86(5):845–52.

39. Schrell UM, Rittig MG, Anders M, et al. Hydroxyurea for treatment of unresectable and recurrent meningiomas. II. Decrease in the size of meningiomas in patients treated with hydroxyurea. J Neurosurg 1997;86(5):840–4.

40. Loven D, Hardoff R, Sever ZB, et al. Non-resectable slow-growing meningiomas treated by hydroxyurea. J Neurooncol 2004;67(1–2):221–6.

41. Smith JS, Lal A, Harmon-Smith M, et al. Association between absence of epidermal growth factor receptor immunoreactivity and poor prognosis in patients with atypical meningioma. J Neurosurg 2007;106(6):1034–40.

42. Norden AD, Raizer JJ, Abrey LE, et al. Phase II trials of erlotinib or gefitinib in patients with recurrent meningioma. J Neurooncol 2010;96(2):211–7.

43. Wen PY, Yung WK, Lamborn KR, et al. Phase II study of imatinib mesylate for recurrent meningiomas (North American Brain Tumor Consortium study 01-08). Neuro Oncol 2009;11(6):853–60.

44. Provias J, Claffey K, delAguila L, et al. Meningiomas: role of vascular endothelial growth factor/vascular permeability factor in angiogenesis and peritumoral edema. Neurosurgery 1997;40(5):1016–26.

45. Kaley TJ, Wen P, Schiff D, et al. Phase II trial of sunitinib for recurrent and progressive atypical and anaplastic meningioma. Neuro Oncol 2015;17(1):116–21.

46. Wahab M, Al-Azzawi F. Meningioma and hormonal influences. Climacteric 2003;6(4):285–92.

47. Kanaan I, Jallu A, Kanaan H. Management strategy for meningioma in pregnancy: a clinical study. Skull Base 2003;13(4):197–203.

48. Goodwin JW, Crowley J, Eyre HJ, et al. A phase II evaluation of tamoxifen in unresectable or refractory meningiomas: a Southwest Oncology Group study. J Neurooncol 1993;15(1):75–7.

49. Grunberg SM, Weiss MH, Spitz IM, et al. Treatment of unresectable meningiomas with the antiprogesterone agent mifepristone. J Neurosurg 1991;74(6):861–6.

50. Lamberts SW, Tanghe HL, Avezaat CJ, et al. Mifepristone (RU 486) treatment of meningiomas.

Journal of neurology, neurosurgery, and psychiatry 1992;55(6):486–90.

51. Norden AD, Drappatz J, Wen PY. Targeted drug therapy for meningiomas. Neurosurg Focus 2007;23(4):E12.

52. Kaley T, Barani I, Chamberlain M, et al. Historical benchmarks for medical therapy trials in surgery- and radiation-refractory meningioma: a RANO review. Neuro Oncol 2014;16(6):829–40.

53. Du Z, Abedalthagafi M, Aizer AA, et al. Increased expression of the immune modulatory molecule PD-L1 (CD274) in anaplastic meningioma. Oncotarget 2015;6(7):4704–16.

Novel Systemic Approaches for the Management of Meningiomas
Immunotherapy and Targeted Therapies

Nazanin Ijad, BSc[a,1], Ashish Dahal, AB[a,1], Albert E. Kim, MD[a],
Hiroaki Wakimoto, MD, PhD[a,b], Tareq A. Juratli, MD[c,2],
Priscilla K. Brastianos, MD[a,d,2,*]

KEYWORDS

- Meningioma • Targeted therapy • Immunotherapy

KEY POINTS

- Significant advances have been made in the characterization of the tumor and immune microenvironment of meningiomas.
- The increased knowledge of the molecular underpinnings of meningioma has led to novel clinical trials of targeted therapies as well as immunotherapies for patients with recurrent or progressive meningiomas.
- Strategies that have shown promising efficacy in trials of patients with recurrent or progressive meningiomas include focal adhesion kinase inhibition, immune checkpoint blockade, and the combination of mammalian target of rapamycin inhibition and octreotide.

INTRODUCTION

Meningiomas, the most prevalent primary intracranial tumor (~35%),[1] arise from the arachnoid cap cells in the meninges, the membranes that surround the brain and the spinal cord. Patients develop neurological symptoms due to the inward growth trajectory of meningiomas, as they can cause pressure on the brain, which manifest in various neurologic symptoms such as headaches, visual disturbances, or seizures. Surgical resection is typically the first-line treatment of patients with symptomatic meningiomas. However, if the mass is not accessible by surgery, radiation therapy is the most common treatment. In cases with small asymptomatic tumors that do not demonstrate rapid growth, clinicians may opt to wait and monitor using serial MRI.

Most meningiomas have a benign natural history after surgical resection. However, a subset of patients with meningiomas experience a progressive course despite treatment, with aggressive regrowth resulting in high morbidity and mortality. The field has long sought effective predictors of meningioma recurrence and malignant transformation, as well as therapeutic targets to guide intensified treatment such as early radiation or systemic therapy. Recent studies, as described later, have shed light into some of these predictors and genetic drivers. Thus, novel and more targeted approaches are currently being tested in numerous clinical trials for

[a] Center for Cancer Research, Massachusetts General Hospital Cancer Center, Harvard Medical School, 55 Fruit Street, Yawkey 9E, Boston, MA 02114, USA; [b] Department of Neurosurgery, Translational Neuro-Oncology Laboratory, Massachusetts General Hospital Cancer Center, Harvard Medical School; [c] Department of Neurosurgery, Carl Gustav Carus University Hospital, TU Dresden, Germany; [d] Broad Institute of Harvard and MIT
[1] Contributed equally.
[2] Jointly co-supervised.
* Corresponding author.
E-mail address: pbrastianos@mgh.harvard.edu

Neurosurg Clin N Am 34 (2023) 447–454
https://doi.org/10.1016/j.nec.2023.02.012
1042-3680/23/

patients who have progressed after surgery and/or radiation.

In this review, the authors discuss relevant molecular drivers that have therapeutic implications and examine recent clinical trial data evaluating targeted therapies and immunotherapies.

NEW MOLECULARLY DRIVEN GRADING OF THE WORLD HEALTH ORGANIZATION CLASSIFICATION OF MENINGIOMAS

Over the last decade, comprehensive molecular studies have led to an improved understanding of the molecular and genetic alterations underlying meningioma development and disease progression. The challenge of previous World Health Organization (WHO) Classification of Tumors of the Central Nervous System[2] was that WHO grade does not always predict recurrence and prognosis for patients with meningiomas.[3] Although most of the treatments are focused on aggressive and malignant high-grade meningiomas, even a subset of low WHO grade meningiomas will develop recurrent tumors despite surgery.[4] This discrepancy between histological grading and the clinical course of meningiomas can be challenging for both clinicians and patients to navigate when deciding on different courses of treatment.[5]

Recent work has now identified novel recurrent somatic genomic alterations that occur more frequently in progressive meningiomas, including hotspot promoter mutations and rearrangements in telomerase reverse transcriptase (TERT), biallelic CDKN2A/B deletions, intragenic deletions in the X-linked dystrophin (DMD), TP53 mutations, and chromosome 1p loss.[3,6–11] Biallelic loss of CDKN2A or CDKN2B and TERT promoter mutations are now considered new criteria for grade 3 (malignant) meningiomas in the fifth edition of the WHO Classification of Tumors of the Central Nervous System.[2] Notably, these genomic alterations identify subsets of progressive meningiomas with poor outcome and can also occur in cases that do not qualify for WHO grade 3 based on histologic features alone.[3,11]

Genomics in Meningiomas

The identification of several molecular alterations in meningiomas has allowed the matching of molecular features of tumors to highly specific targeted therapeutics and thus clinical trials. In the 1990s, seminal studies demonstrated that NF2 is frequently inactivated in meningiomas.[12–14] More recently, actionable hotspot mutations in genes such as AKT1, SMO, and PIK3CA have been identified in a subset of meningiomas.[15–18] These findings hold therapeutic promise, as treatments targeting these specific mutations are currently in clinical use for other cancers. For example, AKT1 and PIK3CA are members of the phosphatidylinositol 3-kinase (PI3K) pathway, which is mutated in a number of other cancers,[19] and can be targeted with kinase inhibitors.[20–22] Indeed, Weller and colleagues[22] published a case report of a patient with a metastatic AKT1-mutant meningioma that had a durable response to the AKT inhibitor AZD5363. Similarly, SMO is a member of the Hedgehog signaling pathway, which is also aberrantly activated in other malignancies such as basal cell carcinoma[23] that are responsive to therapeutic agents targeting SMO.[9]

Furthermore, our improved understanding of meningiomas has recently identified a strong concordance between molecular status and tumor location, as evidenced by the most recent WHO classification of central nervous system tumors. Skull base meningiomas are characterized by mutations including AKT1, SMO, PIK3CA, KLF4, POLR2A, and TRAF7, whereas convexity meningiomas are induced by NF2 or SMARCB1 alterations.[15,16] Similarly, in spinal meningiomas, 2 predominant molecular subgroups were identified: AKT1-mutant meningiomas that originate in the cervical spine ventrally to the spinal cord and NF2-mutant meningiomas that originate most frequently in the thoracic spine dorsally to the spinal cord.[24]

A further important issue in meningiomas that has not received enough attention in the past is tumor heterogeneity. Recent data from our group and others suggest the existence of regionally distinct genomic, epigenomic, transcriptomic, or histologic features within individual patients with meningioma emphasizing inter- and intratumor heterogeneity.[6,25–27] The underlying mechanisms of intratumor heterogeneity in meningiomas have not been thoroughly investigated, in part due to the fact that most analyses thus far have been limited to single tissue samples from individual patients or locally recurrent tumors.

Single-cell analysis serves as a basis for the understanding of heterogeneity in tumors and has proved to be a useful tool to understand how meningiomas develop. Recently, 2 seminal studies reported on single-cell analyses in meningioma. Nassiri and colleagues performed single-nuclear RNA sequencing on 8 tumors across all molecular groups and WHO grades. Most of the cells were neoplastic, whereas 14% were immune cells (T cells and macrophages), 10% were fibroblasts, and 6% were endothelial cells. Further clustering of their neoplastic cells showed that most samples harbored one dominant cluster and a less common second cluster of neoplastic cells with no substantial variability between cells when looking at copy-number profiles of the cells.[28] Also, Wang and colleagues[29] performed single-cell analysis on 3 meningioma samples and demonstrated heterogeneity regarding copy-number variation and gene expression profiles among patient-specific meningioma tumor cell populations. Because only a few cases were characterized in both studies, additional work is required, as tumor heterogeneity can have significant consequences for therapeutic response.

In addition, DNA methylation of meningiomas has become a tool that provides additional diagnostic and prognostic insight.[30] Distinct DNA methylation groups have been found to have different outcomes and therapeutic vulnerabilities.[26,31] Among those, Merlin (encoded by NF2)-intact meningiomas have the best clinical outcomes in contrast to their immune-enriched and hypermitotic counterparts that were associated with a worse clinical outcome. The latter fact was partly explained by loss of merlin or inactivation of FOXM1 causing resistance to cytotoxic therapies and elevated cell proliferation.[26]

EXPLORING THE TUMOR MICROENVIRONMENT AND POTENTIAL VULNERABILITIES

In addition to our improved knowledge of molecular vulnerabilities in meningiomas, significant progress has been made to understand the tumor immune microenvironment (TIME) in meningiomas, which can be exploited for therapeutic benefit. Studies have shown that a subset of high-grade meningiomas possess a high mutation burden (tumor mutational burden), suggesting a greater neoantigen profile and potential susceptibility to immune checkpoint inhibitors (ICI).[32] Regulation of T-cell activity is particularly important within the meningioma microenvironment for enabling tumor growth. One well-defined mechanism is through the immune checkpoint regulatory pathway to downregulate T-cell activity via programmed cell death protein 1 (PD-1)/programmed cell death ligand 1 (PD-L1). Cancers take advantage of this mechanism by upregulating PD-L1 and gain the ability to turn off T cells themselves.[33] Meningiomas were found to express PD-L1 on their cell surface, and higher grade meningiomas expressed significantly higher levels of PD-L1 compared with low-grade tumors, further elucidating the role of immunosuppression in promoting tumor progression.[34] The innate immune system is also important for regulating tumoral activity. Macrophage state and infiltration of the tumor are strong predictors of clinical outcome.

The infiltration of antiinflammatory M2 state macrophages has been correlated with higher rates of recurrence for high-grade meningiomas.[35] Nearly 80% of tumor-associated macrophages in high-grade meningiomas were found to be in the M2 state, and low ratios of M1:M2 cells correlated with increased tumor size and higher WHO grade.[36] Meanwhile, high M1:M2 cell ratios have been associated with higher rates of progression-free survival in other solid tumors.[37]

Recent trials, as described later in this review, have evaluated the efficacy of agents modulating the immune system in patients with meningioma.

Clinical Trials for Progressive or Recurrent Meningiomas

Many systemic treatments have historically had limited efficacy for patients with high-grade meningioma.[38,39] Surgery for recurrent meningioma is associated with higher complication rates and subsequently with increased risk of morbidity,[34-] whereas reirradiation can be associated with significant toxicities.[40] Based on the large body of work aimed at understanding the molecular pathogenesis of high-grade meningiomas and their TIME, a myriad of clinical trials for both targeted therapies and immunotherapies are ongoing. **Tables 1** and **2** delineate some major recently published and ongoing trials.

Targeted Therapy Clinical Trials

Genomically driven approaches are being investigated for the treatment of recurrent or progressive meningioma. For example, Alliance A071401 is a national genomically guided National Cancer Institute (NCI) ongoing trial with multiple drug arms targeting specific genetic alterations for patients with recurrent or progressive meningiomas. The arms of the study include an SMO inhibitor for *SMO*-mutated tumors, an AKT inhibitor for *PIK3CA* or *AKT*-mutated tumors, a cyclin-dependent kinase (CDK) inhibitor for CDK pathway–altered meningiomas, and an focal adhesion kinase (FAK) inhibitor for *NF2*-mutated tumors. FAK inhibition was selected for this trial because of its synthetic lethal relationship with the protein product of *NF2*, merlin.[52] The FAK inhibitor (GSK2256098) arm of the study has now completed accrual and met the primary endpoint of the study.[53] For this study, 36 patients with *NF2* mutations were enrolled, 12 grade 1 and 24 grade 2/3 patients. Among all patients, there was 1 patient with a partial response and 24 patients with stable disease. In grade 1 patients, the observed PFS-6 rate was 83% and in grade 2/3 patients, the observed PFS-6 rate was 33%. GSK2256098 was also well tolerated, with

Table 1
Ongoing or recently completed targeted therapy trials for treating high-grade or progressive meningioma

	Targeted Therapy Trials			
Compound	Meningioma WHO Grades	Number of Patients	PFS-6	Reference
Completed Trials				
Everolimus + Octreotide	2 and 3	20	0.55	Graillon et al,[41] 2021
GSK2256098	1,2,3	24	0.33 (for grade 2–3 patients)	Brastianos et al,[42,53] 2022
Bevacizumab	1,2,3	50	0.73 (for grade 2–3 patients)	Kumthekar et al,[43] 2022
Sunitinib	2 and 3	36	0.42	Kaley et al,[44] 2015
Imatinib + Hydroxyurea	1,2,3	21	0.875 (grade 2) 0.462 (grade 3)	NCT00354913 [45]
Vatalanib	1,2,3	25	0.64 (grade 2) 0.375 (grade 3)	NCT00348790 [46]
Bevacizumab + Everolimus	1,2,3	17	N/A	NCT00972335 [47]
Imatinib	1,2,3	23	0.45	NCT00045734 [48]
Erlotinib	1,2,3	136	N/A	NCT00045110 [49]
AR-42	1,2,3	7	N/A	NCT02282917 [50]
Ongoing Trials				
Vistusertib	2,3	28	0.515	NCT03071874 [51]
Vismodegib, Capivasertib and Abemaciclib	1,2,3	124	N/A	NCT02523014 [42]

only 7 grade 3 adverse events and no grade 4 or 5 adverse events. Given these encouraging results, further study with FAK inhibition as a single agent and in combination with other agents need to be further studied.[53] The other arms of this national precision medicine trial are ongoing.

Given activation of the PI3K/mTOR pathway and expression of SSTR2A receptors in meningiomas, Graillon and colleagues[41] examined the combinatory use of everolimus, an mTOR inhibitor, alongside the somatostatin agonist octreotide to treat patients with aggressive recurrent meningiomas. Both drugs had demonstrated strong antimeningioma properties in previous studies,[54,55] and combinatorial therapy proved successful for inhibiting growth of aggressive meningioma in vitro.[41] The phase II clinical trial enrolled 20 patients with WHO grade 1 to 3 tumors and found a PFS-6 of 55%. A greater than 50% decrease in tumor growth rate was observed at 3 months in 78% of patients, and the median growth rate of tumors decreased from 16.6% to 0.02%. These results highlight a promising efficacy signal of the everolimus/octreotide combination therapy for treating a subset of high-grade meningioma, which should be further explored in future studies.

Another promising approach for meningiomas includes targeting angiogenesis. Preclinical studies have highlighted vascular endothelial growth factor (VEGF) to have a major role in meningioma tumor growth and angiogenesis.[56] A phase II trial of the VEGF-ligand binding monoclonal antibody bevacizumab yielded a PFS-6 of 74% for WHO grade 2/3 meningioma patients who received treatment, highlighting a major improvement in outcome for patients with high-grade tumor.[43] Sunitinib, a small molecule tyrosine kinase inhibitor, is known to have cytostatic, antimigration, and antiangiogenesis activity for meningioma cells due to its targeting primarily of VEGF receptor and platelet-derived growth factor receptor signaling.[44] This drug's efficacy was tested in a trial involving 36 patients with atypical/anaplastic meningioma, and a PFS-6 of 42% was reported.[48] Two patients experienced a significant decrease in their tumor size. However, one major concern involved treatment toxicity, with 7 patients experiencing major complications such as hemorrhage. Overall, however, sunitinib demonstrated antitumoral benefits that warrant further study.

Antibody-mediated targeting of meningioma surface proteins is also an area of investigation for

Table 2
Ongoing or recently completed immunotherapy trials for treating high-grade meningioma

	Immunotherapy Trials			
Compound	Meningioma WHO Grade	Number of Patients	PFS-6	Reference
Completed Trials				
Pembrolizumab	2 and 3	25	0.48	Brastianos et al,[58] 2022
Nivolumab	2 and 3	25	0.424	Bi et al,[64] 2022
Ongoing Trials				
Nivolumab + ipilimumab + radiosurgery	2 and 3	Ongoing	Ongoing	Huang et al,[65] 2022 NCT03604978
Avelumab + proton radiation	2 and 3	Ongoing	Ongoing	NCT03267836

meningiomas. One highly upregulated protein, β1 integrin, was identified as a driver of cellular growth and invasion in high-grade meningiomas.[57,58] Targeting of the β1 integrin proved promising in several cancer histologies for controlling cell growth.[59] In a xenograft mouse study using the anti-β1 monoclonal antibody OS2966 and high-grade patient-derived meningioma cell lines, inhibition of β1 stopped proliferation of meningioma and increased overall survival rates in mice.[58] As studies have demonstrated the safety and tolerability of OS2966 in humans,[60] this is an agent worth exploring for patients with meningiomas.

Evaluating Immunotherapeutic Strategies and Trials for High-Grade Meningiomas

Immunotherapeutic strategies are an exciting avenue of investigation for patients with meningiomas. Our understanding of the meningioma tumor microenvironment has enabled a wide range of promising therapeutic interventions. One set of clinically established immunotherapeutic agents are ICI, which work to disrupt the binding of checkpoint receptors such as PD-1 and CTLA-4 with their respective ligands and prevent tumoral immune escape.[61] This therapeutic strategy has quickly become standard of care for a wide range of solid tumors.[61] The PD-1 inhibitor pembrolizumab was investigated in a phase II study of patients with recurrent/progressive grade 2/3 meningiomas.[62] The trial met primary endpoint and yielded a PFS-6 rate of 48% in a cohort of 25 patients, with 6 individuals experiencing a marked stabilization of their tumor's growth. One patient with metastatic high-grade meningioma had a PFS that lasted for nearly 20 months. Notably, pembrolizumab was very well tolerated in this patient population with 20% percent of

patients experiencing one or more treatment-related adverse events. However, another PD-1 inhibitor drug, nivolumab, was assessed in a trial involving 25 patients but did not meet primary endpoint.[63] Patients on the trial experienced a PFS-6 of 42.2%, less than the study's primary endpoint significance threshold of 51%. However, some patients did benefit, with 2 patients experiencing increased immune infiltration of the tumor while on the nivolumab trial. In a separate case study, a patient with MSH2-deficient meningioma and high tumor mutational burden experienced a strong response to nivolumab.[64] These findings underscore that nivolumab may still be a relevant agent for treating high-grade meningioma, although monotherapy may not be sufficient to yield adequate benefit. Alternatively, improved biomarkers of response are needed to identify the patients who will benefit. Noteworthy, in an ongoing trial, nivolumab was evaluated in combination with the anti-CTLA 4 drug ipilimumab and radiosurgery, demonstrating promising interim results, with a PFS-6 of 62%.[65]

In addition to PD-1 targeting, the inhibitory ligand PD-L1 can also serve as a target for meningioma treatment. Preclinical work has highlighted the potential of the anti-PD-L1 therapy avelumab in meningiomas,[66] and there is an ongoing clinical trial that aims to understand the effect that avelumab/proton radiation therapy has on patient outcomes after surgical resection (Trial: NCT03267836, ongoing).[61] If successful, this trial would offer more immunotherapy options to control treatment-refractory meningioma.

One potential breakthrough in meningioma immunotherapy involves CAR-T cell therapy, a method using genetically engineered T cells to target specific antigens.[67] CAR-T therapy has shown promise in a variety of cancer types, improving both patient outcomes and response to additional treatments.[68,69] A recent study in anaplastic meningioma demonstrated the feasibility of targeting the checkpoint molecule B7-H3 via chimeric T cells, as B7-H3 is highly expressed on the meningioma cell surface.[70] In a first-in-human study of B7-H3 CAR-T cells in a patient with recurrent anaplastic meningioma, administration of CAR-T therapy increased inflammatory cytokine signaling at the tumor site, whereas subsequent IHC analysis supported the antitumor effects of the CAR-T cells.[71] The patient also reported no off-tumor toxicity due to the CAR-T therapy, suggesting that this treatment approach should be further studied in future trials.

SUMMARY

In the last decade, significant advances have been made in understanding the molecular underpinnings of meningioma and its tumor-immune microenvironment. These exciting advances have led to novel clinical trials of targeted therapies as well as immunotherapies for patients with recurrent or progressive meningiomas. Many of these trials are already showing positive results in patients. However, more work is needed to improve outcomes for this patient population. Critically, translating knowledge of these molecular findings into actionable therapeutic strategies requires a better understanding of the underlying mechanisms, intratumor heterogeneity, and associated clinical factors that contribute to the unfavorable prognosis. More studies to characterize the drivers of response and resistance to these novel therapies are also urgently needed.

DISCLOSURES

Outside the scope of this work, P.K. Brastianos has consulted for Angiochem, Genentech-Roche, Lilly, Tesaro, ElevateBio, Pfizer, SK Life Sciences, Advice Connect Inspire, Axiom, Medscape, Kazia, MPM Capital, Sintetica, Voyager Therapeutics, and Dantari; received institutional grant/research support (to MGH) from Merck, BMS, Kinnate, Mirati, and Lilly and honoraria from Merck, Genentech-Roche, Pfizer, and Lilly.

REFERENCES

1. Ostrom QT, Price M, Neff C, et al. CBTRUS statistical report: primary brain and other central nervous system tumors diagnosed in the United States in 2015-2019. Neuro Oncol 2022;24:v1–95.
2. Louis DN, Perry A, Wesseling P, et al. The 2021 WHO classification of tumors of the central nervous system: a summary. Neuro Oncol 2021;23:1231–51.
3. Mirian C, Duun-Henriksen AK, Juratli T, et al. Poor prognosis associated with TERT gene alterations in meningioma is independent of the WHO classification: an individual patient data meta-analysis. J Neurol Neurosurg Psychiatr 2020;91:378–87.
4. Patel B, Desai R, Pugazenthi S, et al. Identification and management of aggressive meningiomas. Front Oncol 2022;12:851758.
5. Pettersson-Segerlind J, Orrego A, Lonn S, et al. Long-term 25-year follow-up of surgically treated parasagittal meningiomas. World Neurosurg 2011;76:564–71.
6. Juratli TA, Thiede C, Koerner MVA, et al. Intratumoral heterogeneity and TERT promoter mutations in progressive/higher-grade meningiomas. Oncotarget 2017;8:109228–37.
7. Juratli TA, Brastianos PK, Cahill DP. TERT Alterations in progressive treatment-resistant meningiomas. Neurosurgery 2018;65:66–8.
8. Juratli TA, McCabe D, Nayyar N, et al. DMD genomic deletions characterize a subset of progressive/higher-grade meningiomas with poor outcome. Acta Neuropathol 2018;136:779–92.
9. Williams EA, Santagata S, Wakimoto H, et al. Distinct genomic subclasses of high-grade/progressive meningiomas: NF2-associated, NF2-exclusive, and NF2-agnostic. Acta Neuropathol Commun 2020;8:171.
10. Goutagny S, Nault JC, Mallet M, et al. High incidence of activating TERT promoter mutations in meningiomas undergoing malignant progression. Brain Pathol 2014;24:184–9.
11. Guyot A, Duchesne M, Robert S, et al. Analysis of CDKN2A gene alterations in recurrent and non-recurrent meningioma. J Neuro Oncol 2019;145:449–59.
12. Lekanne Deprez RH, Bianchi AB, Groen NA, et al. Frequent NF2 gene transcript mutations in sporadic meningiomas and vestibular schwannomas. Am J Hum Genet 1994;54:1022–9.
13. Rouleau GA, Merel P, Lutchman M, et al. Alteration in a new gene encoding a putative membrane-organizing protein causes neuro-fibromatosis type 2. Nature 1993;363:515–21.
14. Ruttledge MH, Sarrazin J, Rangaratnam S, et al. Evidence for the complete inactivation of the NF2 gene in the majority of sporadic meningiomas. Nat Genet 1994;6:180–4.
15. Brastianos PK, Horowitz PM, Santagata S, et al. Genomic sequencing of meningiomas identifies oncogenic SMO and AKT1 mutations. Nat Genet 2013;45:285–9.
16. Clark VE, Erson-Omay EZ, Serin A, et al. Genomic analysis of non-NF2 meningiomas reveals mutations in TRAF7, KLF4, AKT1, and SMO. Science 2013;339:1077–80.

17. Abedalthagafi M, Bi WL, Aizer AA, et al. Oncogenic PI3K mutations are as common as AKT1 and SMO mutations in meningioma. Neuro Oncol 2016;18: 649–55.

18. Sahm F, Bissel J, Koelsche C, et al. AKT1E17K mutations cluster with meningothelial and transitional meningiomas and can be detected by SFRP1 immunohistochemistry. Acta Neuropathol 2013;126: 757–62.

19. Carpten JD, Faber AL, Horn C, et al. A transforming mutation in the pleckstrin homology domain of AKT1 in cancer. Nature 2007;448:439–44.

20. Spencer A, Yoon SS, Harrison SJ, et al. The novel AKT inhibitor afuresertib shows favorable safety, pharmacokinetics, and clinical activity in multiple myeloma. Blood 2014;124:2190–5.

21. Hyman DM, Smyth LM, Donoghue MTA, et al. AKT inhibition in solid tumors With AKT1 mutations. J Clin Oncol 2017;35:2251–9.

22. Weller M, Roth P, Sahm F, et al. Durable control of metastatic AKT1-mutant WHO grade 1 meningothelial meningioma by the AKT inhibitor, AZD5363. J Natl Cancer Inst 2017;109:1–4.

23. Hahn H, Wicking C, Zaphiropoulous PG, et al. Mutations of the human homolog of Drosophila patched in the nevoid basal cell carcinoma syndrome. Cell 1996;85:841–51.

24. Hua L, Alkhatib M, Podlesek D, et al. Two predominant molecular subtypes of spinal meningioma: thoracic NF2-mutant tumors strongly associated with female sex, and cervical AKT1-mutant tumors originating ventral to the spinal cord. Acta Neuropathol 2022;144:1053–5.

25. Magill ST, Vasudevan HN, Seo K, et al. Multiplatform genomic profiling and magnetic resonance imaging identify mechanisms underlying intratumor heterogeneity in meningioma. Nat Commun 2020;11:4803.

26. Choudhury A, Magill ST, Eaton CD, et al. Meningioma DNA methylation groups identify biological drivers and therapeutic vulnerabilities. Nat Genet 2022;54:649–59.

27. Juratli TA, Prilop I, Saalfeld FC, et al. Sporadic multiple meningiomas harbor distinct driver mutations. Acta Neuropathol Commun 2021;9:8.

28. Nassiri F, Liu J, Patil V, et al. A clinically applicable integrative molecular classification of meningiomas. Nature 2021;597:119–25.

29. Wang AZ, Bowman-Kirigin JA, Desai R, et al. Single-cell profiling of human dura and meningioma reveals cellular meningeal landscape and insights into meningioma immune response. Genome Med 2022;14:49.

30. Berghoff AS, Hielscher T, Ricken G, et al. Prognostic impact of genetic alterations and methylation classes in meningioma. Brain Pathol 2022;32:e12970.

31. Maas SLN, Stichel D, Hielscher T, et al. Integrated molecular-morphologic meningioma classification: a multicenter retrospective analysis, retrospectively and prospectively validated. J Clin Oncol 2021;39: 3839–52.

32. Nebot-Bral L, Brandao D, Verlingue L, et al. Hypermutated tumours in the era of immunotherapy: the paradigm of personalised medicine. Eur J Cancer 2017;84:290–303.

33. Han Y, Liu D, Li L. PD-1/PD-L1 pathway: current researches in cancer. Am J Cancer Res 2020;10: 727–42.

34. Varlotto J, Flickinger J, Pavelic MT, et al. Distinguishing grade I meningioma from higher grade meningiomas without biopsy. Oncotarget 2015;6:38421–8.

35. Presta I, Guadagno E, Di Vito A, et al. Innate immunity may play a role in growth and relapse of chordoid meningioma. Int J Immunopathol Pharmacol 2017;30:429–33.

36. Proctor DT, Huang J, Lama S, et al. Tumor-associated macrophage infiltration in meningioma. Neurooncol Adv 2019;1:vdz018.

37. Ma J, Liu L, Che G, et al. The M1 form of tumor-associated macrophages in non-small cell lung cancer is positively associated with survival time. BMC Cancer 2010;10:112.

38. Gupta S, Bi WL, Dunn IF. Medical management of meningioma in the era of precision medicine. Neurosurg Focus 2018;44:E3.

39. Nigim F, Wakimoto H, Kasper EM, et al. Emerging medical treatments for meningioma in the molecular era. Biomedicines 2018;6:86.

40. Toland A, Huntoon K, Dahiya SM. Meningioma: a pathology perspective. Neurosurgery 2021;89:11–21.

41. Graillon T, Sanson M, Campello C, et al. Everolimus and octreotide for patients with recurrent meningioma: results from the phase II CEVOREM trial. Clin Cancer Res 2020;26:552–7.

42. Brastianos PK, Twohy E, Gerstner ER, et al. Alliance A071401: phase II trial of FAK inhibition in meningiomas with somatic NF2 mutations. J Clin Oncol 2020;38:2502.

43. Kumthekar P, Grimm SA, Aleman RT, et al. A multi-institutional phase II trial of bevacizumab for recurrent and refractory meningioma. Neurooncol Adv 2022;4:vdac123.

44. Kaley TJ, Wen P, Schiff D, et al. Phase II trial of sunitinib for recurrent and progressive atypical and anaplastic meningioma. Neuro Oncol 2015;17: 116–21.

45. Reardon DA, Norden AD, Desjardins A, et al. Phase II study of Gleevec(R) plus hydroxyurea (HU) in adults with progressive or recurrent meningioma. J Neuro Oncol 2012;106:409–15.

46. Raizer JJ, Grimm SA, Rademaker A, et al. A phase II trial of PTK787/ZK 222584 in recurrent or progressive radiation and surgery refractory meningiomas. J Neuro Oncol 2014;117:93–101.

47. Shih KC, Chowdhary S, Rosenblatt P, et al. A phase II trial of bevacizumab and everolimus as treatment

for patients with refractory, progressive intracranial meningioma. J Neuro Oncol 2016;129:281–8.

48. Wen PY, Yung WK, Lamborn KR, et al. Phase II study of imatinib mesylate for recurrent meningiomas (North American Brain Tumor Consortium study 01-08). Neuro Oncol 2009;11:853–60.

49. Raizer JJ, Abrey LE, Lassman AB, et al. A phase I trial of erlotinib in patients with nonprogressive glioblastoma multiforme postradiation therapy, and recurrent malignant gliomas and meningiomas. Neuro Oncol 2010;12:87–94.

50. Welling DB, Collier KA, Burns SS, et al. Early phase clinical studies of AR-42, a histone deacetylase inhibitor, for neurofibromatosis type 2-associated vestibular schwannomas and meningiomas. Laryngoscope Investig Otolaryngol 2021;6:1008–19.

51. Plotkin SR, Kumthekar P, Wen PY, et al. Multi-center, single arm phase II study of the dual mTORC1/mTORC2 inhibitor vistusertib for patients with recurrent or progressive grade II-III meningiomas. J Clin Oncol 2021;39:2024.

52. Shapiro IM, Kolev VN, Vidal CM, et al. Merlin deficiency predicts FAK inhibitor sensitivity: a synthetic lethal relationship. Sci Transl Med 2014;6:237ra68.

53. Brastianos PK, Twohy E, Gerstner ER, et al. Alliance A071401: Phase II Trial of Focal Adhesion Kinase Inhibition in Meningiomas With Somatic NF2 Mutations. J Clin Oncol 2023;41:618–28.

54. Puchner MJA, Hans VH, Harati A, et al. Bevacizumab-induced regression of anaplastic meningioma. Ann Oncol 2010;21:2445–6.

55. Bertolini F, Pecchi A, Stefani A, et al. Everolimus effectively blocks pulmonary metastases from meningioma. Neuro Oncol 2015;17:1301–2.

56. Machein MR, Plate KH. VEGF in brain tumors. J Neuro Oncol 2000;50:109–20.

57. Figarella-Branger D, Roche PH, Daniel L, et al. Cell-adhesion molecules in human meningiomas: correlation with clinical and morphological data. Neuropathol Appl Neurobiol 1997;23:113–22.

58. Nigim F, Kiyokawa J, Gurtner A, et al. A monoclonal antibody against beta1 integrin inhibits proliferation and increases survival in an orthotopic model of high-grade meningioma. Target Oncol 2019;14:479–89.

59. Carbonell WS, DeLay M, Jahangiri A, et al. beta1 integrin targeting potentiates antiangiogenic therapy and inhibits the growth of bevacizumab-resistant glioblastoma. Cancer Res 2013;73:3145–54.

60. Nwagwu CD, Immidisetti AV, Bukanowska G, et al. Convection-enhanced delivery of a first-in-class anti-beta1 integrin antibody for the treatment of high-grade glioma utilizing real-time imaging. Pharmaceutics 2020;13:40.

61. Darvin P, Toor SM, Sasidharan Nair V, et al. Immune checkpoint inhibitors: recent progress and potential biomarkers. Exp Mol Med 2018;50:1–11.

62. Brastianos PK, Kim AE, Giobbie-Hurder A, et al. Phase 2 study of pembrolizumab in patients with recurrent and residual high-grade meningiomas. Nat Commun 2022;13:1325.

63. Bi WL, Nayak L, Meredith DM, et al. Activity of PD-1 blockade with nivolumab among patients with recurrent atypical/anaplastic meningioma: phase II trial results. Neuro Oncol 2022;24:101–13.

64. Dunn IF, Du Z, Touat M, et al. Mismatch repair deficiency in high-grade meningioma: a rare but recurrent event associated with dramatic immune activation and clinical response to PD-1 blockade. JCO Precis Oncol 2018;2018.

65. Huang J, Gao F, Shimony J, et al. The interim result of a phase I/II study of nivolumab with or without ipilimumab in combination with multi-fraction stereotactic radiosurgery for recurrent, high-grade, radiation-relapsed meningioma. J Clin Oncol 2022;40:2068.

66. Giles AJ, Hao S, Padget M, et al. Efficient ADCC killing of meningioma by avelumab and a high-affinity natural killer cell line, haNK. JCI Insight 2019;4:e130688.

67. Sterner RC, Sterner RM. CAR-T cell therapy: current limitations and potential strategies. Blood Cancer J 2021;11:69.

68. Garfall AL, Maus MV, Hwang WT, et al. Chimeric antigen receptor T Cells against CD19 for multiple myeloma. N Engl J Med 2015;373:1040–7.

69. Kantarjian H, Stein A, Gokbuget N, et al. Blinatumomab versus Chemotherapy for advanced acute lymphoblastic leukemia. N Engl J Med 2017;376:836–47.

70. Deng J, Ma M, Wang D, et al. Expression and clinical significance of immune checkpoint regulator B7-H3 (CD276) in human meningioma. World Neurosurg 2020;135:e12–8.

71. Tang X, Liu F, Liu Z, et al. Bioactivity and safety of B7-H3-targeted chimeric antigen receptor T cells against anaplastic meningioma. Clin Transl Immunology 2020;9:e1137.

Stereotactic Radiosurgery for Intracranial Meningiomas

Stylianos Pikis, MD[1], Georgios Mantziaris, MD, Chloe Dumot, MD, PhD[2],
Zhiyuan Xu, MD, Jason Sheehan, MD, PhD*

KEYWORDS

- Meningioma • Radiosurgery • Outcomes • Complications

KEY POINTS

- Intracranial meningiomas are extra-axial, well-demarcated tumors that often constitute ideal targets for stereotactic radiosurgery (SRS).
- Prescription doses of 12 to 16 Gy provide high and long-lasting control of WHO Grade I meningiomas with low complication rates. WHO Grade II and III intra-cranial meningiomas are treated with prescription doses greater than 16 Gy when feasible.
- SRS may be offered as an alternative to observation in patients with newly diagnosed asymptomatic meningiomas and should be recommended when growth is documented on follow-up neuroimaging.

INTRODUCTION

Meningiomas are thought to originate from the meningothelial cells of the arachnoid mater and are the most common primary brain tumor in adults. Histologically confirmed meningiomas occur with an incidence of 9.12/100,000 population and account for 39% of all primary brain tumors and 54.5% of all non-malignant brain tumors.[1] Risk factors for meningioma include age 65 years and older,[1] female gender,[1] African-American race,[1] history of exposure to head and neck ionizing radiation,[2] and certain genetic disorders such as neurofibromatosis II.[3] Intracranial meningiomas are the most commonly benign, WHO Grade I neoplasms. Atypical (ie, WHO Grade II) and anaplastic (ie, WHO Grade III meningiomas) are considered malignant lesions.

Management decisions should take into consideration tumor size, location, and, if present, severity of symptoms attributed to the meningioma. Observation is often chosen for small, asymptomatic meningiomas,[4] and maximum safe resection is frequently the treatment of choice for the majority of growing or symptomatic meningiomas.[5] Ionizing radiation delivered as single fraction stereotactic radiosurgery, as hypofractionated stereotactic radiosurgery in 2 to 5 fractions, and as fully fractionated stereotactic radiotherapy provides long-lasting control of WHO Grade I meningiomas as primary treatment, as adjuvant treatment following subtotal resection, and as salvage treatment at tumor recurrence.[6] Moreover, radiotherapy or radiosurgery is also indicated as adjuvant treatment for Grade II and III meningiomas and as salvage treatment at recurrence.

Stereotactic radiosurgery of intracranial lesions involves the administration of a single, ablative dose of ionizing radiation to an intracranial target. The rapid dose falloff outside the radiosurgical target allows for sparing of the surrounding normal tissue from the radiation adverse effects. Most meningiomas are well-circumscribed, slow

Department of Neurological Surgery, University of Virginia Health System, Charlottesville, VA 22908, USA
[1] Present address: Mpotsary 3, Egkomi 2415, Nicosia, Cyprus.
[2] Present address: 43 rue Thomas Blanchet, 69,008 Lyon, France.
* Corresponding author.
E-mail address: jsheehan@virginia.edu

Neurosurg Clin N Am 34 (2023) 455–462
https://doi.org/10.1016/j.nec.2023.02.010
1042-3680/23/© 2023 Elsevier Inc. All rights reserved.

growing, extra-axial lesions, therefore they often represent ideal targets for stereotactic radiosurgery (SRS). However, owing to the lack of randomized studies, the most appropriate patients, treatment parameters, and tumor characteristics for meningioma SRS are still uncertain.

STEREOTACTIC RADIOSURGERY FOR WHO GRADE I MENINGIOMAS
Indications for Radiosurgery

- Primary SRS is indicated for asymptomatic or minimally symptomatic intracranial meningiomas of less than 3 cm in diameter or less than 10 cc in volume, particularly when growth is documented on follow-up neuro-image, the surgical risk is high due to tumor location, in patients with contraindications to surgery, and in those who deny surgery.
- After sub-total resection of a WHO Grade I meningioma, as either adjuvant therapy or when growth of the residual is documented on follow-up.
- At small-to-moderate volume meningioma recurrence after gross total resection (GTR).
- Hypo-fractionated SRS can often be used for larger volume meningiomas, previously irradiated meningiomas, and ones situated next to radiation-sensitive critical structures.

Clinical Outcomes for Stereotactic Radiosurgery

SRS has been demonstrated as a safe alternative to Simpson Grade I surgical resection in patients with small and medium sized (<3 cm) meningiomas.[7] A European multi-center study evaluating 4565 patients with SRS-treated intracranial meningiomas, reported 5 and 10 year PFS rates of 95.2% and 88.5%, respectively. The permanent morbidity rate at last follow-up was 6.6% and was disabling (Grade 3) in 1.2%[8] (**Table 1**). A systematic review and meta-analysis by the International Stereotactic Radiosurgery Society included 27 studies with 3654 patients harboring 3750 benign, non-cavernous sinus meningiomas treated with SRS. The median patient age at SRS and follow-up period was 57 years and 60 months, respectively. The median tumor volume for single fraction SRS was 5.6 cc, and for hypo-fractionated SRS was 6.4 cc. The median margin dose for single fraction SRS was 14 Gy (range 11–17 Gy), and the most common regimen for hypofractionated SRS of meningiomas was 25 Gy in 5 fractions. Eight- to 10 year progression-free survival (PFS) rates were available in 10 of the included studies reporting on 1146 patients and ranged between 55% and

97% (median 85%). Neurologic deterioration rate ranged from 0% to 13.3%, and the reported radiation toxicity rate ranged from 2.5% to 34.6%.[9] In a systematic review of 49 retrospective studies, evaluating SRS for benign cavernous sinus meningiomas, Lee and colleagues reported 10 year PFS rate ranging from 69% to 97%. Preservation of neurologic function was noted in 80% to 100% of patients with long-term follow-up. Improvement of pre-SRS deficits was reported in 39% of patients 5 years after SRS and was more likely in patients who underwent primary SRS. Improved cavernous sinus meningioma control was associated with a single fraction margin dose greater than 14 Gy, medium to small sized meningioma, primary SRS, presence of cranial nerve deficits less than 12 months, female gender, younger age, and less conformal plans.[10]

Radiosurgical Technique and Treatment Parameters

Frame-based, single-session and mask-based hypo-fractionated radiosurgery procedures utilize thin slice (1 mm), 3D T2- and pre- and post-contrast enhanced, T1-weighted brain MRI and/or head computed tomography for treatment planning (**Fig. 1**). Hypo-fractionated, frameless SRS is usually performed for meningiomas larger than 3 cm in maximum diameter and for those tumors at close proximity to critical neurovascular structures. The prescription volume should include the entire tumor volume and often any nodular thickened part of the dura.

During single-session SRS, single fraction prescription doses of 12 to 15 Gy seem to provide adequate control of non-cavernous sinus meningiomas. A prescription dose of at least 14 Gy is advisable for single-session SRS (level III recommendation).[9] Single-session SRS using prescription doses of 11 to 16 Gy is associated with 5 year meningioma control rate equal to or greater than 90% (level III evidence).[11] Kolova and colleagues reported a higher SRS failure rate when using prescription doses of 12 Gy or less and a higher rate of SRS-induced edema when doses greater than 16 Gy are used.[12] Kondziolka and colleagues reported similar tumor control with prescription dose equal to or greater than 15 Gy versus less than 15 Gy.[13] In a study by Stafford and colleagues, prescription doses less than 16 Gy afforded similar local tumor control rate to prescription doses ≥ 16 Gy.[14] In hypo-fractionated SRS for meningioma, 25 Gy in 5 fractions is the most commonly preferred regimen. Higher doses are usually delivered for Grade II and III meningiomas.

Table 1
Selected studies including more than 200 patients on Radiosurgery for WHO Grade I meningiomas

Author/year	Setting	Patient Number	Median/Mean Tumor Volume (cm³)	Mean/Median Prescription Dose (Gy)	Mean/Median Follow-up (months)	10-y LC (%)	Complications (%)
Flickinger et al, 2003	Image defined	219	5	14	29	93.2	8.8
Kreil et al, 2005	Image defined (n = 101), Residual/recurrent (n = 99)	200	6.5	12	76	97	5.7
Feigl et al, 2007	Residual (n = 123) Image defined (n = 91)	214	6.46	13.6	24	N/R	6.7%
Kollova et al, 2007	Image defined (n = 259), Residual/recurrent (109)	368	4.4	12.55	60	90	10.2% temporary 5.7% permanent
Kondziolka et al,[34] 2008	Image defined (n = 536) Residual (n = 384)	920	7.4	14	48	87.2	7.7
Santacroce et al,[8] 2012	Residual/recurrent	3854	4.8	14	63	82	6.6
Pollock et al, 2012	Image defined (n = 252) Residual (n = 164)	416	7.3	16	60	89	11
Starke et al, 2012	Image defined (n = 109) Residual (n = 146)	255	5	14	78	79	10 neurologic deterioration
Kano et al, 2013	Image defined (n = 173) Residual (n = 99)	272 CSM	7.9	13	62	86	11
Sheehan et al, 2014	Image defined (n = 408) Residual (n = 355)	763	8.8	13.2	66.7	82	New/worsened endocrinopathy in 1.8%

(continued on next page)

Table 1
(continued)

Author/year	Setting	Patient Number	Median/Mean Tumor Volume (cm³)	Mean/Median Prescription Dose (Gy)	Mean/Median Follow-up (months)	10-y LC (%)	Complications (%)
Kondziolka et al, 2016	Image defined (n = 132) Residual (n = 136) Recurrent (n = 22)	290	5.5	15	56	87.7	17.9
Park et al,[33] 2019	Image defined (n = 120) Residual (n = 46) Recurrent (n = 34)	200 CSM	7.5	13	48.9	84	7.5% CN complications 1.5% pituitary dysfunction
Sheehan et al, 2022	Image defined (n = 727)	727	4.3	13	57.2	NR	2.5

Abbreviations: CSM, cavernous sinus meningiomaand; NR, not reported.

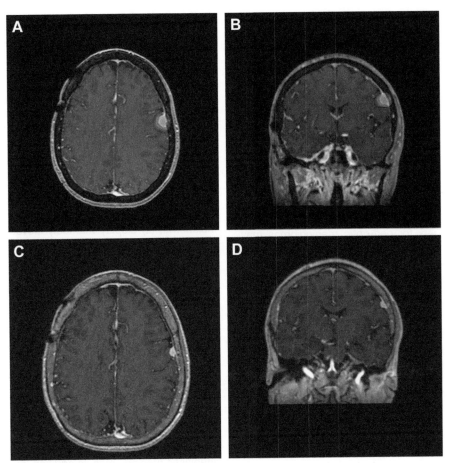

Fig. 1. Procedural, T1-weighted, post-contrast axial (*A*), and coronal (*B*), brain MRI demonstrating the radiosurgical target at the left frontal convexity (yellow highlighted area). Axial (*C*) and coronal (*D*), T1-weighted contrast-enhanced brain MRI 76 months after SRS significant for decrease in the size of the tumor.

Asymptomatic Meningiomas

Asymptomatic, incidentally discovered meningiomas occur with a prevalence of 0.9% in the general population[15] and account for 30% of newly diagnosed meningiomas.[16] Though observation is initially recommended,[5] 24% to 92% of small to medium sized meningiomas will demonstrate growth after observation periods of 4 or more years,[11] and 20% of the patients will develop meningioma-related symptoms.[17] The international Multicenter Matched Cohort Analysis of Incidental Meningioma Progression During Active Surveillance or After Stereotactic Radiosurgery (IMPASSE) study evaluated the safety and efficacy of radiosurgery as compared with observation for the management of asymptomatic meningiomas. Meningioma control was 99.4% in the SRS cohort and 62% in the observation cohort. New neurologic deficits occurred in 2.3% and 3.2% in the SRS and observation cohort, respectively.[11] Focused, matched cohort and single arm analyses

from the IMPASSE study further confirmed the superior meningioma control of SRS as compared with observation without an increased risk for new neurologic deficits for asymptomatic skull base,[18–21] convexity,[22] and parasagittal/parafalcine[23] asymptomatic meningiomas.

Complications of Stereotactic Radiosurgery for Intracranial Meningiomas

The main complications of meningioma SRS are adverse radiation effects such as peri-tumoral edema, radiation-induced optic-neuropathy and other cranial nerve neuropathies, and radiation-associated malignancies.

Peri-tumoral edema usually occurs within 2 years of SRS for meningioma in 2% to 50% of the patients and is symptomatic in 5% to 46%[24] manifesting with seizures, focal neurologic deficits, and/or signs and symptoms of high intracranial pressure. Factors reported to be associated with an increased risk for peri-tumoral edema after meningioma SRS include pre-SRS peri-tumoral edema,[25] increasing meningioma–brain contact interface area,[25] maximum dose,[26,27] prescription dose,[27] meningioma volume,[27,28] and non-skull base location.[27,29] The reported volume thresholds for increasing risk of post-SRS adverse radiation effect (AREs) vary in the literature from 4.2 cm[3] to 10 cm[3].[27,28] Management of post-SRS peri-tumoral edema includes an initial course of oral corticosteroids. Patients with refractory symptoms or those who develop corticosteroid side effects are usually managed with bevacizumab. In cases refractory to medical treatment or those who develop life-threatening symptoms, resection can be considered.

Radiosurgery for peri-optic meningiomas may be limited by the sensitivity of the anterior visual pathways (AVP) to radiation. In a multicenter study of 438 patients managed with SRS for a peri-optic meningioma, 10% of patients experienced visual decline. The actuarial 5 year and 10 year post-SRS visual decline rates of 9% and 21%, respectively. Tumor progression and maximum dose to the optic apparatus of 10 Gy or higher were associated with visual decline after SRS.[30] In patients without a history of prior radiotherapy, the risk of developing radiation-induced optic neuropathy (RION) is dose-dependent and cumulative. In radiation naïve patients, the risk of RION is less than 1% when the maximum point dose to the AVP is less than 10 Gy, 20 Gy, and 25 Gy in 1, 3, and 5 fraction SRS, respectively. In patients with a prior history of radiation therapy, the risk of RION increases to greater than 10%.[31]

SRS attributed cranial nerve neuropathies have been reported in 6.3% to 7.5% of patients managed with SRS for cavernous sinus meningioma.[32–34] They most commonly manifest as diplopia and trigeminal neuropathy and approximately 50% of these are transient and recover spontaneously or after corticosteroid treatment.[32,34]

Radiosurgery-associated intracranial malignancies have been rarely reported after SRS.[35–37] In a retrospective study, Pollock and colleagues reported malignant transformation in 7 of 316 (2.2%) patients managed with SRS for WHO Grade I meningioma.[37] In the series by Malik and colleagues, reported 1 of 306 patients with WHO Grade I meningioma developed a higher grade meningioma after radiosurgery.[32] Radiosurgery-induced glioblastoma has been reported in three case reports in 18,[38] 36[39], and 84[40] months after meningioma SRS. In a multicenter study that evaluated the incidence of radiosurgery-associated intracranial malignancies, none of the 1490 patients with meningioma treated with SRS developed radiation-associated malignancies.[36]

Radiosurgery for Atypical and Anaplastic Meningiomas

Atypical meningiomas account for 20% to 35% of all meningiomas and are defined by WHO as intermediate-grade meningioma characterized by > 4 to less than 20 mitoses per 10 HPF, brain invasion, and/or at three or more of the following: high cellularity, small cells with a high nuclear:cytoplasmic ratio, prominent nucleoli, sheeting, and focal necrosis. Anaplastic meningiomas account for 1% to 3% of all meningiomas and are defined by WHO as high-grade meningiomas with overtly malignant cytomorphology (anaplasia) that can (1) resemble carcinoma, high-grade sarcoma, or melanoma; (2) display markedly elevated mitotic activity; (3) harbor a TERT promoter mutation; and/or (4) have homozygous deletion of CDKN2A and/or CDKN2B.

Maximum safe resection is the initial treatment of choice for atypical and anaplastic meningiomas.[5] Adjuvant, fractionated radiotherapy is recommended for anaplastic meningiomas[5] and has been associated with improved survival of patients with grade II meningioma[41] and is currently recommended after STR and should be considered after GTR of an atypical meningioma.[5]

Reported data on SRS for atypical and anaplastic meningiomas are mainly limited to the residual and recurrent settings. Typically, doses greater than 16 Gy are given for atypical and anaplastic meningiomas. In addition, available series are limited by small patient numbers, and by the inclusion of patients treated prior to the 2016 revision of the WHO classification of central nervous system tumors, which included brain invasion as a criterion for grade II meningioma diagnosis. Nevertheless, the reported 5 year PFS rates of SRS for Grade II and for Grade III meningiomas range from 25% to 83% and from 0% to 72%, respectively.[42] The reported complication rates of SRS for atypical and anaplastic meningiomas range from 0% to 62%.[42] In a multicenter study, Shepard and colleagues reported outcomes of 233 patients with atypical and of 38 patients with anaplastic meningiomas, managed with adjuvant SRS of stable residual, salvage SRS for residual tumor progression and at recurrence. The median OS for atypical meningiomas was 187.4 months and for anaplastic meningiomas it was 70 months. The 2 and 5 year PFS rates for atypical meningiomas were 67.8%, and 36.4% and for anaplastic meningiomas the 2 and 5 year PFS rates were 59.9% and 20.4%.[43] In a retrospective study of 68 patients with atypical meningioma, Hasegawa and colleagues reported 3, 5, and 10 year PFS of 52%, 35%, and 25%, respectively.[44] In conclusion, SRS is primarily indicated as a salvage therapy for recurrent, small volume atypical meningiomas.

SUMMARY

Stereotactic radiosurgery typically affords tumor control and neurologic preservation in the vast majority of patients with WHO grade I meningiomas. It is frequently used in the setting of recurrent or residual meningiomas. However, SRS can also be used in the upfront setting and even for asymptomatic meningiomas. For higher grade meningiomas, SRS plays a valuable role in the management of patients with recurrent or residual Grade II or III meningiomas.

CONFLICT OF INTEREST

The authors report no conflict of interest.

REFERENCES

1. Ostrom Quinn T, Gino C, Waite K, et al. CBTRUS Statistical Report: Primary Brain and Other Central Nervous System Tumors Diagnosed in the United States in 2014–2018. Neuro Oncol 2021;23(Supplement_3). iii1–105.

2. Joseph W, Margaret W, Claus Elizabeth B. Epidemiology and etiology of meningioma. J Neuro Oncol 2010;99(3):307–14.

3. Mohammed N, Hung Yi-C, Xu Z, et al. Neurofibromatosis type 2–associated meningiomas: an international multicenter study of outcomes after Gamma Knife stereotactic radiosurgery. J Neurosurg 2021; 136(1):109–14.

4. Agarwal V, McCutcheon Brandon A, Hughes Joshua D, et al. Trends in management of intracranial meningiomas: analysis of 49,921 Cases from Modern Cohort. World Neurosurgery 2017;106: 145–51.

5. Roland G, Pantelis S, Jenkinson Michael D, et al. EANO guideline on the diagnosis and management of meningiomas. Neuro Oncol 2021;23(11):1821–34.

6. Hirsch M, Abel S, Yu A, et al. Trends in the use of radiation for meningioma across the United States. Radiat Oncol J 2022;40(1):29–36.

7. Pollock Bruce E, Stafford Scott L, Utter A, et al. Stereotactic radiosurgery provides equivalent tumor control to Simpson Grade 1 resection for patients with small- to medium-size meningiomas. Int J Radiat Oncol Biol Phys 2003;55(4):1000–5.

8. Antonio S, Walier M, Régis J, et al. Long-term Tumor Control of Benign Intracranial Meningiomas After Radiosurgery in a Series of 4565 Patients. Neurosurgery 2012;70(1):32–9.

9. Marcello M, Sahgal A, De Salles Antonio AF, et al. Stereotactic Radiosurgery for Intracranial Noncavernous Sinus Benign Meningioma: International Stereotactic Radiosurgery Society Systematic Review, Meta-Analysis and Practice Guideline. Neurosurgery 2020;87(5):879–90.

10. Cheng-Chia L, Trifiletti Daniel M, Sahgal A, et al. Stereotactic Radiosurgery for Benign (World Health Organization Grade I) Cavernous Sinus Meningiomas-International Stereotactic Radiosurgery Society (ISRS) Practice Guideline: A Systematic Review. Neurosurgery 2018;83(6):1128–42.

11. Sheehan J, Stylianos P, Islim A, et al. An International Multicenter Matched Cohort Analysis of Incidental Meningioma Progression During Active Surveillance or After Stereotactic Radiosurgery: The IMPASSE Study. Neuro Oncol 2021. https://doi.org/10.1093/neuonc/noab132. noab132.

12. Kollová A, Roman L, Novotný J, et al. Gamma Knife surgery for benign meningioma. J Neurosurg 2007; 107(2):325–36.

13. Douglas K, John C F, Bernardo P, et al. Judicious Resection and/or Radiosurgery for Parasagittal Meningiomas: Outcomes from a Multicenter Review. Neurosurgery 1998;43(3):405–13.

14. Stafford Scott L, Pollock Bruce E, Foote Robert L, et al. Meningioma Radiosurgery: Tumor Control, Outcomes, and Complications among 190 Consecutive Patients. Neurosurgery 2001;49(5):1029–38.

15. Vernooij Meike W. Incidental Findings on Brain MRI in the General Population. N Engl J Med 2007;8.

16. Stylianos P, Adomas B, Sheehan J. Outcomes from treatment of asymptomatic skull base meningioma with stereotactic radiosurgery. Acta Neurochir 2021;163(1):83–8.

17. Romani R, Ryan G, Christian B, et al. Non-operative meningiomas: long-term follow-up of 136 patients. Acta Neurochir 2018;160(8):1547–53.

18. Georgios M, Stylianos P, Adomas B, et al. Stereotactic radiosurgery for asymptomatic petroclival region meningiomas: a focused analysis from the IMPASSE study. Acta Neurochir 2022;164(1):273–9.

19. Stylianos P, Georgios M, Yavuz S, et al. Stereotactic Radiosurgery for Incidentally Discovered Cavernous Sinus Meningiomas: A Multi-institutional Study. World Neurosurgery 2022;158:e675–80.

20. Georgios M, Stylianos P, Yavuz S, et al. Stereotactic radiosurgery versus active surveillance for asymptomatic, skull-based meningiomas: an international, multicenter matched cohort study. J Neuro Oncol 2022;156(3):509–18.

21. Islim Abdurrahman I, Georgios M, Stylianos P, et al. Comparison of Active Surveillance to Stereotactic Radiosurgery for the Management of Patients with an Incidental Frontobasal Meningioma-A Sub-Analysis of the IMPASSE Study. Cancers 2022;14(5): 1300.

22. Stylianos P, Georgios M, Islim Abdurrahman I, et al. Stereotactic radiosurgery versus active surveillance

for incidental, convexity meningiomas: a matched cohort analysis from the IMPASSE study. J Neuro Oncol 2022;157(1):121–8.

23. Stylianos P, Georgios M, Adomas B, et al. Stereotactic Radiosurgery Compared With Active Surveillance for Asymptomatic, Parafalcine, and Parasagittal Meningiomas: A Matched Cohort Analysis From the IMPASSE Study. Neurosurgery 2022;90(6):750–7.

24. Milano Michael T, Sharma M, Soltys Scott G, et al. Radiation-Induced Edema After Single-Fraction or Multifraction Stereotactic Radiosurgery for Meningioma: A Critical Review. Int J Radiat Oncol Biol Phys 2018;101(2):344–57.

25. Cai R, Barnett Gene H, Novak Eric, et al. Principal Risk of Peritumoral Edema After Stereotactic Radiosurgery for Intracranial Meningioma Is Tumor-Brain Contact Interface Area. Neurosurgery 2010;66(3): 513–22.

26. Sheehan Jason P, Cheng-Chia L, Xu Zhiyuan, et al. Edema following Gamma Knife radiosurgery for parasagittal and parafalcine meningiomas. J Neurosurg 2015;123(5):1287–93.

27. Sheehan Jason P, Cohen-Inbar Or, Rawee R, et al. Post-radiosurgical edema associated with parasagittal and parafalcine meningiomas: a multicenter study. J Neuro Oncol 2015;125(2):317–24.

28. Yeon Hoe. Choi Young Jae., Kim Jeong Hoon., et al. Peritumoral Brain Edema after Stereotactic Radiosurgery for Asymptomatic Intracranial Meningiomas: Risks and Pattern of Evolution. J Korean Neurosurg Soc 2015;58(4):379–84.

29. Chang J, Chang J, Choi J, et al. Complications after gamma knife radiosurgery for benign meningiomas. J Neurol Neurosurg Psychiatry 2003;74(2):226–30.

30. Adomas B, Kormath AR, Mohanad S, et al. Stereotactic Radiosurgery for Perioptic Meningiomas: An International, Multicenter Study. Neurosurgery 2021;88(4):828–37.

31. Milano Michael T, Grimm J, Soltys Scott G, et al. Single- and Multi-Fraction Stereotactic Radiosurgery Dose Tolerances of the Optic Pathways. Int J Radiat Oncol Biol Phys 2021;110(1):87–99.

32. Malik I, Rowe JG, Walton L, et al. The use of stereotactic radiosurgery in the management of meningiomas. Br J Neurosurg 2005;19(1):13–20.

33. Park K-J, Kano H, Iyer A, et al. Gamma Knife stereotactic radiosurgery for cavernous sinus meningioma:

long-term follow-up in 200 patients. J Neurosurg 2018;130(6):1799–808.

34. Douglas K, Mathieu D, Dade LL, et al. Radiosurgery as definitive management of intracranial meningiomas. Neurosurgery 2008;62(1):53–60.

35. Adomas B, Styllianos P, Schlesinger D, et al. Editorial: Radiosurgical induced malignancy associated with stereotactic radiosurgery. Acta Neurochir 2021;163(4):969–70.

36. Wolf A, Naylor K, Tam M, et al. Risk of radiation-associated intracranial malignancy after stereotactic radiosurgery: a retrospective, multicentre, cohort study. Lancet Oncol 2019;20(1):159–64.

37. Pollock Bruce E, Link MJ, Stafford Scott L, et al. The Risk of Radiation-Induced Tumors or Malignant Transformation After Single-Fraction Intracranial Radiosurgery: Results Based on a 25-Year Experience. Int J Radiat Oncol Biol Phys 2017;97(5):919–23.

38. Labuschagne Jason J, Chetty D. Glioblastoma multiforme as a secondary malignancy following stereotactic radiosurgery of a meningioma: case report. Neurosurg Focus 2019;46(6):E11.

39. Lee HS, Kim Jong H, Jung-Il L. Glioblastoma Following Radiosurgery for Meningioma. J Korean Neurosurg Soc 2012;51(2):98–101.

40. Yu John S, Wilson D, Black Keith L, et al. Glioblastoma induction after radiosurgery for meningioma. Lancet 2000;356(9241):1576–7.

41. Rydzewski Nicholas R, Lesniak Maciej S, Chandler James P, et al. Gross total resection and adjuvant radiotherapy most significant predictors of improved survival in patients with atypical meningioma. Cancer 2018;124(4):734–42.

42. Ding D, Starke Robert M, Hantzmon J, et al. The role of radiosurgery in the management of WHO Grade II and III intracranial meningiomas. Neurosurg Focus 2013;35(6):E16.

43. Shepard Matthew J, Xu Z, Kearns K, et al. Stereotactic Radiosurgery for Atypical (World Health Organization II) and Anaplastic (World Health Organization III) Meningiomas: Results From a Multicenter, International Cohort Study. Neurosurgery 2021;88(5):980–8.

44. Hasegawa H, Vakharia K, Link MJ, et al. The role of single-fraction stereotactic radiosurgery for atypical meningiomas (WHO grade II): treatment results based on a 25-year experience. J Neuro Oncol 2021;155(3):335–42.

The Role of Radiotherapy in the Treatment of Higher-Grade Meningioma

Grace Lee, MD[a,b], Helen A. Shih, MD[a,b],*

KEYWORDS

- Meningioma • Atypical • Anaplastic • Malignant • WHO grade 2 • WHO grade 3
- Radiation therapy

KEY POINTS

- High-grade meningiomas (atypical and anaplastic/malignant) are associated with higher rates of recurrence following first-line treatment with maximum safe surgical resection.
- Currently, adjuvant radiation therapy (RT) is advised for incompletely resected atypical and all anaplastic meningiomas regardless of resection extent with improved local control and progression-free survival.
- In completely resected atypical meningiomas, the role of adjuvant RT is debated, and the potential benefits of RT should be carefully balanced with the risks of toxicity.
- The results from randomized trials ROAM/EORTC-1308 and NRG Oncology BN003 may help guide optimal postoperative management in completed resected atypical meningiomas.

BACKGROUND

Although most (70%–80%) meningiomas are benign and indolent, there is a subset of tumors that are more aggressive and associated with higher rates of recurrence (6- to 8-fold increased risk) affecting morbidity and mortality.[1,2] The World Health Organization (WHO) classifies such high-grade meningiomas as WHO grade 2 (atypical) and 3 (anaplastic/malignant), based on specific histopathologic features and subtypes.[3–7] The prevalence of high-grade meningiomas has increased from less than 10% to now up to approximately 25% to 30% of all meningiomas (25%–30% atypical, 1%–3% anaplastic) with changes in the WHO criteria defining atypical and anaplastic meningiomas (**Table 1**).[3–8] Under the most recent WHO 2021 update on grading system, meningiomas are categorized as a single tumor type with 15 subtypes, and malignancy grading is within-tumor grading regardless of subtype (**Table 2**).[4] The WHO 2021 also introduced several molecular biomarkers associated with the classification and grading of meningiomas (ie, SMARCE1 in clear cell subtype, BAP1 in rhabdoid and papillary subtypes, KLF4/TRAF7 in secretory subtype mutations, and TERT promoter mutation and/or homozygous deletion of CDKN2A/B in anaplastic meningiomas).[4,8]

High-grade meningiomas are more likely to recur following initial treatment (surgery and/or radiation therapy [RT]) with approximate 10-year progression-free survival (PFS) and overall survival (OS) of 23% to 78% and 50% to 79%, respectively, for atypical meningiomas and 0% and 14% to 34%, respectively, for anaplastic meningiomas.[9–11] Management requires a balance between optimizing disease control and minimizing treatment toxicity. Maximum safe surgical resection is the preferred first-line treatment when meningioma is in an accessible location. The extent of resection, with gross total resection (GTR) defined as typically Simpson grade 1 to 2, sometimes inclusive of grade 3 resection, and subtotal

a Harvard Medical School, 25 Shattuck Street, Boston, MA 02115, USA; b Department of Radiation Oncology, Massachusetts General Hospital, 30 Fruit Street, Boston, MA 02114, USA
* Corresponding author.
E-mail address: hshih@mgh.harvard.edu

Neurosurg Clin N Am 34 (2023) 463–478
https://doi.org/10.1016/j.nec.2023.02.013

Table 1
Summary of histopathologic criteria of World Health Organization classification of meningiomas from 1993 to 2016

WHO Grade	1993	2000	2007	2016
1 (Benign)	Without features of grade 2 & 3	Without features of grade 2 & 3	Without features of grade 2 & 3	Without features of grade 2 & 3
2 (Atypical)	Several of the following features: (I) frequent mitoses; (II) increased cellularity; (III) small cells with high n:c ratio and/or prominent nucleoli; (IV) uninterrupted patternless or sheetlike growth; (V) foci of spontaneous or geographic necrosis	4–19 mitoses per 10 hpf and/or 3 or more of the following: (I) increased cellularity; (II) high n:c ratio; (III) prominent nucleoli; (IV) uninterrupted patternless or sheetlike growth; (V) foci of spontaneous necrosis	4–19 mitoses per 10 hpf and/or 3 or more of the following: (I) increased cellularity; (II) small cells with high n:c ratio; (III) prominent nucleoli; (IV) uninterrupted patternless or sheetlike growth; (V) foci of spontaneous or geographic necrosis; (VI) brain invasion	4–19 mitoses per 10 hpf and/or brain invasion and/or 3 or more of the following: (I) increased cellularity; (II) small cells with high n:c ratio; (III) prominent nucleoli; (IV) uninterrupted patternless or sheetlike growth; (V) foci of spontaneous or geographic necrosis
3 (Anaplastic/malignant)	Features of frank malignancy far in excess of the abnormalities noted in atypical meningiomas	≥20 mitoses per 10 hpf and/or malignant characteristics resembling carcinoma, sarcoma, or melanoma	≥20 mitoses per 10 hpf and/or malignant characteristics resembling carcinoma, sarcoma, or melanoma	≥20 mitoses per 10 hpf and/or malignant characteristics resembling carcinoma, sarcoma, or melanoma

Abbreviations: hpf, high-power field; n:c, nuclear:cytoplasmic (3–5).

Table 2
Meningioma histologic subtypes and grades based on World Health Organization 2021 update

Histologic Type	Histologic Malignancy Grade[a]
Meningothelial	1, 2
Fibrous	1, 2
Transitional	1, 2
Angiomatous	1, 2
Psammomatous	1, 2
Secretary	1, 2
Microcystic	1, 2
Lymphoplasmacyte-rich	1, 2
Atypical (including brain invasive)	2
Chordoid	2
Clear cell	2
Anaplastic/malignant	3

[a] Malignancy grading within-tumor grading regardless of subtype.

tumor resection (STR) defined as Simpson grade 4 to 5,[12] is a significant prognostic factor for PFS and OS. Rates of recurrence are substantial with STR and even following GTR in high-grade meningiomas.

The available evidence on the role of RT in high-grade meningiomas are based on retrospective studies and limited number of prospective trials, with challenges in interpreting the outcomes of studies with serial WHO classification changes in defining atypical and anaplastic/malignant meningiomas over the past few decades. Nevertheless, based on prior studies, there is consensus that RT has an important role for high-grade meningiomas in both the adjuvant and salvage settings (**Fig. 1**). Adjuvant RT is currently standard in initial management of anaplastic and incompletely resected atypical meningiomas. The role of adjuvant RT in completely resected atypical meningiomas, however remains, a topic of controversy.

DISCUSSION
Adjuvant Radiation Therapy in Atypical (World Health Organization Grade 2) Meningiomas

Atypical or WHO grade 2 meningiomas represent a heterogeneous group comprising 25% to 30% of all meningiomas with variable outcomes at intermediate range between benign and anaplastic meningiomas. Reported 10-year PFS rates range from

23% to 78%, and 10-year OS rates range between 50% to 79%.[9,10,11] The extent of resection is an important prognostic factor,[12] with recurrence/progression rates of 60% to 100% with STR only and 30% to 50% with GTR only.[13–17] The routine utilization of adjuvant RT in atypical meningiomas is supported by multiple retrospective series and 2 recent phase 2 nonrandomized trials (selected studies summarized in **Table 3**).[1,13–16,18–41] The optimal timing of RT in completely resected atypical meningiomas remains in debate.

Gross total resected tumors
Several retrospective series on atypical meningiomas support disease control benefit of adjuvant RT irrespective of resection extent. The OS benefit of adjuvant RT is less clear in most studies because of insufficient follow-up length and/or number of patients. A recent meta-analysis by Song and colleagues[42] included 3078 patients with atypical meningioma from 24 studies published between 2010 and February 2021 and showed that adjuvant RT was associated with reduced tumor recurrence (hazard ratio [HR] = 0.70; $P<.001$). When stratified by GTR and STR, adjuvant RT was associated with significant improvement in PFS (HR = 0.69; P = .01; HR = 0.41; $P<.001$) and OS (HR = 0.55; P = .007; HR = 0.47; P = .01) for both groups.[42] In a recent single-institution retrospective study from Massachusetts General Hospital of 230 patients with atypical meningiomas (151 GTR, 79 STR) resected between 2000 and 2015, 51 (22%) patients underwent upfront adjuvant RT (median, 59.4 Gy; 57% proton therapy), whereas 179 (78%) underwent surveillance. Those who received upfront adjuvant RT had a better PFS (5-year PFS 79% vs 62%; P = .03), irrespective of resection extent, but there was no difference in OS (5-year OS 91% vs 94%; P = .95) with a median follow-up of nearly 7 years.[14] Receipt of adjuvant RT was associated with approximately one-fifth lower risk for recurrence (HR = 0.21; $P<.01$).[14] In another retrospective study by Aizer and colleagues[16] of 91 patients with atypical meningioma treated between 1997 and 2011 among which most (81%) underwent GTR and 34 (37%) underwent adjuvant RT (60 Gy; interquartile range [IQR] 55.8–64 Gy), the propensity score model showed that adjuvant RT was associated with improved local control (LC) in those who underwent GTR (5-year LC 83% vs 68%; HR = 0.25; P = .04), although there was no difference in OS. In contrast, in a series of 133 patients with atypical meningioma diagnosed between 2001 and 2010 reported by Jenkinson and colleagues,[26] among 113 (85%) of patients who

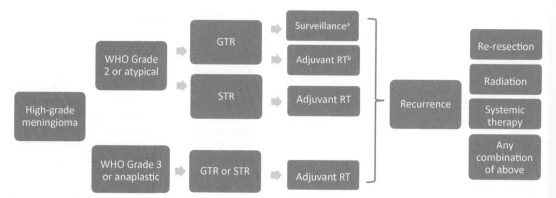

Fig. 1. RT in high-grade meningiomas. [a]Consider for patients concerned about and/or at increased risk of RT toxicity with older age, comorbidities, large radiation field, and close proximity of target to critical structures. [b]Consider for patients with high-risk clinicopathologic features, such as less than Simpson grade 1, nonconvexity tumor location, presence of brain invasion, high number of mitoses per 10 high-power fields, and/or prominent nucleoli. Also, for patients who are willing to accept risk of RT-related complications and minimal risk of recurrence.

achieved GTR, 28% underwent early adjuvant RT (median, 60 Gy; range, 54–60 Gy), and there was no significant difference in PFS (5-year PFS, 77% vs 76%; $P = .784$) or OS (5-year OS 82% vs 79%; $P = .808$) compared with those who underwent surveillance. The difference in 5-year outcomes across studies suggests additional nuanced differences in either diagnoses or treatment of studied patients; for example, lack of stratification of Simpson grade of GTR, residual tumor volume of STR, nuances in RT and dose constraints, and subsequent salvage therapies.

In addition to retrospective institutional reports, several population-based studies using cancer data registries have also attempted to examine the impact of adjuvant RT in atypical meningiomas.[43–46] In one of the largest studies by Rydzewski and colleagues[44] based on National Cancer Data Base query, which included 7811 atypical meningioma cases, adjuvant RT was found to be significantly associated with improved OS, both independently (HR = 0.70; $P = .010$) and in unison with GTR (HR = 0.47; $P = .002$).

Two prospective phase 2 nonrandomized trials (NRG Oncology/RTOG-0539 and EORTC 22042-26042) investigating the outcomes of adjuvant RT in completely resected atypical meningiomas have been recently published, with both demonstrating improved PFS rates of 89% to 94% compared with expected rate of 70% based on historical controls, with acceptable toxicity rates.[18,19] Initial outcomes from NRG Oncology/RTOG-0539 for 48 evaluable patients in the intermediate-risk cohort, which included 32 patients with newly diagnosed WHO grade 2 meningioma and GTR (Simpson grade 1–3) treated to

54 Gy, were reported with 3-year local failure (LF), PFS, and OS rates of 4%, 94%, and 96%, respectively (median follow-up of 3.7 years).[29] Adverse events were limited to grade 1 or 2. In the EORTC 22042-26042 trial, 56 patients with gross totally resected (Simpson grade 1–3) WHO grade 2 meningioma received adjuvant RT to 60 Gy. At a median of 5.1 years, the reported 3-year LF, PFS, and OS were 14%, 89%, and 98%.[18] Late treatment-related symptoms of grade 3 or greater were observed in 14% of patients, and no grade 5 events were observed.[18]

Subtotally resected tumors

Adjuvant RT improves LC and may improve OS in patients with incompletely resected atypical meningiomas who remain at high risk of recurrence/progression without any adjuvant therapy. Retrospective studies have consistently demonstrated improved LC and sometimes improved OS with adjuvant RT (typical doses of 54–60 Gy).[14,17,22,42,47–49] Recently reported outcomes for the high-risk cohort from NRG Oncology/RTOG-0539 included 11 patients with initial WHO grade 2 meningioma and STR treated with intensity-modulated radiation therapy (IMRT) to 60 Gy and reported a 3-year PFS of 73%.[18] Accurate delineation of residual tumor and surgical bed is crucial in achieving optimal LC.

Overall, most prior studies support that adjuvant RT (54–60 Gy) improves clinical outcomes (LC, PFS) in atypical meningiomas after STR, and several also suggest benefit of adjuvant RT even after GTR. Patient and clinicopathologic factors should be considered to balance the tumor control benefit and potential treatment toxicities with adjuvant RT.

Table 3
Summary of selected major prior studies on adjuvant radiation therapy for atypical (World Health Organization grade 2) meningiomas

Publication	Study Design	N	Treatment	Resection	Median RT Dose (Gy)	Median FU (mo)	PFS	OS (%)	Toxicity
Aghi et al,[15] 2009	Retrospective	108	Surgery (n = 100) Surgery + RT (n = 8)	GTR (n = 108)	CRT 60.2 Gy	39	44% vs 100% at 5 y (P = .1)	NA	13% radionecrosis requiring surgery
Mair et al,[20] 2011	Retrospective	114	Surgery (n = 84) Surgery + RT (n = 30)	GTR (n = 66) STR (n = 48)	CRT 51.8 Gy	NA	40% vs 60% at 5 y (NS)	NA	NA
Komotar et al,[21] 2012		45	Surgery (n = 32) Surgery + RT (n = 13)	GTR (n = 45)	CRT 59.4 Gy	44	Crude recurrence rates 41% vs 8% (P = .085)	NA	Minimal short term grade 1–2
Hardesty et al,[13] 2013	Retrospective	228	Surgery (n = 157) Surgery + RT (n = 71)	GTR (n = 149) STR (n = 79)	IMRT 54 Gy (n = 39) SRS (n = 32)	52	Crude recurrence rates 23% surgery alone vs 18% IMRT vs 25% SRS (NS)	NA	3% cranial wound breakdown requiring surgery in IMRT cohort
Park et al,[22] 2013	Retrospective	83	Surgery (n = 56) Surgery + RT (n = 27)	GTR (n = 55) STR (n = 25)	CRT 61.2 Gy	43	44% vs 59% at 5 y (P = .029)	90% at 5 y for all (NS)	No severe acute
Bagshaw et al,[23] 2014	Retrospective	59	Surgery (n = 42) Surgery + RT (n = 17)	GTR (n = 52) STR (n = 11)	CRT 54 Gy SRS 15 Gy (n = 3)	42	Median time to LF 46 vs 180 mo (P = .02)	88% alive at time of analysis (NS)	Grade 3 (n = 2) Grade 4 (n = 1)
Aizer et al,[16] 2014	Retrospective	91	Surgery (n = 57) Surgery + RT (n = 34)	GTR (n = 74) STR (n = 17)	CRT 60 Gy (n = 33) SRS 16 Gy (n = 1)	57	68% vs 83% at 5 y in GTR (P = .04)	NA	NA
Hammouche et al,[24] 2014	Retrospective	79	Surgery (n = 43) Surgery + RT (n = 36)	GTR (n = 34) STR (n = 45)	CRT 56 Gy	50	Crude recurrence rates 33% vs 28% (HR = 0.96; P = .91)	81% at 5 y for all (NS)	NA

(continued on next page)

Table 3
(continued)

Publication	Study Design	N	Treatment	Resection	Median RT Dose (Gy)	Median FU (mo)	PFS	OS (%)	Toxicity
Yoon et al,[25] 2015	Retrospective	158	Surgery (n = 135) Surgery + RT (n = 23)	GTR (n = 109) STR (n = 42)	CRT 57 Gy SRS 14 Gy (n = 11)	32	Median PFS 88 vs 59 mo (P = .2)	83% vs 89% at 5 y (P = .59)	NA
Jenkinson et al,[26] 2016	Retrospective	133	Surgery (n = 97) Surgery + RT (n = 36)	GTR (n = 113) STR (n = 19)	CRT 60 Gy	57	76% vs 72% at 5 y (P = .68)	73% vs 68% at 5 y (P = .48)	NA
Dohm et al,[27] 2017	Retrospective	115	Surgery (n = 52) Surgery + early RT (n = 31)	GTR (n = 78) STR (n = 37)	CRT 55.7 Gy SRS 14.5 Gy (n = 16)	37	27% vs 59% at 5 y (P = .003)	55% vs 71% at 5 y (P = .012)	Grade 3 (n = 7) Grade 4 (n = 1)
Champeaux et al,[28] 2017	Retrospective	215[a]	Surgery (n = 150) Surgery + RT (n = 65)	GTR (n = 165) STR (n = 49)	CRT 54 Gy (n = 56) SRS 16 Gy (n = 9)	54	82% at 5 y (NS)	Cause-specific survival 88% at 5 y (NS)	NA
Weber et al,[19] 2018 (EORTC 22042-26042)	Phase 2, nonrandomized	56	Surgery + RT (n = 56)	GTR (n = 56)	CRT 60 Gy	61	89% at 3 y (significantly >70% based on historical controls)	98% at 3 y	14% grade 3–4
Rogers et al,[29] 2018 (RTOG 0539)	Phase 2, nonrandomized	56[b]	Surgery (n = 4) Surgery + RT (n = 52)	GTR (n = 32)	IMRT 54 Gy (n = 44) 3DCRT 54 Gy (n = 8)	44	94% at 3 y (significantly >70% based on historical controls)	96% at 3 y	No grade 3
Masalha et al,[30] 2018	Retrospective	161	Surgery (n = 128) Surgery + RT (n = 33)	GTR (n = 102) STR (n = 59)	CRT 55–57 Gy	NA	73% vs 64% at 5 y (P = .22)	NA	NA

Study	Type	N	Treatment	Resection	RT		Outcome	LC/OS	Toxicity
Chen et al,[31] 2018	Retrospective	182	Surgery (n = 140) Surgery + RT (n = 42)	GTR (n = 114) STR (n = 68)	CRT 59.4 Gy (n = 36) SRS (n = 6)	52	65% vs 82% at 5 y (P = .08)	87% vs 85% at 5 y (P = .64)	12% grade 2+ (5% radionecrosis)
Budohoski et al,[32] 2018	Retrospective	220	Surgery (n = 205) Surgery + RT (n = 57)	GTR (n = 143) STR (n = 62)	NA	24	59% at 5 y (OR = 0.38; P = .046)	87% at 5 y	NA
Zhi et al,[1] 2019	Retrospective	149	Surgery (n = 96) Surgery + RT (n = 53)	GTR (n = 98) STR (n = 51)	CRT 59.4 Gy	74	54% vs 76% at 5 y (P = .011)	80% vs 86% at 5 y (P = .621)	NA
Li et al,[33] 2019	Retrospective	302	Surgery (n = 227) Surgery + RT (n = 75)	GTR (n = 201) STR (n = 101)	CRT 54 Gy (n = 71) SRS (n = 4)	42	48% at 5 y (HR = 0.66; P = .079)	79% at 5 y (HR = 0.54; P = .022)	NA
Zeng et al,[34] 2019	Retrospective	1014	Surgery (n = 727) Surgery + RT (n = 315)	GTR (n = 727) STR (n = 315)	NA	NA	NA	77% vs 83% at 5 y (P = .071)	NA
Hemmati et al,[35] 2019	Retrospective	99	Surgery (n = 80) Surgery + RT (n = 19)	GTR (n = 60) STR (n = 12)	CRT 59.4 Gy SRS (n = 1)	37	Median 64 vs 37 mo (P = .009)	HR = 0.709; P = .661	NA
Keric et al,[36] 2020	Retrospective	258	Surgery (n = 212) Surgery + RT (n = 46)	GTR (n = 194) STR (n = 53)	IMRT 56.6 Gy (n = 41) SRS 23 Gy (n = 2)	31	69% vs 71% at 5 y (HR = 0.71; P = .44)	NA	No grade 3
Poulen et al,[37] 2020	Retrospective	88	Surgery (n = 81) Surgery + early RT (n = 7)	GTR (n = 76) STR (n = 7)	CRT 56 Gy SRS (n = 1)	69	56% at 5 y (median 60 vs 69 mo, P = .52)	90% at 5 y (P = .93)	NA

(continued on next page)

Table 3
(continued)

Publication	Study Design	N	Treatment	Resection	Median RT Dose (Gy)	Median FU (mo)	PFS	OS (%)	Toxicity
Rogers et al,[18] 2020 (RTOG 0539)	Phase 2, nonrandomized	53[c]	Surgery + RT (n = 53)	GTR (n = 21) STR (n = 11)	IMRT 60 Gy (n = 52) 3DCRT 60 Gy (n = 1)	48	59% at 3 y for all 73% at 3 y for 11 patients with initial WHO grade 2 and STR	79% at 3 y for all	Most patients with grade 1–3 toxicity Necrosis related grade 5 event (n = 1)
Lee et al,[14] 2021	Retrospective	230	Surgery (n = 179) Surgery + RT (n = 51)	GTR (n = 151) STR (n = 79)	CRT 59.4 Gy (n = 48) SRS 13 Gy (n = 3)	81	62% vs 79% at 5 y (P = .03)	94% vs 91% at 5 y (0.95)	NA
Torres-Bayona et al,[38] 2021	Retrospective	32	Surgery (n = 10) Surgery + RT (n = 22)	GTR (n = 28) STR (n = 4)	CRT 59.4 Gy (n = 20) SRS 15 Gy (n = 2)	50	Recurrence rates 60% vs 45% Median 51 vs 38 mo (P = .555)	Median 55 vs 53 mo (P = .597)	NA
Unterberger et al,[39] 2021	Retrospective	43	Surgery (n = 19) Surgery + RT (n = 24)	GTR (n = 28) STR (n = 11)	CRT 55.8 Gy	44	39% vs 71% at 5 y (P = .004)	NA	2% radionecrosis, 2% seizures
Bray et al,[40] 2021	Retrospective	162	Surgery (n = 54) Surgery + RT (n = 108)	GTR (n = 118) STR (n = 44)	CRT 18–60 Gy (n = 105) SRS (n = 3)	59	49% vs 94% at 5 y (P<.001)	NA	4% radionecrosis, 1% wound breakdown requiring surgery, 1% seizure
Kent et al,[41] 2022	Retrospective	66[d]	Surgery (n = 36) Surgery + RT (n = 28)	GTR (n = 25) STR (n = 28)	CRT 55.8 Gy	149	12% vs 58% at 10 y (SS)	41% vs 49% at 10 y (P = .30)	NA

Abbreviations: 3DCRT, 3-dimensional conformal radiation therapy; CRT, conventional radiation therapy; FU, follow-up; NA, not assessed; NS, not statistically significant; SS, statistically significant; STR, subtotal resection.

[a] Eighteen patients had prior WHO grade 1 meningiomas.
[b] Thirty-two patients with initial WHO grade 2 and GTR, as series includes recurrent grade 1 meningiomas.
[c] Eleven patients with WHO grade 2 and STR; series also includes initial grade 3 and recurrent grade 2 or 3 meningiomas.
[d] Fifty-two patients with WHO grade 2 and 14 with WHO grade 3; 2 had RT alone for unresectable disease.

Adjuvant Radiation Therapy in Anaplastic/Malignant (World Health Organization Grade 3) Meningiomas

Anaplastic/malignant or WHO grade 3 meningiomas are rare (1%–3% of all meningiomas) but very aggressive and associated with high rates of recurrence irrespective of their resection extent. Reported recurrence rates range from 50% to 94%, and median survival is between 3 and 6 years.[43,47,50–53] Small retrospective studies and 1 recent prospective observational study demonstrate an important role for adjuvant RT in anaplastic meningiomas of any resection extent. There have been no randomized controlled trials to date.

Several retrospective studies with relatively small size cohorts of anaplastic meningiomas have demonstrated the benefit of adjuvant RT in LC, PFS, and possibly OS, regardless of extent of surgical resection (selected studies summarized in **Table 4**).[18,54–62] In a retrospective study by Dziuk and colleagues,[54] which included 38 patients with malignant meningioma treated between 1984 and 1992, adjuvant RT (median, 54 Gy; range, 30.6–63 Gy) following initial resection was associated with a significantly better 5-year PFS of 80% versus 15% with surgery alone ($P = .002$). In a multicenter retrospective study by Champeaux and colleagues[57] that included 178 patients with WHO grade 3 meningiomas treated between 1989 and 2017, median OS was 2.9 years, and adjuvant RT (median, 59.4 Gy; IQR, 50.4–60 Gy) was an independent prognostic factor for survival (HR = 0.64; $P = .039$). In a retrospective study by Zhu and colleagues[60] from China of 63 anaplastic meningiomas among which 38 were newly diagnosed and treated between 2003 and 2008 (33 GTR, 5 STR), adjuvant RT (mean, 54 Gy; range 30–63 Gy) was found to be an independent factor associated with better PFS (HR = 0.198; $P = .002$). In their subgroup analysis of GTR and STR cohorts, adjuvant RT was associated with longer OS for both cohorts (HR = 0.193; $P = .003$; HR = 0.223; $P = .013$, respectively). In a Surveillance Epidemiology and End Results database (2000–2015) analysis by Li and colleagues,[61] which included 530 patients with high-grade meningiomas, adjuvant RT was associated with better OS in both WHO grade 3 meningioma patients (n = 178) who underwent GTR ($P<.0001$) and STR ($P = .022$).

Initial outcomes from NRG Oncology/RTOG-0539 of 53 patients in the high-risk meningioma cohort treated with adjuvant IMRT (60 Gy in 30 fractions) included 17 patients with initial WHO grade 3 meningiomas who underwent either GTR or STR, and their reported 3-year PFS and OS rates were 65% and 82%, respectively.[18] Most recurrences/progression observed in the study were either in-field or in-field and marginal with respect to RT planning target volume. Acute and late adverse events were limited to grades 1 to 3, except for a single necrosis-related grade 5 event.

In summary, based on prior retrospective studies as well as initial results of the recent RTOG-0539 trial, there is consensus that all anaplastic/malignant or WHO grade 3 meningiomas should undergo adjuvant RT, irrespective of surgical resection extent, with benefit in LC and PFS, and possibly OS. The optimal RT dose for anaplastic meningiomas is not well established, with several studies supporting LC benefit with greater than 60 Gy.[54,63,64] In general, based on the maximal safe dose deliverable to the surrounding brain structure, a minimum dose of 60 Gy is recommended in treating anaplastic meningiomas. Prospective studies investigating safe dose escalation techniques are needed, as tumor recurrence rates remain high even with 60 Gy in anaplastic meningiomas.

Radiation therapy in progressive/recurrent high-grade meningiomas after treatment

Clinicopathologic features associated with increased risk of recurrence include older age, nonconvexity tumor location, less than Simpson grade 1 resection, presence of brain invasion, a high number of mitoses per 10 high-power fields, and prominent nucleoli.[15,50,51,65] Studies suggest that meningiomas that recur following initial treatment (surgery and/or RT) behave more aggressively and are resistant to treatment compared with primary tumors, thus more difficult to control with salvage therapy.[14,23,31,60,66] Salvage therapy modalities generally include surgery, RT (fractionated, stereotactic radiosurgery [SRS], or brachytherapy), systemic therapy, or any combination of these, with treatment of choice dependent on patient symptoms, prior treatments, location, and extent of recurrent disease. In patients who previously had surgical resection alone, salvage RT is often used. In patients who received prior RT, reirradiation may be considered in certain cases, although there may be increased risk of toxicity, such as radionecrosis.

The recently published NRG Oncology/RTOG-0539 trial included 8 patients with recurrent WHO grade 2 and 5 patients with recurrent WHO grade 3 meningiomas of any resection extent treated with adjuvant RT (IMRT 60 Gy in 30 fractions). In the recurrent grade 2 cohort, the 3-year PFS and OS were 45% and 71%, respectively. In the recurrent grade 3 cohort, the 3-year PFS was 40%.

Table 4
Summary of selected major studies on adjuvant radiation therapy for anaplastic (World Health Organization grade 3) meningiomas

Author, y	Study Design	N	Treatment	Median RT Dose	Median FU (mo)	PFS	OS	Toxicity
Dziuk et al,[54] 1998	Retrospective	38	Surgery (n = 19) Surgery + RT (n = 19)	CRT 54 Gy	3–144	15% vs 80% at 5 y (P = .002)	NA	NA
Sughrue et al,[55] 2010	Retrospective	63	Surgery + RT (n = 63)	NA	60	57% at 5 y 40% at 10 y	61% at 5 y 40% at 10 y	19% neurologic morbidity
Sumner et al,[56] 2017	Retrospective	190	Surgery (n = 101) Surgery + RT (n = 89)	NA	56	NA	63% vs 79% at 5 y (P = .01)	NA
Champeux et al,[57] 2019	Retrospective	178[a]	Surgery + RT (n = 53)	CRT 59.4 Gy	54	NA	40% at 5 y 28% 10 y Adjuvant RT was an independent prognostic factor for OS (HR = 0.64; P = .039)	NA
Masalha et al,[58] 2019	Retrospective	36	Surgery (n = 8) Surgery + RT (n = 21)	CRT 59.4 Gy	49	25% vs 52% at 1 y 13% vs 19% at 3 y (P = .01)	63% vs 71% at 1 y 13% vs 19% at 3 y (P = .16)	NA
Zhou et al,[59] 2019	Retrospective	254	Surgery (n = 103) Surgery + RT (n = 151)	CRT 56 Gy	35	NA	38% vs 58% at 5 y (P = .011)	NA
Zhu et al,[60] 2019	Retrospective	63[b]	Surgery (n = 20) Surgery + RT (n = 43)	CRT 54 Gy SRS 14 Gy	77	Adjuvant RT associated with better PFS with HR = 0.198 (P = .002)	In subgroup analysis, adjuvant RT associated with longer OS in WHO grade 3 with GTR (HR = 0.193; P = .003) and STR (HR = 0.223; P = .013)	Acute grade 1–3 toxicities in 18 patients No late toxicities

Li et al,[61] 2019	Retrospective (SEER)	178[c]	Surgery (n = 58) Surgery + RT (n = 120)	NA	144	NA	Adjuvant RT associated with better OS in WHO grade 3 with GTR (P<.001) and STR (P = .002)	NA
Alhourani et al,[62] 2019	Retrospective (NCDB)	178	Surgery (n = 98) Surgery + RT (n = 80)	IMRT 54 Gy (n = 73) SRS (n = 7)	120	NA	Median OS 38.5 vs 32.8 mo (P = .57)	NA
Rogers et al,[18] 2020 (RTOG 0539)	Phase 2, nonrandomized	53[d]	Surgery + RT (n = 120)	IMRT 60 Gy (n = 52) 3DCRT 60 Gy (n = 1)	48	59% at 3 y for all 65% at 3 y for 17 patients with initial WHO grade 3	79% at 3 y for all 82% at 3 y for 17 with initial WHO grade 3	Most patients with grade 1–3 toxicity Necrosis-related grade 5 event (n = 1)

Abbreviation: NCDB, National Cancer Data Base.

a Sixty-seven patients had prior WHO grade 1 or 2 meningiomas.

b Study includes 162 patients among which 63 were WHO grade 3 and 38 had newly diagnosed WHO grade 3.

c Study includes 530 patients among which 178 patients had biopsy-confirmed WHO grade 3 meningiomas.

d Seventeen patients with initial WHO grade 3 as series includes recurrent grade 3, new grade 2 with subtotal resection, and recurrent grade 2 meningiomas.

Both of the recurrent grade 2 and 3 cohorts had inferior outcomes compared with the cohort with newly diagnosed WHO grade 3, which had 3-year PFS of 65% and 3-year OS of 82%.[18]

Few retrospective studies have reported the feasibility of reirradiation for recurrent meningiomas previously treated with RT. In a retrospective study by Lin and colleagues,[67] which included 43 patients receiving a second course of RT after prior SRS or fractionated RT, with very short 2-year results reported, LC, PFS, and OS rates were 70%, 43%, and 68%, respectively, with no significant difference between fractionated RT versus SRS. Toxicity of reirradiation was thought to be acceptable with grade 2 to 4 radionecrosis in 15% of patients. Other studies have shown that longer interval between prior RT and reirradiation may be associated with less cumulative radiation-associated toxicity, which would be in keeping with general irradiation principles.[1] Clinicians should be cautious, as most significant radiation toxicity arises over many years postirradiation.

Radiation Techniques

Conventional dosing for fractionated RT is typically 54 to 60 Gy in 1.8- to 2.0-Gy fractions. Prior studies suggest that dose-escalated external beam radiation therapy (EBRT) using cross-section imaging with CT or MRI improves clinical outcomes in high-grade meningiomas. EBRT techniques using IMRT or volumetric modulated arc therapy, which allow for highly conformal dose distribution, are preferred over 3-dimensional conformal RT.[68,69] Studies have shown that total dose greater than or equal to 60 Gy improves LC, whereas dose less than 50 to 54 Gy is associated with reduced or no benefits.[15,18,19,47,63,64,70] Studies have also looked at combined photon and proton RT to greater than 60 Gy (RBE), which may improve LC and possibly OS compared with lower doses with photon-based RT alone.[63]

SRS may be an alternative form of RT that can be convenient and effective for tumor size less than 10 cc, maximum diameter less than 3 to 4 cm, and sufficient distance from critical tissues at risk. SRS allows for delivery of high-dose RT in a single or few fractions with a steep dose fall-off at the edge of the target volume, sparing dose exposure to the surrounding brain structures. Techniques such as Gamma Knife, linear accelerator, or Cyber-Knife are commonly used to deliver SRS. With single-fraction SRS, typical doses used are 14 to 20 Gy. SRS is increasingly used in either adjuvant or, more frequently, salvage settings. A recent large retrospective multicenter study by Kowalchuk and colleagues[71] included 223 atypical meningiomas (with high-risk criteria per RTOG-0539) treated with SRS (median dose, 15 Gy; volume, 6.1 cc) and reported a 3-year PFS of 54%, comparable to the rate of 59% reported in the high-risk RTOG-0539 cohort. Another international, multi-center retrospective study by Shepard and colleagues,[72] which included 223 atypical and 38 anaplastic meningiomas patients treated with Gamma Knife SRS (median dose, 15 Gy; volume, 7.5 cc), reported a 5-year PFS of 34%. A smaller study by Kano and colleagues[73] of 12 patients with high-grade meningioma with 30 lesions treated by SRS (mean dose, 18 Gy; volume, 4.4 cc) showed that marginal dose less than 20 Gy was a significant predictor of short-term progression with an inferior 5-year PFS of 29% compared with 63% in lesions treated with 20 Gy. Although LC within treated tumor volume has been acceptable with SRS, marginal failures remain a challenge with SRS.[74]

There have been a limited number of small studies reporting the outcomes of particle therapy using proton and/or carbon ion therapy for high-grade meningiomas. Proton and carbon ion RT both offer the advantages of highly localized deposition of energy in the tumor target while minimizing dose to surrounding nontarget structures owing to the Bragg peak phenomenon, allowing for overall higher-dose delivery to the target with less collateral damage to adjacent healthy tissue. Prior studies have reported comparable rates of LC to conventional photon-based RT. A systemic review by Coggins and colleagues,[75] which reviewed 12 published works on particle therapy RT for high-grade meningiomas, reported a mean LC rate of 60% at 5 years with proton therapy (mean, 64 Gy [RBE]; range, 52 to 72 Gy [RBE]) and LC rates of 95% and 63% at 2 years with carbon ion therapy (mean, 57.6 Gy; range, 30–68.4 Gy) for grade 2 and 3 meningiomas, respectively.

Other forms of local RT include interstitial brachytherapy, which can be an effective adjunct to surgery, and EBRT for aggressive and/or recurrent tumors. However, interstitial brachytherapy is associated with high rates of complications. A study by Ware and colleagues,[76] including 21 patients with recurrent high-grade meningiomas, reported a 27% rate of wound complications requiring surgical intervention and 27% rate of radionecrosis with 13% requiring surgery. Salvage brachytherapy with I-125 or Cs-131 seeds for recurrent, previously irradiated high-grade meningiomas has also been associated with a high reoperation rate of 40% owing to wound complications.[77]

Radiation Toxicity

Adjuvant RT with conventional fractionated doses of 54 to 60 Gy is generally associated with modest toxicity, and reported significant adverse events range from 0% to 17%, including radionecrosis (0%–15%), visual disturbances (2%–5%), hypopituitarism (5%–30%), and cognitive impairment (2%–17%).[78] With SRS, up to 27% rates of toxicity have been reported, although this rate can be less than 10% when limited volumes are treated.[73,74,79–82] Factors that may increase one's risk of radiation-related toxicities include older age, poor performance status at baseline, large treatment volume, and proximity of target to critical structures, such as the optic pathways or pituitary gland.[83–85] In patients with symptomatic radiation-induced edema or necrosis, initial management generally includes moderate dose glucocorticoid with a taper course over several weeks. For patients who fail to achieve symptomatic response to conservative management, various other treatment options including bevacizumab, surgical resection, and laser interstitial therapy (LITT) may be considered.[86] Potential RT toxicity and morbidity must be balanced with tumor control benefit of RT, taking into consideration patient and tumor characteristics.

Clinical Trials and Future Directions

Several prospective trials aim to further define the role and clinical outcomes of RT in high-grade meningiomas. To address the main controversy regarding the role of adjuvant RT in gross totally resected atypical meningiomas, there are 2 cooperative group randomized controlled trials currently underway comparing adjuvant RT versus surveillance that will help guide optimal postoperative management of such patients. The ROAM/EORTC-1308 trial recently closed in 2021, and results from the study are anticipated in 2025. Another trial, NRG Oncology BN003, is currently accruing patients. Outcomes of interest include PFS, treatment toxicity, quality of life, neurocognitive function, time to second-line treatment, and OS. In addition, secondary analyses investigating clinicopathologic and molecular features that predict most benefit from adjuvant RT will be important. Furthermore, clinical trials investigating ion beam RT including proton (NCT02693990, NCT01117844, NCT02978677 [proton dose escalation]) and carbon ion therapy (NCT01166321) in high-grade meningiomas are currently underway to better define the efficacy and clinical outcomes of ion beam RT compared with photon RT.

With regards to future directions, as molecularly based classifications are emerging in various central nervous system tumors, such classification in meningioma, which allows for better understanding of tumor biology, response to RT, and potential targeted treatment, will be crucial.

SUMMARY

In summary, high-grade meningiomas (WHO grade 2 and 3) are at increased risk for recurrence following initial treatment with maximum safe surgical resection. Evidence from retrospective data and few prospective nonrandomized studies supportS an important role of RT in both adjuvant and salvage settings. Currently, adjuvant RT is advised for subtotally resected grade 2 and all grade 3 meningiomas irrespective of resection extent given LC, PFS, and potential OS benefit. For gross totally resected grade 2 meningiomas, the timing of adjuvant RT remains controversial with some divergent results from retrospective studies, although 2 recent prospective observational studies (RTOG-0539 and EORTC 22042-26042) have demonstrated excellent outcomes in such patients receiving adjuvant RT. Although upfront adjuvant RT may be considered for these patients given the aggressive and resistant nature of meningiomas at recurrence, potential treatment toxicity and clinicopathologic characteristics as well as individual patient preference should be factored in deciding between adjuvant RT versus close surveillance. The results from ROAM/EORTC-1308 and NRG Oncology BN003 are anticipated to be practice-changing and guide optimal postoperative management in completed resected atypical meningiomas.

CLINICS CARE POINTS

- Subtotally resected World Health Organization grade 2 and all grade 3 meningiomas irrespective of resection extent should be treated with adjuvant radiation therapy.
- In completely resected World Health Organization grade 2 (atypical) meningiomas, the probable disease control benefit of adjuvant radiation therapy should be weighed against the risks of radiation therapy.
- Clinicopathologic features and patient preferences should be considered in identifying patients who best benefit from adjuvant radiation therapy.

DISCLOSURE

All authors have indicated they have no financial relationships relevant to this article to disclose.

REFERENCES

1. Zhi M, Girvigian MR, Miller MJ, et al. Long-term outcomes of newly diagnosed resected atypical meningiomas and the role of adjuvant radiotherapy. World Neurosurgery 2019;122:e1153–61.
2. Rogers L, Barani I, Chamberlain M, et al. Meningiomas: knowledge base, treatment outcomes, and uncertainties. A RANO review. J Neurosurg 2015; 122(1):4–23.
3. Louis DN, Perry A, Reifenberger G, et al. The 2016 World Health Organization classification of tumors of the central nervous system: a summary. Acta Neuropathol 2016;131(6):803–20.
4. Louis DN, Perry A, Wesseling P, et al. The 2021 WHO classification of tumors of the central nervous system: a summary. Neuro Oncol 2021;23(8):1231–51.
5. Louis DN, Ohgaki H, Wiestler OD, et al. The 2007 WHO classification of tumours of the central nervous system. Acta Neuropathol 2007;114(2):97–109.
6. Hwang KL, Hwang WL, Bussière MR, et al. The role of radiotherapy in the management of high-grade meningiomas. Chin Clin Oncol 2017;6(Suppl 1):S5.
7. Kleihues P, Burger PC, Scheithauer BW. Histological typing of tumours of the central nervous system. Springer Berlin Heidelberg 1993. https://doi.org/10.1007/978-3-642-84988-6.
8. Torp SH, Solheim O, Skjulsvik AJ. The WHO 2021 classification of central nervous system tumours: a practical update on what neurosurgeons need to know—a minireview. Acta Neurochir 2022;164(9):2453–64.
9. Ostrom QT, Cioffi G, Waite K, et al. CBTRUS statistical report: primary brain and other central nervous system tumors diagnosed in the United States in 2014–2018. Neuro Oncol 2021;23(Supplement_3). https://doi.org/10.1093/neuonc/noab200. iii1-iii105.
10. Bi WL, Zhang M, Wu WW, et al. Meningioma genomics: diagnostic, prognostic, and therapeutic applications. Front Surg 2016;3. https://doi.org/10.3389/fsurg.2016.00040.
11. Smith SJ, Boddu S, Macarthur DC. Atypical meningiomas: WHO moved the goalposts? Br J Neurosurg 2007;21(6):588–92.
12. Simpson D. The recurrence of intracranial meningiomas after surgical treatment. J Neurol Neurosurg Psychiatry 1957;20(1):22–39.
13. Hardesty DA, Wolf AB, Brachman DG, et al. The impact of adjuvant stereotactic radiosurgery on atypical meningioma recurrence following aggressive microsurgical resection. J Neurosurg 2013;119(2):475–81.
14. Lee G, Lamba N, Niemierko A, et al. Adjuvant radiation therapy versus surveillance after surgical resection of atypical meningiomas. Int J Radiat Oncol Biol Phys 2021;109(1):252–66.
15. Aghi MK, Carter BS, Cosgrove GR, et al. Long-term recurrence rates of atypical meningiomas after gross total resection with or without postoperative adjuvant radiation. Neurosurgery 2009;64(1):56–60 [discussion: 60].
16. Aizer AA, Arvold ND, Catalano P, et al. Adjuvant radiation therapy, local recurrence, and the need for salvage therapy in atypical meningioma. Neuro Oncol 2014;16(11):1547–53.
17. Park H, Kim I, Jung H. Atypical meningioma: outcomes and prognostic factors. Int J Radiat Oncol Biol Phys 2009;75(3):S238.
18. Rogers CL, Won M, Vogelbaum MA, et al. High-risk meningioma: initial outcomes from NRG Oncology/RTOG 0539. Int J Radiat Oncol Biol Phys 2020; 106(4):790–9.
19. Weber DC, Ares C, Villa S, et al. Adjuvant postoperative high-dose radiotherapy for atypical and malignant meningioma: A phase-II parallel nonrandomized and observation study (EORTC 22042-26042). Radiother Oncol 2018;128(2):260–5.
20. Mair R, Morris K, Scott I, et al. Radiotherapy for atypical meningiomas. J Neurosurg 2011;115(4):811–9.
21. Komotar RJ, Iorgulescu JB, Raper DMS, et al. The role of radiotherapy following gross-total resection of atypical meningiomas. J Neurosurg 2012;117(4):679–86.
22. Park HJ, Kang HC, Kim IH, et al. The role of adjuvant radiotherapy in atypical meningioma. J Neuro Oncol 2013;115(2):241–7.
23. Bagshaw HP, Burt LM, Jensen RL, et al. Adjuvant radiotherapy for atypical meningiomas. J Neurosurg 2017;126(6):1822–8.
24. Hammouche S, Clark S, Wong AHL, et al. Long-term survival analysis of atypical meningiomas: survival rates, prognostic factors, operative and radiotherapy treatment. Acta Neurochir 2014;156(8):1475–81.
25. Yoon H, Mehta M, Perumal K, et al. Atypical meningioma: Randomized trials are required to resolve contradictory retrospective results regarding the role of adjuvant radiotherapy. J Can Res Ther 2015;11(1):59.
26. Jenkinson MD, Waqar M, Farah JO, et al. Early adjuvant radiotherapy in the treatment of atypical meningioma. J Clin Neurosci 2016;28:87–92.
27. Dohm A, McTyre ER, Chan MD, et al. Early or late radiotherapy following gross or subtotal resection for atypical meningiomas: Clinical outcomes and local control. J Clin Neurosci 2017;46:90–8.
28. Champeaux C, Houston D, Dunn L. Atypical meningioma. A study on recurrence and disease-specific survival. Neurochirurgie 2017;63(4):273–81.
29. Rogers L, Zhang P, Vogelbaum MA, et al. Intermediate-risk meningioma: initial outcomes from NRG Oncology RTOG 0539. J Neurosurg 2018;129(1):35–47.
30. Masalha W, Heiland DH, Franco P, et al. Atypical meningioma: progression-free survival in 161 cases treated at our institution with surgery versus surgery and radiotherapy. J Neuro Oncol 2018;136(1):147–54.

31. Chen WC, Hara J, Magill ST, et al. Salvage therapy outcomes for atypical meningioma. J Neuro Oncol 2018;138(2):425–33.

32. Budohoski KP, Clerkin J, Millward CP, et al. Predictors of early progression of surgically treated atypical meningiomas. Acta Neurochir 2018;160(9):1813–22.

33. Li H, Zhang YS, Zhang GB, et al. Treatment protocol, long-term follow-up, and predictors of mortality in 302 cases of atypical meningioma. World Neurosurgery 2019;122:e1275–84.

34. Zeng Q, Shi F, Guo Z. Effectiveness of postoperative radiotherapy on atypical meningioma patients: a population-based study. Front Oncol 2019;9:34.

35. Hemmati SM, Ghadjar P, Grün A, et al. Adjuvant radiotherapy improves progression-free survival in intracranial atypical meningioma. Radiat Oncol 2019;14(1):160.

36. Keric N, Kalasauskas D, Freyschlag CF, et al. Impact of postoperative radiotherapy on recurrence of primary intracranial atypical meningiomas. J Neuro Oncol 2020;146(2):347–55.

37. Poulen G, Vignes JR, Le Corre M, et al. WHO grade II meningioma: Epidemiology, survival and contribution of postoperative radiotherapy in a multicenter cohort of 88 patients. Neurochirurgie 2020;66(2):73–9.

38. Torres-Bayona S, Gil-Durán M, Rodríguez-Hernández P, et al. Radiotherapy versus observation after surgical resection of atypical meningiomas. Interdisciplinary Neurosurgery 2021;25:101201.

39. Unterberger A, Ng E, Pradhan A, et al. Adjuvant radiotherapy for atypical meningiomas is associated with improved progression free survival. J Neurol Sci 2021;428:117590.

40. Bray DP, Quillin JW, Press RH, et al. Adjuvant radiotherapy versus watchful waiting for World Health Organization grade II atypical meningioma: a single-institution experience. Neurosurgery 2021;88(5):E435–42.

41. Kent CL, Mowery YM, Babatunde O, et al. Long-term outcomes for patients with atypical or malignant meningiomas treated with or without radiation therapy: a 25-year retrospective analysis of a single-institution experience. Advances in Radiation Oncology 2022;7(3):100878.

42. Song D, Xu D, Han H, et al. Postoperative adjuvant radiotherapy in atypical meningioma patients: a meta-analysis study. Front Oncol 2021;11:787962.

43. Stessin AM, Schwartz A, Judanin G, et al. Does adjuvant external-beam radiotherapy improve outcomes for nonbenign meningiomas? A Surveillance, Epidemiology, and End Results (SEER)-based analysis. J Neurosurg 2012;117(4):669–75.

44. Rydzewski NR, Lesniak MS, Chandler JP, et al. Gross total resection and adjuvant radiotherapy most significant predictors of improved survival in patients with atypical meningioma: Resection and RT for Atypical Meningioma. Cancer 2018;124(4):734–42.

45. Brown DA, Goyal A, Kerezoudis P, et al. Adjuvant radiation for WHO grade II and III intracranial meningiomas: insights on survival and practice patterns from a National Cancer Registry. J Neuro Oncol 2020;149(2):293–303.

46. Aizer AA, Bi WL, Kandola MS, et al. Extent of resection and overall survival for patients with atypical and malignant meningioma: Extent of Resection and Recurrence in Meningioma. Cancer 2015;121(24):4376–81.

47. Goldsmith BJ, Wara WM, Wilson CB, et al. Postoperative irradiation for subtotally resected meningiomas. A retrospective analysis of 140 patients treated from 1967 to 1990. J Neurosurg 1994;80(2):195–201.

48. Wang C, Kaprealian TB, Suh JH, et al. Overall survival benefit associated with adjuvant radiotherapy in WHO grade II meningioma. Neuro Oncol 2017;19(9):1263–70.

49. Unterberger A, Nguyen T, Duong C, et al. Meta-analysis of adjuvant radiotherapy for intracranial atypical and malignant meningiomas. J Neuro Oncol 2021;152(2):205–16.

50. Palma L, Celli P, Franco C, et al. Long-term prognosis for atypical and malignant meningiomas: a study of 71 surgical cases. J Neurosurg 1997;86(5):793–800.

51. Pasquier D, Bijmolt S, Veninga T, et al. Atypical and malignant meningioma: outcome and prognostic factors in 119 irradiated patients. a multicenter, retrospective study of the rare cancer network. Int J Radiat Oncol Biol Phys 2008;71(5):1388–93.

52. Perry A, Scheithauer BW, Stafford SL, et al. "Malignancy" in meningiomas: A clinicopathologic study of 116 patients, with grading implications. Cancer 1999;85(9):2046–56.

53. Perry A, Stafford SL, Scheithauer BW, et al. Meningioma grading: an analysis of histologic parameters. Am J Surg Pathol 1997;21(12):1455–65.

54. Dziuk TW, Woo S, Butler EB, et al. Malignant meningioma: An indication for initial aggressive surgery and adjuvant radiotherapy. J Neuro Oncol 1998;37(2):177–88.

55. Sughrue ME, Sanai N, Shangari G, et al. Outcome and survival following primary and repeat surgery for World Health Organization Grade III meningiomas. J Neurosurg 2010;113(2):202–9.

56. Sumner WA, Amini A, Hankinson TC, et al. Survival benefit of postoperative radiation in papillary meningioma: Analysis of the National Cancer Data Base. Rep Practical Oncol Radiother 2017;22(6):495–501.

57. Champeaux C, Jecko V, Houston D, et al. Malignant meningioma: an international multicentre retrospective study. Neurosurg 2019;85(3):E461–9.

58. Masalha W, Heiland DH, Delev D, et al. Survival and prognostic predictors of anaplastic meningiomas. World Neurosurgery 2019;131:e321–8.

59. Zhou H, Bai HX, Chan L, et al. Survival benefit of adjuvant radiotherapy in elderly patients with WHO grade III meningioma. World Neurosurgery 2019;131:e303–11.

60. Zhu H, Bi WL, Aizer A, et al. Efficacy of adjuvant radiotherapy for atypical and anaplastic meningioma. Cancer Med 2019;8(1):13–20.

61. Li D, Jiang P, Xu S, et al. Survival impacts of extent of resection and adjuvant radiotherapy for the modern management of high-grade meningiomas. J Neuro Oncol 2019;145(1):125–34.

62. Alhourani A, Aljuboori Z, Yusuf M, et al. Management trends for anaplastic meningioma with adjuvant radiotherapy and predictors of long-term survival. Neurosurg Focus 2019;46(6):E4.

63. Hug EB, Devries A, Thornton AF, et al. Management of atypical and malignant meningiomas: role of high-dose, 3D-conformal radiation therapy. J Neuro Oncol 2000;48(2):151–60.

64. Milosevic MF, Frost PJ, Laperriere NJ, et al. Radiotherapy for atypical or malignant intracranial meningioma. Int J Radiat Oncol Biol Phys 1996;34(4):817–22.

65. Yang SY, Park CK, Park SH, et al. Atypical and anaplastic meningiomas: prognostic implications of clinicopathological features. J Neurol Neurosurg Psychiatry 2008;79(5):574–80.

66. Lubgan D, Rutzner S, Lambrecht U, et al. Stereotactic radiotherapy as primary definitive or postoperative treatment of intracranial meningioma of WHO grade II and III leads to better disease control than stereotactic radiotherapy of recurrent meningioma. J Neuro Oncol 2017;134(2):407–16.

67. Lin AJ, Hui C, Dahiya S, et al. Radiologic response and disease control of recurrent intracranial meningiomas treated with reirradiation. Int J Radiat Oncol Biol Phys 2018;102(1):194–203.

68. MacDonald SM, Ahmad S, Kachris S, et al. Intensity modulated radiation therapy versus three-dimensional conformal radiation therapy for the treatment of high grade glioma: a dosimetric comparison. J Appl Clin Med Phys 2007;8(2):47–60.

69. Wagner D, Christiansen H, Wolff H, et al. Radiotherapy of malignant gliomas: Comparison of volumetric single arc technique (RapidArc), dynamic intensity-modulated technique and 3D conformal technique. Radiother Oncol 2009;93(3):593–6.

70. Kaur G, Sayegh ET, Larson A, et al. Adjuvant radiotherapy for atypical and malignant meningiomas: a systematic review. Neuro Oncol 2014;16(5):628–36.

71. Kowalchuk RO, Shepard MJ, Sheehan K, et al. Treatment of WHO Grade 2 Meningiomas With Stereotactic Radiosurgery: Identification of an Optimal Group for SRS Using RPA. Int J Radiat Oncol Biol Phys 2021;110(3):804–14.

72. Shepard MJ, Xu Z, Kearns K, et al. Stereotactic radiosurgery for atypical (World Health Organization II) and anaplastic (World Health Organization III) meningiomas: results from a multicenter, international cohort study. Neurosurgery 2021;88(5):980–8.

73. Kano H, Takahashi JA, Katsuki T, et al. Stereotactic radiosurgery for atypical and anaplastic meningiomas. J Neuro Oncol 2007;84(1):41–7.

74. Attia A, Chan MD, Mott RT, et al. Patterns of failure after treatment of atypical meningioma with gamma knife radiosurgery. J Neuro Oncol 2012;108(1):179–85.

75. Coggins WS, Pham NK, Nguyen AV, et al. A systematic review of ion radiotherapy in maintaining local control regarding atypical and anaplastic meningiomas. World Neurosurgery 2019;132:282–91.

76. Ware ML, Larson DA, Sneed PK, et al. Surgical resection and permanent brachytherapy for recurrent atypical and malignant meningioma. Neurosurgery 2004;54(1):55–63 [discussion: 63-64].

77. Koch MJ, Agarwalla PK, Royce TJ, et al. Brachytherapy as an adjuvant for recurrent atypical and malignant meningiomas. Neurosurg 2019;85(5):E910–6.

78. Vagnoni L, Aburas S, Giraffa M, et al. Radiation therapy for atypical and anaplastic meningiomas: an overview of current results and controversial issues. Neurosurg Rev 2022. https://doi.org/10.1007/s10143-022-01806-3.

79. Pollock BE, Stafford SL, Link MJ, et al. Stereotactic radiosurgery of World Health Organization grade II and III intracranial meningiomas: Treatment results on the basis of a 22-year experience. Cancer 2012;118(4):1048–54.

80. Helis CA, Hughes RT, Cramer CK, et al. Stereotactic radiosurgery for atypical and anaplastic meningiomas. World Neurosurgery 2020;144:e53–61.

81. Kondziolka D, Mathieu D, Lunsford LD, et al. Radiosurgery as definitive management of intracranial meningiomas. Neurosurgery 2008;62(1):53–60.

82. El-Khatib M, El Majdoub F, Hoevels M, et al. Stereotactic LINAC radiosurgery for incompletely resected or recurrent atypical and anaplastic meningiomas. Acta Neurochir 2011;153(9):1761–7.

83. Darzy KH, Shalet SM. Hypopituitarism following radiotherapy. Pituitary 2009;12(1):40–50.

84. Farzin M, Molls M, Kampfer S, et al. Optic toxicity in radiation treatment of meningioma: a retrospective study in 213 patients. J Neuro Oncol 2016;127(3):597–606.

85. Smart D. Radiation toxicity in the central nervous system: mechanisms and strategies for injury reduction. Semin Radiat Oncol 2017;27(4):332–9.

86. Vellayappan B, Tan CL, Yong C, et al. Diagnosis and Management of Radiation Necrosis in Patients With Brain Metastases. Front Oncol 2018;8:395.

Modeling Meningiomas
Optimizing Treatment Approach

Majid Khan, BS[a], Chadwin Hanna, BS[b], Matthew Findlay, BS[c],
Brandon Lucke-Wold, MD, PhD[b], Michael Karsy, MD, PhD, MSc[d],*,
Randy L. Jensen, MD, PhD, MHPE[d]

KEYWORDS

- Preclinical models • Meningiomas • Emerging treatments • Subclassification

KEY POINTS

- Current models of meningioma include in vitro cell culture, heterotopic animal flank models, orthotopic intracranial animal models, and genetically engineered mouse models.
- Preclinical models have been limited in translating treatment findings into clinical use.
- More recent understanding of meningioma driver mutations and advances in CRISPR/Cas9 technology may allow for more refined preclinical meningioma models.
- Artificial intelligence and radiomics may aid characterizing meningiomas and offer noninvasive methods to differentiate tumors.

INTRODUCTION

One of the key barriers for developing systemic treatments for meningiomas has been the lack of preclinical models.[1] Although meningiomas are among the most abundant brain and spinal tumors, no systemic agent exists to limit tumor growth or selectively target tumor cells. Recently, the ability to establish preclinical models has begun to shift the field as technology improves. Cultured human meningioma cells have been used successfully for testing pharmaceutical agents of interest, and several agents are now advancing to clinical trials.[2] There are some shortcomings in cell culture technology, namely the limited number of passages that can be obtained and the difficulty in optimizing the specific culture medium milieu that is required.[3] Mouse models have therefore been established using xenograft human cell lines or genetically engineered mouse models (GEMM).[4] NF2 tumor suppressor gene modifications in murine models have also yielded spontaneous meningeal tumorigenesis.[5] Yet questions remain about the accuracy of predicting actual tumor mechanisms and microenvironments with these approaches.

Some preclinical models now provide important insights into the molecular basis for tumor growth and overall tumor aggressiveness.[6] Next-generation sequencing of these cultured tumor cells offers insight into which meningioma subtypes may be amenable to radiation.[7] For example, trabectedin and histone deacetylase inhibitors have emerged as prime candidates for aborting tumor growth and are now in clinical trials.[8] Beyond the bench, artificial intelligence (AI) is offering new tools for investigation. Neural networks have aided in quicker classification and automated histologic interpretation.[9] Because the field has rapidly expanded, a systematic review overviewing preclinical model type, proposed areas of utility, and recent advances in technology is warranted. Here, we provide a clearer understanding of the preclinical models used in meningioma research.

[a] Reno School of Medicine, University of Nevada, Reno, NV, USA; [b] Department of Neurosurgery, University of Florida, Gainesville, FL, USA; [c] School of Medicine, University of Utah, Salt Lake City, UT, USA; [d] Department of Neurosurgery, Clinical Neurosciences Center, University of Utah, 175 North Medical Drive East, Salt Lake City, UT 84132, USA
* Corresponding author.
E-mail address: neuropub@hsc.utah.edu

Neurosurg Clin N Am 34 (2023) 479–492
https://doi.org/10.1016/j.nec.2023.02.014
1042-3680/23/© 2023 Elsevier Inc. All rights reserved.

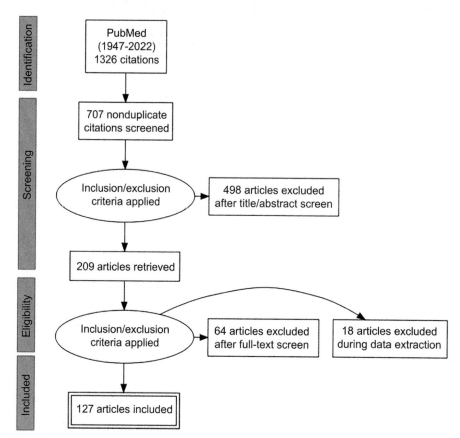

Fig. 1. PRISMA flow diagram.

METHODS

A systematic review of the literature identified from the PubMed database was performed in accordance with the PRISMA guidelines. A comprehensive search using the search ["meningioma" AND ("preclinical models" OR "mouse models" OR "model" OR "vitro" OR "vivo" OR "artificial intelligence" OR "machine learning" OR "AI" OR "ML")] was conducted, including all studies from database inception until May 2022. Publications describing modeling of meningiomas in vivo or in vitro and using cell culture, animal, machine learning, AI, or preclinical entities were included. Reviews, retrospective studies, trials, case reports, incomplete papers, and non-English studies were excluded.

RESULTS
Article Selection

A total of 1326 articles were screened from the literature search (**Fig. 1**). After removal of duplicates, 707 of these studies were then assessed for evaluation of inclusion/exclusion criteria. Of these, 498 studies were excluded for the following reasons: review article, cohort study, retrospective

study, clinical trial, meta-analysis, case report, cross-sectional study, retraction, or non-English. A further 82 articles were excluded during article full-text and data screening. Ultimately, 127 studies were included in this review. The various approaches for modeling meningiomas are summarized in **Fig. 2**.

In Vitro Modeling

In vitro modeling of meningiomas uses cell techniques using tissue culture obtained from human meningioma patients.[1] These cell lines and their characteristics are summarized in **Table 1**. The Ben-Men-1 cell line, which exhibits similar cytologic, immunocytochemical, structural, and genetic features to most meningiomas, is derived from a benign World Health Organization (WHO) grade 1 meningioma tumor.[10,11] However, the Ben-Men-1 cell line does not account for immortalization because of cell senescence, and thus other cell lines have been developed to prevent this (ie, SF-4422 and Me3TSC).[4,12,13] The variety of meningioma cell lines, from less aggressive WHO grade I primary tumor samples (eg, Ben-Men-1 and HBL-52) to more aggressive WHO grade III primary tumors (eg, IOMM-Lee, CH157-

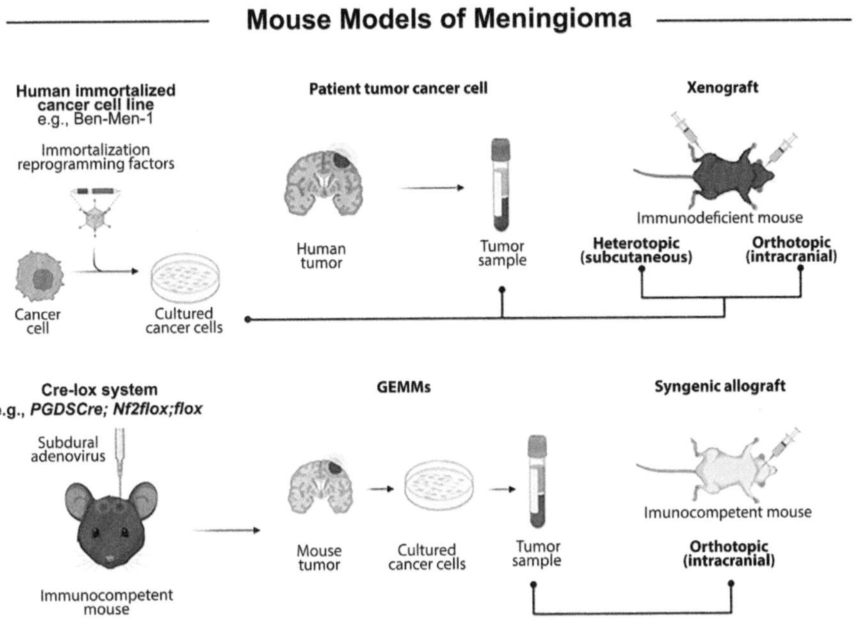

Mouse Models of Meningioma

Fig. 2. Comparison of various mouse models of meningioma. Several in vitro–derived meningioma cancer cell lines currently exist along with the potential for immortalization of new lines. Patient-derived tumor cell lines remain challenging to generate. Xenograft models can involve injections of tumor cells or tissue into animal flanks (heterotopic) or cranial cavity (orthotopic). Several methods for genetically engineered mouse models (GEMMs) can include use of the Cre-lox system for targeted germline mutation and the introduction of genetically modified cells into immunocompromised animals.

MN, KT21), allows for greater modeling capabilities.[11,14] Although IOMM-Lee initially lacked the NF2 mutation, which is the primary cause of malignancy in meningiomas in vivo, an NF2 mutant cell line (CH157-MN) and a Clustered Regularly Interspaced Short Palindromic Repeats (CRISPR)/CRISPR-associated protein 9 (Cas9) NF2 mutation gene edited cell line (IOMM-Lee) have been generated to improve insight into the role of this mutation.[15–17] Furthermore, a WHO grade II meningioma cell line (MENII-1) is available.[18]

In vitro preclinical models have been used in study of the therapeutic efficacy of radiation,[19] chemotherapy,[20–23] anti-platelet-derived growth

Table 1
Summary of meningioma cell line characteristics

Name	Phenotype	Immortalization	Genetics	References
BenMen1	Grade I, meningothelial	hTERT	22q loss NF2 mutant	Puttman et al,[10] 2005
Me3TSC	Grade I, meningothelial	hTERT + SV40	—	Cargioli et al,[13] 2007
SF4433	Grade I, meningothelial	hTERT + HPV E6/E7	No 22q loss	Baia et al,[12] 2006
HBL-52	Grade I, meningothelial	—	TRAF7 mutant	Mei et al,[11] 2017, Akat et al,[128] 2008
IOMM-Lee	Grade III	—	No 22q loss	Lee WH,[14] 1999
CH157-MN	Grade III	—	22q loss *NF2* mutant	Tsai et al,[129] 1995
MENII-1	Grade II	hTERT + HPV E6/E7	22q loss	Striedinger et al,[18] 2008
KT 21	Grade III	—	22q loss C-myc	Tanaka et al,[130] 1989

factor (PDGF) and anti-vascular endothelial growth factor (VEGF) targeting,[24–26] and other gene and monoclonal antibody therapies.[24,27–30] Furthermore, these cell lines provide insight into cellular characteristics, such as receptor expression and activity,[31–33] cellular and molecular profiles,[34] genetics,[35,36] molecular signaling,[37–39] and metabolite levels.[40,41] Three-dimensional in vitro cell culture and organoid models of meningioma cell lines are also recently feasible platforms for studying meningiomas.[42] Recent technological advancements have also allowed for CRISPR and Cas9 gene editing in meningioma cell lines, which allow for cell clone generation, gene knock-out/In studies, and new cell-line generation.[15,43]

In Vivo Modeling

In vivo modeling of meningiomas involves the injection of meningioma cells or virus into animals, inducing meningioma.[1] These in vivo models are characterized as xenograft models (eg, heterotopic and orthotropic models) (**Table 2**),[44–46] GEMMs (**Table 3**),[1,4,46] and further syngeneic allograft models (ie, animals with intact immune systems).[4] Heterotopic modeling of meningiomas uses primary cells or generated cell lines in nonneural locations, such as the flank, to induce development of tumor.[47] The tumor is injected subcutaneously, with induction rates (ie, tumor take) around 60%.[4,48] Furthermore, tumor formation in this model system is improved with compounds simulating a tumor microenvironment (eg, Matrigel, Corning Life Sciences, Pittston, PA).[44,48] On the other hand, orthotopic modeling involves intracranial tumor injection.[45,49,50] The injection site, number of cells, and injection volumes are commonly adjusted, allowing for study flexibility and increased outcomes assessments.[45,49,51] Thus, higher rates of tumor induction (mean, 97%) are seen in orthotopic technique as a result of direct brain targeting and bypassing the blood-brain barrier.[4,10,13,49,50,52–58] Both heterotopic and orthotopic models allow for evaluation of tumor inhibition treatments, such as chemotherapeutics and monoclonal antibodies, with the understanding that the animal is immunodeficient (ie, little to no primary host immune system effect on experiment/treatment), and gene manipulation studies.[28,30,37,38,51,59]

GEMMs mimic their human meningioma counterparts and further allow for increased experimental control through gene manipulation.[1,46,60] Compared with xenograft models, meningioma prevalence is lower (mean, 42%).[17,61–65] The Cre-loxP system, which was first used to modulate the NF2 gene, initially pioneered the understanding of murine meningioma tumorigenesis and has since further allowed for generation of higher-grade tumorigenesis.[61,66] NF2 knockout mutations do not initially produce tumors, but altering chromosome 21, which controls tumor suppressor genes, can result in meningioma development and proliferation. However, these mutations have variable responses in tumor grade alteration. In addition, p53 mutations do not promote murine meningioma tumorigenesis alone.[62] Ultimately, NF2 inactivation combined with tumor suppressor (CDKN2AB) deletion has been necessary for tumor generation, resulting in grade II and III meningiomas.[17] The meningeal promotor (prostaglandin-D2-synthase [PGDS]) allows for induction of oncogenic mutations and has led to development of second-generation meningioma GEMMs (PGDSCre-SmoM2).[65,67] The RCAS-TVA system has also been evaluated in GEMMs.

The CRISPR/Cas9 system allows for genetic manipulation of animal models at a low cost.[15,60] This, in conjunction with the methods mentioned previously, allows for increased accessibility for scientists and clinicians studying meningiomas. GEMMs and CRISPR technologies allow study of specific somatic mutations found in human meningiomas and the ability to explore the impact of new promotor targets through generating germline mutations.[68,69] Development of stable models for reproducible further study or re-creation of a clinical phenotype seems reasonable via the use of CRISPR/Cas9. Moreover, TRAF7, AKT1, PIK3CA, and other meningiomas with driver mutations have yet to be generated and fully investigated.

Artificial Intelligence/Machine Learning/Imaging Technologies

Advances in noninvasive monitoring of meningiomas have greatly improved the use of animal models. The main methods of monitoring tumor induction, growth, and treatment efficacy are via bioluminescence and small-animal MRI (see later).[45,50,70] Recently, a fluorescently guided imaging technique was introduced that allows for the possibility of selective meningioma identification in vivo and in vitro.[34] These tools improve the evaluation of novel tumor models and preclinical treatments in a more cost-effective manner.

With recent advances in AI, there has been a surge of research dedicated to the use of AI models for predicting disease diagnoses and treatment outcomes.[71,72] In meningioma research, AI models are being integrated into MRI radiomics modalities to preoperatively differentiate meningiomas from other intracranial masses and to accurately predict important diagnostic variables, such as grade,

Table 2
Summary of orthotopic xenograft models

Mouse Strain/ Age of Injection (wk)	Injected Cell Types (WHO Grade)/ Numbers/Volume (µL)	Site of Injection	Tumor Take (%)	Treatment	Clinical Results	References
Athymic/6	IOMM-Lee (III); human tumor/106/10	WM/TF floor	85–100	—	—	Jensen et al,[49] 1998
Athymic/6-8	IOMM-Lee (III)/106/3	TF floor	100	Verotoxin	Inhibition of TG	Salhia et al,[52] 2002
Athymic/6	BenMenI (I)	Convexity	100	—	—	Puttmann et al,[10] 2005
Athymic/6-8	IOMM-Lee (III)/5.105	Brain	100	siRNA	Inhibition of TG	Kondraganti et al,[131] 2006
Athymic/4	Me3TSC (I)-Me10 T (I)/106/5	Convexity (SDS)	100	—	—	Baia et al,[12] 2006 & Cargioli et al,[13] 2007
Athymic/3	CH-157-MN (III); IOMM-Lee (III)/104-106/3	TF floor/SDS convexity	90	Lb100 + RT	Increased survival compared with RT alone	Ragel et al,[54] 2008 & Ho et al,[59] 2018
Athymic/5-6	IOMM-Lee (III)/5.104/0.5	Skull base	100	Temozolomide	Inhibition of TG; increased survival	Baia et al,[45] 2008
Athymic/5	KT21-DEP1 loss (III)	Convexity	100	—	—	Petermann et al,[132] 2011
Athymic/5	PD grade I/106/10	Convexity (prefrontal cortex)	90–100	Celecoxib	No effect	Friedrich et al,[51] 2013 & Friedrich et al,[133] 2012
Athymic/8-10	IOMM-Lee (III)/2.5 × 105/5	Convexity	100	Cilengitide + RT Sorafenib Temsirolimus	Inhibition of TG	38,55,134
Athymic/6-8	BenMen1(I)/106/3	Skull base	100	Histone deacetylase inhibitor AR-42	Affect cell cycle progression; inhibition of TG	Burns et al,[110] 2013
NOD/SCID/gamma null mouse/8	IOMM-Lee (III)/5.104/3	Skull base (Pgi)	100	Peripheral blood mononuclear cells	Inhibition of TG	Iwami et al,[56] 2013

(continued on next page)

Table 2
(continued)

Mouse Strain/Age of Injection (wk)	Injected Cell Types (WHO Grade)/Numbers/Volume (μL)	Site of Injection	Tumor Take (%)	Treatment	Clinical Results	References
Athymic/6–8	BenMenI (I)-KT21-MG1 (III)/106/5	Skull base	100	Group 1 Pak inhibitor	Inhibition of TG	Chow et al,[135] 2015
Athymic/NA	PD grade I/106/10	Convexity	100	—	—	Michelhaugh et al,[136] 2015
Athymic/5–6	Primary malignant meningioma *NF2*-mutant MN3/tumorsphere 50,000/3–5	Convexity	100	Oncolytic HSV OS2966	Increased survival Increased survival	Nigim et al,[28] 2019 & Nigim et al,[137] 2016
Athymic/NA	CH-157 MN (III)	Convexity	100	Hydroxyurea + verapamil	No effect	Karsy et al,[57] 2016
Athymic/5–6	CH-157 MN (III)/5.104/5	Convexity/skull base	55–80	—	—	La Cava et al,[50] 2019
Athymic/6–8	IOMM-Lee (III)/104	Skull base	100	—	—	Giles et al,[27] 2019
Athymic/6	KT21-MG1/50,000/	Convexity	100	Mebendazole ± RT	Inhibition of TG; increased survival	Skibinski et al,[138] 2018
SCID mice/4–6	IOMM-Lee (III)/106/3–10	Skull base	100	Ganoderic acid DM	Inhibition of TG Increased survival	Das et al,[139] 2020
SCID mice/4–6	IOMM-Lee (III)-BenMen1 (I)	Skull base	100	Palbiciblib + RT	Inhibition of TG; increased survival	Das et al,[58] 2020

Abbreviations: HSV, herpes simplex virus; NOD, nonobese diabetic; PD, patient-derived; Pgi, postglenoid injection; RT, radiotherapy; SCID, severe combined immunodeficient; SDS, subdural space; TF, temporal fossa; TG, tumor growth; WM, white matter.
Modified from MDPI via an open access Creative Commons CC BY 4.0 license (Boetto et al. 2021).[4]

Table 3
Summary of GEMM models

Construction	Genetics	Temporal Window of Activation	Phenotype (Grade)	Meningioma Prevalence (%)	References
AdCre; Nf2flox/flox	Nf2 loss	PN2-PN3	M/F (I)	29 (TO), 19 (SD)	Kalamarides et al,[61] 2001
AdCre; Nf2flox/flox; Ink4a*/*	Nf2 loss + homozygous P16Ink4a mutation	PN2-PN3	M/F/T (I)	38 (TO), 36 (SD)	Kalamarides et al,[62] 2008
AdCre; Nf2flox/flox; Ink4ab−/−	Nf2 + CDKN2AB loss	PN2-PN3	66% (I), 31% (II), 3% (III)	72	Peyre et al,[17] 2013
PGDSCre; Nf2flox:flox	Nf2 loss in PGDS+ cells	E12.5-PN2	M (I), F (I)	38, 38	Kalamarides et al,[63] 2011
PGDSCre; Nf2flox/flox; p16ink4a-	Nf2 loss + P16ink4a mutation in PGDS+ cells	E12.5-PN2	M (I), F (I)	50, 50	
PGDSCre; Nf2flox/flox; p53flox/flox	Nf2 loss + p53 nullizygosity in PGDS+ cells	E12.5-PN2	F (I)	43	
PGDStv-a; PDGF-B	PDGF overexpression in PGDS+ cells	E12.5-PN2	(I)	27	Peyre et al,[64] 2015
PGDStv-a; PDGF-B; AdCre; Nf2flox/flox	PDGF overexpression + Nf2 loss in PGDS+ cells	E12.5-PN7	Grade I (60%), Grade II (40%)	52	
PGDStv-a; PDGF-B; AdCre; Nf2flox/flox; Cdkn2ab−/−	PDGF overexpression + nf2 loss + Cdkn2ab loss	E12.5-PN7	Grade I (33%), Grade II (47%), Grade III (20%)	79	
PGDSCre; SmoM2	Activating mutation of Smo in PGDS+ cells	E12.5-PN2	M (I)	21	Boetto et al,[65] 2018

Abbreviations: F, fibroblastic; M, meningothelial; PDGF, platelet-derived growth factor; PGDS, prostaglandin-D2-synthase; PN, postnatal day; SD, subdural; T, transitional; TO, transorbital.
Modified from MDPI via an open access Creative Commons CC BY 4.0 license (Boetto et al. 2021).

histologic subtype, or tumor firmness.[73–77] After a radiologic diagnosis of meningioma, these variables are usually not determined for most patients until after resection of the meningioma.[78] Computer-aided diagnosis systems using machine-learning radiomics models have the potential to revolutionize presurgical meningioma diagnosis and clinical planning by giving physicians accurate answers without the need for surgery.[74,77,79]

In contrast to conventional radiomics models that use predefined mathematical equations for feature extraction, machine-learning radiomics models can handle massive amounts of data and can directly extract and calculate a plethora of radiomic features in relation to the specific task (eg, meningioma grading).[80,81] Regardless of the task, each AI-integrated radiomics model has to process an image through similar steps in order for the model to output a predictive response. MRI is the imaging modality of choice for meningioma analysis because of its superior soft tissue contrast differentiation. T1-weighted, T2-weighted, T1 contrast-enhanced, and occasionally fluid-attenuated inversion recovery MRI sequences are used to radiologically diagnose meningioma.[82,83] Given sequence variability, differences in image quality, and cross-institutional hardware heterogeneity, AI-integrated radiomics models must be trained on diverse image datasets to be effective in the clinical environment.[74,76,84] Training, validation, and testing image datasets for research purposes are typically retrospectively acquired from clinical databases containing preoperative MRI scans of meningiomas.[79,85,86] For supervised learning, these images are classified and labeled by a model task variable based on postoperative tumor analysis (eg, grade 2 vs grade 3, or angiomatous vs anaplastic).[80] Unsupervised learning, which is rarely used in the radiomics pipeline, would not require image labeling.[80]

Researchers are using the previously described methods and training machine-learning radiomics models to be used as tools for physicians. For example, tumor firmness is an important factor in the operative strategy of meningioma resection. Despite attempts at workflow-guided predictions and the creation of new grading schemes, there are currently no validated techniques to predict meningioma firmness through preoperative imaging.[87,88] Recently, however, AlKubeyyer and colleagues developed a model able to classify meningiomas as "firm" or "soft" using T2-weighted MRI scans, achieving an area under the receiver operating characteristic curve of 0.87 during validation.[77] Clinical application of this model can assist physicians in surgical planning and inform their preoperative counseling of patients.

There are further examples of researchers creating high-accuracy, AI-integrated radiomics models for differentiating meningiomas, gliomas, and pituitary tumors and differentiating meningioma grades using various MRI sequences.[74,89,90] Additionally, Aurna and colleagues[74] have created a user interface for real-time validation of images.

Machine-learning radiomics models are also being used for more than tumor differentiation. In nomograms and models used for clinical outcome prediction, radiomic features are sometimes analyzed along with other clinical variables, such as presurgical leukocyte count.[72,91] The combination of radiomics and other tumor-independent clinical features has been shown to increase the accuracy of models that predict tumor recurrence in squamous cell carcinoma.[92,93] However, there are currently no predictive models for meningioma recurrence.[94] As further research reveals biomarkers and clinical features that correlate with meningioma outcomes, it is expected that more accurate nomograms will be developed for prediction of clinical outcomes including progression-free survival.[95,96]

DISCUSSION
Treatment Innovations

Current in vitro treatment innovations are attractive because they involve the study of various treatment modalities, meningiomas tumor cell lines, and novel basic science techniques. Genomic profiling of human meningioma cell lines allows for identification of novel pharmacologic and molecular targets in meningiomas, including understanding the effects of genetic mutations.[11] In grade I meningioma cell lines (HBL-52 and Ben-Men1), the tyrosine kinase inhibitor sunitinib, which is effective in gliomas, resulted in reduced tumor survival and migration.[25] Dovitinib (TK1258), an angiokinase inhibitor, was evaluated in grade III meningioma cell lines (CH 157 MN and IOMM-Lee) that were codeleted or mutated for CHEK2/NF2.[97] This interesting approach allowed rapid testing of a therapeutic modality against several cell lines and mutation profiles. Monoclonal antibody therapy is also being evaluated in vitro and in vivo (eg, beta1 integrin mAb).[14,27–29] Radiation treatment effects are also evaluated in cell cultures of meningioma, some with combined molecular protein/gene target therapy (eg, LB-100).[19,59,98–102]

mRNA and protein expression levels (eg, HuR, CLDN6, hENT1, dCK, RLIP76)[103–107] are being evaluated in meningioma cell lines, in addition to patient-obtained meningioma patient samples, and compared for evaluation of diagnostic and prognostic markers. Histone-modifying agents (eg, AR-42),[70] transcription factors (eg, FOXM1, GATA-4, TERT),[37,108,109] tumor-suppressor genes, and growth factors are also being evaluated as potential targets for treatment modalities for meningiomas.[18,22,110–121]

In vivo meningioma modeling has allowed for more robust and clinically applicable treatment innovations. The application of verotoxin was one of the earliest treatments performed on a xenograft model (IOMM-Lee, orthotopic) in the effect of tumor growth inhibition.[52] Genetic treatments have also been evaluated (eg, siRNA and LB-100), as well as combination gene/radiation therapy survival outcomes evaluation.[53,59] Chemotherapeutics and other pharmaceuticals (eg, nonsteroidal anti-inflammatory drugs) have also been investigated in these models.[4,45,51] Advances in the last decade mainly include assessment of gene-modulating pharmaceutical therapy, viral, monoclonal antibody, and even noncancer therapeutics, in combination or without radiotherapy.[28,57,58,110,122] Most outcomes in recent meningioma treatments have resulted in inhibition of tumor growth in vivo in combination with increased animal survival, which suggest promising results for human clinical trial studies.

Limitations of In Vitro Models

Reproduction of a true tumor microenvironment and tumor behavior are the limitations of any meningioma model. Cell senescence is a concern for cultured in vitro modeling because low/no innate telomerase activity results in limited cell growth and passaging.[123,124] Transduction techniques have arisen as a workaround to induce expression of the telomerase subunit and thus allow for continued cell passage.[12] However, these induced expressed genes have not been associated with naturally occurring meningiomas in vivo and may alter growth and behavior from parent tumors. Another limitation involves long-term culture, where cell-line karyotypes can increase in complexity and make it difficult to generalize findings to original tumors.[125]

Limitations of In Vivo Models

Several limitations for in vivo models exist. Although heterotopic injection of meningioma cell lines or tumor culture in animal flanks can induce meningioma with classical histopathologic features, these lesions may not generalize well to human meningiomas.[126] Orthotopic models of meningiomas using stereotaxic injection of patient-derived tumor compared with cultured cell samples may lead to lower rates of tumor induction (20%–100%).[4] A large limitation lies in requiring the host animal's immune system to be immunocompromised, which does not allow for study of tumor cells in relation to the immune system. Meningioma tumorigenesis is not ideally studied in xenograft models because of strong selective pressures during cell culture and variabilities in tumor take and growth rate; thus, these models are better suited for preclinical testing of therapeutic treatments than studying biomolecular events and pathways.[127] Studying drug delivery to tumors in animals also differs from human pharmacodynamics and pharmacokinetics.[57] Time to model generation is another limitation, which in addition to costs, can be prohibitive for study. Tumor induction rates for GEMMs range from 30% to 80%, much lower than other xenograft model techniques.[4] GEMM generation can often yield nonmeningioma tumor generation, which can result in early animal death.

Limitations of Artificial Intelligence/Machine Learning/Imaging Technologies

Cost and availability of these technologies remain the biggest limitation to imaging technologies. Bioluminescence is inexpensive and can be integrated into experiments through grafting of luciferase expression in cell lines or crossing of luciferase reporter and then using Cre-loxP-dependent tumorigenesis.[54] MRI requires continued sequential following of tumor, which incurs cost and experimental burden.

SUMMARY

This systematic review has provided insight into the development of preclinical models for meningioma, including cell culture, in vivo animal work, and artificial neural networks. Each unique tool has utility, and advancements are being made by combining the different approaches for emerging clinical trials. These models need to be refined and expanded to advance the understanding of molecular dynamics and aid in the discovery of effective therapeutic targets.

CLINICS CARE POINTS

- Various preclinical models for meningioma include immortalized cell lines, patient-derived cell lines, heterotopic and orthotopic xenograft models, and genetically engineered mouse models.

- Different preclinical tumor models have variable strengths and weaknesses in predicting human treatment response.

REFERENCES

1. Choudhury A, Raleigh DR. Preclinical models of meningioma: cell culture and animal systems. Handb Clin Neurol 2020;169:131–6.
2. Horbinski C, Xi G, Wang Y, et al. The effects of palbociclib in combination with radiation in preclinical models of aggressive meningioma. Neurooncol Adv 2021;3(1):vdab085.
3. Zhang H, Qi L, Du Y, et al. Patient-derived orthotopic xenograft (PDOX) mouse models of primary and recurrent meningioma. Cancers 2020;12(6):1478.
4. Boetto J, Peyre M, Kalamarides M. Mouse models in meningioma research: a systematic review. Cancers 2021;13(15):3712.
5. Kalamarides M, Peyre M, Giovannini M. Meningioma mouse models. J Neuro Oncol 2010;99(3):325–31.
6. Suppiah S, Nassiri F, Bi WL, et al. Molecular and translational advances in meningiomas. Neuro Oncol 2019;21(Suppl 1):i4–17.
7. Nigim F, Wakimoto H, Kasper EM, et al. Emerging medical treatments for meningioma in the molecular era. Biomedicines 2018;6(3):86.
8. Vranic A, Peyre M, Kalamarides M. New insights into meningioma: from genetics to trials. Curr Opin Oncol 2012;24(6):660–5.
9. Khayat Kashani HR, Azhari S, Nayebaghayee H, et al. Prediction value of preoperative findings on meningioma grading using artificial neural network. Clin Neurol Neurosurg 2020;196:105947.
10. Puttmann S, Senner V, Braune S, et al. Establishment of a benign meningioma cell line by hTERT-mediated immortalization. Lab Invest 2005;85(9):1163–71.
11. Mei Y, Bi WL, Greenwald NF, et al. Genomic profile of human meningioma cell lines. PLoS One 2017;12(5):e0178322.
12. Baia GS, Slocum AL, Hyer JD, et al. A genetic strategy to overcome the senescence of primary meningioma cell cultures. J Neuro Oncol 2006;78(2):113–21.
13. Cargioli TG, Ugur HC, Ramakrishna N, et al. Establishment of an in vivo meningioma model with human telomerase reverse transcriptase. Neurosurgery 2007;60(4):750–9 [discussion: 759-760].
14. Lee WH. Characterization of a newly established malignant meningioma cell line of the human brain: IOMM-Lee. Neurosurgery. 1990;27(3):389–95 [discussion: 396].
15. Waldt N, Kesseler C, Fala P, et al. Crispr/Cas-based modeling of NF2 loss in meningioma cells. J Neurosci Methods 2021;356:109141.
16. Leone PE, Bello MJ, de Campos JM, et al. NF2 gene mutations and allelic status of 1p, 14q and 22q in sporadic meningiomas. Oncogene 1999;18(13):2231–9.
17. Peyre M, Stemmer-Rachamimov A, Clermont-Taranchon E, et al. Meningioma progression in mice triggered by Nf2 and Cdkn2ab inactivation. Oncogene 2013;32(36):4264–72.
18. Striedinger K, VandenBerg SR, Baia GS, et al. The neurofibromatosis 2 tumor suppressor gene product, merlin, regulates human meningioma cell growth by signaling through YAP. Neoplasia 2008;10(11):1204–12.
19. Pinzi V, Bisogno I, Ciusani E, et al. In vitro assessment of radiobiology of meningioma: a pilot study. J Neurosci Methods 2019;311:288–94.
20. Taut FJ, Zeller WJ. In vitro chemotherapy of steroid receptor positive human meningioma low-passage primary cultures with nitrosourea-methionine-steroid conjugates. Clin Neuropharmacol 1996;19(6):520–5.
21. Tsuchida T, Matsudaira T, Yoshimura K, et al. [Chemosensitivity of cultured meningiomas]. Hum Cell 1995;8(4):155–6.
22. Puduvalli VK, Li JT, Chen L, et al. Induction of apoptosis in primary meningioma cultures by fenretinide. Cancer Res 2005;65(4):1547–53.
23. Preusser M, Spiegl-Kreinecker S, Lotsch D, et al. Trabectedin has promising antineoplastic activity in high-grade meningioma. Cancer 2012;118(20):5038–49.
24. Yu T, Cao J, Alaa Eddine M, et al. Receptor-tyrosine kinase inhibitor ponatinib inhibits meningioma growth in vitro and in vivo. Cancers 2021;13(23):5898.
25. Andrae N, Kirches E, Hartig R, et al. Sunitinib targets PDGF-receptor and Flt3 and reduces survival and migration of human meningioma cells. Eur J Cancer 2012;48(12):1831–41.
26. Ragel BT, Jensen RL, Gillespie DL, et al. Celecoxib inhibits meningioma tumor growth in a mouse xenograft model. Cancer 2007;109(3):588–97.
27. Giles AJ, Hao S, Padget M, et al. Efficient ADCC killing of meningioma by avelumab and a high-affinity natural killer cell line, haNK. JCI Insight 2019;4(20):e130688.
28. Nigim F, Kiyokawa J, Gurtner A, et al. A monoclonal antibody against beta1 integrin inhibits proliferation and increases survival in an orthotopic model of high-grade meningioma. Target Oncol 2019;14(4):479–89.
29. Konstantinidou A, Korkolopoulou P, Patsouris E, et al. Apoptosis detected with monoclonal antibody

to single-stranded DNA is a predictor of recurrence in intracranial meningiomas. J Neuro Oncol 2001; 55(1):1–9.

30. Nakano T, Fujimoto K, Tomiyama A, et al. Eribulin prolongs survival in an orthotopic xenograft mouse model of malignant meningioma. Cancer Sci 2022; 113(2):697–708.

31. Kunert-Radek J, Stepien H, Radek A, et al. Somatostatin suppression of meningioma cell proliferation in vitro. Acta Neurol Scand 1987;75(6):434–6.

32. Glick RP, Gettleman R, Patel K, et al. Insulin and insulin-like growth factor I in brain tumors: binding and in vitro effects. Neurosurgery 1989;24(6): 791–7.

33. Tichomirowa MA, Theodoropoulou M, Daly AF, et al. Toll-like receptor-4 is expressed in meningiomas and mediates the antiproliferative action of paclitaxel. Int J Cancer 2008;123(8):1956–63.

34. Linsler S, Ketter R, Oertel J, et al. Fluorescence imaging of meningioma cells with somatostatin receptor ligands: an in vitro study. Acta Neurochir 2019;161(5):1017–24.

35. Kajikawa H, Kawamoto K, Herz F, et al. Flow-through cytometry of meningiomas and cultured meningioma cells. Acta Neuropathol 1978;44(3): 183–7.

36. Ironside JW, Battersby RD, Lawry J, et al. DNA in meningioma tissues and explant cell cultures. A flow cytometric study with clinicopathological correlates. J Neurosurg 1987;66(4):588–94.

37. Kim H, Park KJ, Ryu BK, et al. Forkhead box M1 (FOXM1) transcription factor is a key oncogenic driver of aggressive human meningioma progression. Neuropath Appl Neuro 2020;46(2):125–41.

38. Tuchen M, Wilisch-Neumann A, Daniel EA, et al. Receptor tyrosine kinase inhibition by regorafenib/sorafenib inhibits growth and invasion of meningioma cells. Eur J Cancer 2017;73:9–21.

39. Koehorst SG, Spapens ME, Van Der Kallen CJ, et al. Progesterone receptor synthesis in human meningiomas: relation to the estrogen-induced proteins pS2 and cathepsin-D and influence of epidermal growth factor, Forskolin and phorbol ester in vitro. Int J Biol Markers 1998;13(1):16–23.

40. Jensen RL, Origitano TC, Lee YS, et al. In vitro growth inhibition of growth factor-stimulated meningioma cells by calcium channel antagonists. Neurosurgery 1995;36(2):365–73 [discussion: 373-374].

41. Ragel BT, Gillespie DL, Kushnir V, et al. Calcium channel antagonists augment hydroxyurea- and ru486-induced inhibition of meningioma growth in vivo and in vitro. Neurosurgery 2006;59(5): 1109–20 [discussion: 1120-1121].

42. Chan HSC, Ng HK, Chan AK, et al. Establishment and characterization of meningioma patient-derived organoid. J Clin Neurosci 2021;94:192–9.

43. Magill ST, Vasudevan HN, Seo K, et al. Multiplatform genomic profiling and magnetic resonance imaging identify mechanisms underlying intratumor heterogeneity in meningioma. Nat Commun 2020; 11(1):4803.

44. Malham GM, Thomsen RJ, Synek BJ, et al. Establishment of primary human meningiomas as subcutaneous xenografts in mice. Brit J Neurosurg 2001; 15(4):328–34.

45. Baia GS, Dinca EB, Ozawa T, et al. An orthotopic skull base model of malignant meningioma. Brain Pathol 2008;18(2):172–9.

46. Mawrin C. Animal models of meningiomas. Chin Clin Oncol 2017;6(Suppl 1):S6.

47. Rana MW, Pinkerton H, Thornton H, et al. Hetero-transplantation of human glioblastoma multiforme and meningioma to nude mice. Proc Soc Exp Biol Med 1977;155(1):85–8.

48. Jensen RL, Leppla D, Rokosz N, et al. Matrigel augments xenograft transplantation of meningioma cells into athymic mice. Neurosurgery 1998;42(1): 130–5 [discussion: 135-136].

49. McCutcheon IE, Friend KE, Gerdes TM, et al. Intracranial injection of human meningioma cells in athymic mice: an orthotopic model for meningioma growth. J Neurosurg 2000;92(2):306–14.

50. La Cava F, Fringuello Mingo A, Irrera P, et al. Orthotopic induction of CH157MN convexity and skull base meningiomas into nude mice using stereotactic surgery and MRI characterization. Animal Model Exp Med 2019;2(1):58–63.

51. Friedrich S, Schwabe K, Grote M, et al. Effect of systemic celecoxib on human meningioma after intracranial transplantation into nude mice. Acta Neurochir 2013;155(1):173–82.

52. Salhia B, Rutka JT, Lingwood C, et al. The treatment of malignant meningioma with verotoxin. Neoplasia 2002;4(4):304–11.

53. Kondraganti S, Gondi CS, McCutcheon I, et al. RNAi-mediated downregulation of urokinase plasminogen activator and its receptor in human meningioma cells inhibits tumor invasion and growth. Int J Oncol 2006;28(6):1353–60.

54. Ragel BT, Elam IL, Gillespie DL, et al. A novel model of intracranial meningioma in mice using luciferase-expressing meningioma cells. J Neurosurg 2008;108(2):304–10.

55. Pachow D, Andrae N, Kliese N, et al. mTORC1 inhibitors suppress meningioma growth in mouse models. Clin Cancer Res 2013;19(5):1180–9.

56. Iwami K, Natsume A, Ohno M, et al. Adoptive transfer of genetically modified Wilms' tumor 1-specific T cells in a novel malignant skull base meningioma model. Neuro Oncol 2013;15(6):747–58.

57. Karsy M, Hoang N, Barth T, et al. Combined hydroxyurea and verapamil in the clinical treatment of refractory meningioma: human and orthotopic

xenograft studies. World Neurosurg 2016;86: 210–9.

58. Das A, Alshareef M, Martinez Santos JL, et al. Evaluating anti-tumor activity of palbociclib plus radiation in anaplastic and radiation-induced meningiomas: pre-clinical investigations. Clin Transl Oncol 2020;22(11):2017–25.

59. Ho WS, Sizdahkhani S, Hao S, et al. LB-100, a novel protein phosphatase 2A (PP2A) inhibitor, sensitizes malignant meningioma cells to the therapeutic effects of radiation. Cancer Lett 2018;415: 217–26.

60. Castle KD, Chen M, Wisdom AJ, et al. Genetically engineered mouse models for studying radiation biology. Transl Cancer Res 2017;6(Suppl 5): S900–13.

61. Kalamarides M, Niwa-Kawakita M, Leblois H, et al. Nf2 gene inactivation in arachnoidal cells is rate-limiting for meningioma development in the mouse. Genes Dev 2002;16(9):1060–5.

62. Kalamarides M, Stemmer-Rachamimov AO, Takahashi M, et al. Natural history of meningioma development in mice reveals: a synergy of Nf2 and p16(Ink4a) mutations. Brain Pathol 2008; 18(1):62–70.

63. Kalamarides M, Stemmer-Rachamimov AO, Niwa-Kawakita M, et al. Identification of a progenitor cell of origin capable of generating diverse meningioma histological subtypes. Oncogene 2011; 30(20):2333–44.

64. Peyre M, Salaud C, Clermont-Taranchon E, et al. PDGF activation in PGDS-positive arachnoid cells induces meningioma formation in mice promoting tumor progression in combination with Nf2 and Cdkn2ab loss. Oncotarget 2015;6(32):32713–22.

65. Boetto J, Apra C, Bielle F, et al. Selective vulnerability of the primitive meningeal layer to prenatal Smo activation for skull base meningothelial meningioma formation. Oncogene 2018;37(36):4955–63.

66. Waldt N, Scharnetzki D, Kesseler C, et al. Loss of PTPRJ/DEP-1 enhances NF2/Merlin-dependent meningioma development. J Neurol Sci 2020;408: 116553.

67. Castellil MG, Butti G, Chiabrando C, et al. Arachidonic acid metabolic profiles in human meningiomas and gliomas. J Neuro Oncol 1987;5(4):369–75.

68. Lah TT, Nanni I, Trinkaus M, et al. Toward understanding recurrent meningioma: the potential role of lysosomal cysteine proteases and their inhibitors. J Neurosurg 2010;112(5):940–50.

69. de Ridder LI, Calliauw LJ. Invasiveness in in vitro and clinical evaluation of meningiomas. Surg Neurol 1992;37(4):269–73.

70. Bush ML, Oblinger J, Brendel V, et al. AR42, a novel histone deacetylase inhibitor, as a potential therapy for vestibular schwannomas and meningiomas. Neuro Oncol 2011;13(9):983–99.

71. Kumar Y, Koul A, Singla R, et al. Artificial intelligence in disease diagnosis: a systematic literature review, synthesizing framework and future research agenda. J Ambient Intell Humaniz Comput 2022; 1–28.

72. Lin Y, Dai P, Lin Q, et al. A predictive nomogram for atypical meningioma based on preoperative magnetic resonance imaging and routine blood tests. World Neurosurg 2022;163:e610–6.

73. Li X, Lu Y, Xiong J, et al. Presurgical differentiation between malignant haemangiopericytoma and angiomatous meningioma by a radiomics approach based on texture analysis. J Neuroradiol 2019;46(5): 281–7.

74. Aurna NF, Yousuf MA, Taher KA, et al. A classification of MRI brain tumor based on two stage feature level ensemble of deep CNN models. Comput Biol Med 2022;146:105539.

75. Yang L, Xu P, Zhang Y, et al. A deep learning radiomics model may help to improve the prediction performance of preoperative grading in meningioma. Neuroradiology 2022;64(7):1373–82.

76. Vassantachart A, Cao Y, Gribble M, et al. Automatic differentiation of grade I and II meningiomas on magnetic resonance image using an asymmetric convolutional neural network. Sci Rep 2022;12(1): 3806.

77. AlKubeyyer A, Ben Ismail MM, Bchir O, et al. Automatic detection of the meningioma tumor firmness in MRI images. J X Ray Sci Technol 2020;28(4):659–82.

78. Apra C, Peyre M, Kalamarides M. Current treatment options for meningioma. Expert Rev Neurother 2018;18(3):241–9.

79. Park YW, Oh J, You SC, et al. Radiomics and machine learning may accurately predict the grade and histological subtype in meningiomas using conventional and diffusion tensor imaging. Eur Radiol 2019;29(8):4068–76.

80. Wagner MW, Namdar K, Biswas A, et al. Radiomics, machine learning, and artificial intelligence: what the neuroradiologist needs to know. Neuroradiology 2021;63(12):1957–67.

81. Gillies RJ, Kinahan PE, Hricak H. Radiomics: images are more than pictures, they are data. Radiology 2016;278(2):563–77.

82. Watts J, Box G, Galvin A, et al. Magnetic resonance imaging of meningiomas: a pictorial review. Insights Imaging 2014;5(1):113–22.

83. Tamrazi B, Shiroishi MS, Liu CS. Advanced imaging of intracranial meningiomas. Neurosurg Clin N Am 2016;27(2):137–43.

84. Park YW, Shin SJ, Eom J, et al. Cycle-consistent adversarial networks improves generalizability of radiomics model in grading meningiomas on external validation. Sci Rep 2022;12(1):7042.

85. Laukamp KR, Thiele F, Shakirin G, et al. Fully automated detection and segmentation of meningiomas

using deep learning on routine multiparametric MRI. Eur Radiol 2019;29(1):124–32.

86. Lu Y, Liu L, Luan S, et al. The diagnostic value of texture analysis in predicting WHO grades of meningiomas based on ADC maps: an attempt using decision tree and decision forest. Eur Radiol 2019; 29(3):1318–28.

87. Shiroishi MS, Cen SY, Tamrazi B, et al. Predicting meningioma consistency on preoperative neuroimaging studies. Neurosurg Clin N Am 2016;27(2):145–54.

88. Zada G, Yashar P, Robison A, et al. A proposed grading system for standardizing tumor consistency of intracranial meningiomas. Neurosurg Focus 2013;35(6):E1.

89. Chen H, Li S, Zhang Y, et al. Deep learning-based automatic segmentation of meningioma from multiparametric MRI for preoperative meningioma differentiation using radiomic features: a multicentre study. Eur Radiol 2022;32(10):7248–59.

90. Duan CF, Li N, Li Y, et al. Comparison of different radiomic models based on enhanced T1-weighted images to predict the meningioma grade. Clin Radiol 2022;77(4):e302–7.

91. Gennatas ED, Wu A, Braunstein SE, et al. Preoperative and postoperative prediction of long-term meningioma outcomes. PLoS One 2018;13(9): e0204161.

92. Keek S, Sanduleanu S, Wesseling F, et al. Computed tomography-derived radiomic signature of head and neck squamous cell carcinoma (peri)tumoral tissue for the prediction of locoregional recurrence and distant metastasis after concurrent chemoradiotherapy. PLoS One 2020;15(5):e0232639.

93. Qiu Q, Duan J, Deng H, et al. Development and validation of a radiomics nomogram model for predicting postoperative recurrence in patients with esophageal squamous cell cancer who achieved pCR after neoadjuvant chemoradiotherapy followed by surgery. Front Oncol 2020;10:1398.

94. Chen WC, Hara J, Magill ST, et al. Salvage therapy outcomes for atypical meningioma. J Neuro Oncol 2018;138(2):425–33.

95. Erkan EP, Strobel T, Dorfer C, et al. Circulating tumor biomarkers in meningiomas reveal a signature of equilibrium between tumor growth and immune modulation. Front Oncol 2019;9:1031.

96. de Carvalho GTC, da Silva-Martins WC, de Magalhaes K, et al. Recurrence/regrowth in grade I meningioma: how to predict? Front Oncol 2020; 10:1144.

97. Das A, Martinez Santos JL, Alshareef M, et al. In vitro effect of dovitinib (TKI258), a multi-target angiokinase inhibitor on aggressive meningioma cells. Cancer Invest 2020;38(6):349–55.

98. Colvett KT, Hsu DW, Su M, et al. High PCNA index in meningiomas resistant to radiation therapy. Int J Radiat Oncol Biol Phys 1997;38(3):463–8.

99. Yamamoto M, Sanomachi T, Suzuki S, et al. Gemcitabine radiosensitization primes irradiated malignant meningioma cells for senolytic elimination by navitoclax. Neurooncol Adv 2021;3(1):vdab148.

100. Jiang C, Song T, Li J, et al. RAS promotes proliferation and resistances to apoptosis in meningioma. Mol Neurobiol 2017;54(1):779–87.

101. Rao Gogineni V, Kumar Nalla A, Gupta R, et al. Radiation-inducible silencing of uPA and uPAR in vitro and in vivo in meningioma. Int J Oncol 2010;36(4): 809–16.

102. Velpula KK, Gogineni VR, Nalla AK, et al. Radiation-induced hypomethylation triggers urokinase plasminogen activator transcription in meningioma cells. Neoplasia 2013;15(2):192–203.

103. Gauchotte G, Hergalant S, Vigouroux C, et al. Cytoplasmic overexpression of RNA-binding protein HuR is a marker of poor prognosis in meningioma, and HuR knockdown decreases meningioma cell growth and resistance to hypoxia. J Pathol 2017; 242(4):421–34.

104. Yamamoto M, Sanomachi T, Suzuki S, et al. Roles for hENT1 and dCK in gemcitabine sensitivity and malignancy of meningioma. Neuro Oncol 2021; 23(6):945–54.

105. Fan SY, Jiang JD, Qian J, et al. Overexpression of RLIP76 required for proliferation in meningioma is associated with recurrence. PLoS One 2015; 10(5):e0125661.

106. Wang M, Deng X, Ying Q, et al. MicroRNA-224 targets ERG2 and contributes to malignant progressions of meningioma. Biochem Biophys Res Commun 2015;460(2):354–61.

107. Yang A, Yang X, Wang J, et al. Effects of the tight junction protein CLDN6 on cell migration and invasion in high-grade meningioma. World Neurosurg 2021;151:e208–16.

108. Negroni C, Hilton DA, Ercolano E, et al. GATA-4, a potential novel therapeutic target for high-grade meningioma, regulates miR-497, a potential novel circulating biomarker for high-grade meningioma. EBioMedicine 2020;59:102941.

109. Spiegl-Kreinecker S, Lotsch D, Neumayer K, et al. TERT promoter mutations are associated with poor prognosis and cell immortalization in meningioma. Neuro Oncol 2018;20(12):1584–93.

110. Burns SS, Akhmametyeva EM, Oblinger JL, et al. Histone deacetylase inhibitor AR-42 differentially affects cell-cycle transit in meningeal and meningioma cells, potently inhibiting NF2-deficient meningioma growth. Cancer Res 2013;73(2):792–803.

111. Nalla AK, Gogineni VR, Gupta R, et al. Suppression of uPA and uPAR blocks radiation-induced MCP-1 mediated recruitment of endothelial cells in meningioma. Cell Signal 2011;23(8):1299–310.

112. Liu ZY, Wang JY, Liu HH, et al. Retinoblastoma protein-interacting zinc-finger gene 1 (RIZ1)

dysregulation in human malignant meningiomas. Oncogene 2013;32(10):1216–22.

113. Johnson MD, Reeder JE, O'Connell M. MKP-3 regulates PDGF-BB effects and MAPK activation in meningioma cells. J Clin Neurosci 2015;22(4): 752–7.

114. von Spreckelsen N, Waldt N, Poetschke R, et al. KLF4(K409Q)-mutated meningiomas show enhanced hypoxia signaling and respond to mTORC1 inhibitor treatment. Acta Neuropathol Commun 2020;8(1):41.

115. Tang H, Zhu H, Wang X, et al. KLF4 is a tumor suppressor in anaplastic meningioma stem-like cells and human meningiomas. J Mol Cell Biol 2017; 9(4):315–24.

116. Hu D, Wang X, Mao Y, et al. Identification of CD105 (endoglin)-positive stem-like cells in rhabdoid meningioma. J Neuro Oncol 2012;106(3):505–17.

117. Magrassi L, De-Fraja C, Conti L, et al. Expression of the JAK and STAT superfamilies in human meningiomas. J Neurosurg 1999;91(3):440–6.

118. Jensen RL, Soleau S, Bhayani MK, et al. Expression of hypoxia inducible factor-1 alpha and correlation with preoperative embolization of meningiomas. J Neurosurg 2002;97(3):658–67.

119. Kanno H, Nishihara H, Wang L, et al. Expression of CD163 prevents apoptosis through the production of granulocyte colony-stimulating factor in meningioma. Neuro Oncol 2013;15(7):853–64.

120. Saydam O, Shen Y, Wurdinger T, et al. Downregulated microRNA-200a in meningiomas promotes tumor growth by reducing E-cadherin and activating the Wnt/beta-catenin signaling pathway. Mol Cell Biol 2009;29(21):5923–40.

121. Johnson MD, O'Connell MJ, Walter K. Cucurbitacin I blocks cerebrospinal fluid and platelet derived growth factor-BB stimulation of leptomeningeal and meningioma DNA synthesis. BMC Complement Altern Med 2013;13:303.

122. Wilisch-Neumann A, Pachow D, Wallesch M, et al. Re-evaluation of cytostatic therapies for meningiomas in vitro. J Cancer Res Clin Oncol 2014; 140(8):1343–52.

123. Dezamis E, Sanson M. [The molecular genetics of meningiomas and genotypic/phenotypic correlations]. Rev Neurol (Paris) 2003;159(8–9):727–38.

124. Maes L, Kalala JP, Cornelissen R, et al. Telomerase activity and hTERT protein expression in meningiomas: an analysis in vivo versus in vitro. Anticancer Res 2006;26(3B):2295–300.

125. Zankl H, Ludwig B, May G, et al. Karyotypic variations in human meningioma cell cultures under different in vitro conditions. J Cancer Res Clin Oncol 1979;93(2):165–72.

126. Ragel BT, Couldwell WT, Gillespie DL, et al. A comparison of the cell lines used in meningioma research. Surg Neurol 2008;70(3):295–307 [discussion: 307].

127. Florian CL, Preece NE, Bhakoo KK, et al. Cell type-specific fingerprinting of meningioma and meningeal cells by proton nuclear magnetic resonance spectroscopy. Cancer Res 1995;55(2):420–7.

128. Akat K, Bleck CK, Lee YM, et al. Characterization of a novel type of adherens junction in meningiomas and the derived cell line HBL-52. Cell Tissue Res 2008;331(2):401–12.

129. Tsai JC, Goldman CK, Gillespie GY. Vascular endothelial growth factor in human glioma cell lines: induced secretion by EGF, PDGF-BB, and bFGF. J Neurosurg 1995;82(5):864–73.

130. Tanaka K, Sato C, Maeda Y, et al. Establishment of a human malignant meningioma cell line with amplifiedc-myc oncogene. Cancer 1989;64(11): 2243–9.

131. Kondraganti S, Gondi CS, Gujrati M, et al. Restoration of tissue factor pathway inhibitor inhibits invasion and tumor growth in vitro and in vivo in a malignant meningioma cell line. Int J Oncol 2006; 29(1):25–32.

132. Petermann A, Haase D, Wetzel A, et al. Loss of the protein-tyrosine phosphatase DEP-1/PTPRJ drives meningioma cell motility. Brain Pathol 2011;21(4): 405–18.

133. Friedrich S, Schwabe K, Klein R, et al. Comparative morphological and immunohistochemical study of human meningioma after intracranial transplantation into nude mice. J Neurosci Methods 2012; 205(1):1–9.

134. Wilisch-Neumann A, Kliese N, Pachow D, et al. The integrin inhibitor cilengitide affects meningioma cell motility and invasion. Clin Cancer Res 2013;19(19): 5402–12.

135. Chow HY, Dong B, Duron SG, et al. Group I Paks as therapeutic targets in NF2-deficient meningioma. Oncotarget 2015;6(4):1981–94.

136. Michelhaugh SK, Guastella AR, Varadarajan K, et al. Development of patient-derived xenograft models from a spontaneously immortal low-grade meningioma cell line, KCI-MENG1. J Transl Med 2015;13:227.

137. Nigim F, Esaki S, Hood M, et al. A new patient-derived orthotopic malignant meningioma model treated with oncolytic herpes simplex virus. Neuro Oncol 2016;18(9):1278–87.

138. Skibinski CG, Williamson T, Riggins GJ. Mebendazole and radiation in combination increase survival through anticancer mechanisms in an intracranial rodent model of malignant meningioma. J Neuro Oncol 2018;140(3):529–38.

139. Das A, Alshareef M, Henderson F Jr, et al. Ganoderic acid A/DM-induced NDRG2 over-expression suppresses high-grade meningioma growth. Clin Transl Oncol 2020;22(7):1138–45.

High-Value Care Outcomes of Meningiomas

Adrian E. Jimenez, BS, Debraj Mukherjee, MD, MPH*

KEYWORDS

- High-value care • Meningioma • Neuro-oncology

KEY POINTS

- High-value meningioma outcomes research focuses on optimizing hospital length of stay, discharge disposition, charges, and readmission.
- Improving outcomes in one domain of high-value care will likely have positive influences on other outcomes.
- Optimizing high-value care outcomes in meningiomas should focus on this population specifically, considering the disparate prognoses and treatments for different types of brain tumors.

INTRODUCTION

Meningiomas are the most common form of primary central nervous system tumor, and they are estimated to comprise between 10% and 20% of all intracranial neoplasms. The large number of patients presenting with meningiomas, combined with the expected increase in the prevalence of this disease due to an aging population, makes optimization of meningioma postoperative outcomes an excellent high-value care target.[1–4] Given the relatively broad definition of high-value care as optimizing resource expenditures relative to patient outcomes, an operationalized definition of high-value care research that be applied to studying meningiomas specifically is research, which seeks to minimize unnecessary length of stay (LOS), avoid nonhome discharge disposition when unnecessary, minimize hospital costs/charges, and avoid hospital readmission after discharge. Although outcomes may influence each other (ie, longer LOS leads to higher charges), each of the 4 aforementioned outcomes has unique causes and effects that are best conceptualized separately. This review will explore the current body of literature specifically describing each outcome among patients with meningioma (**Table 1**). Given the differences in baseline health states and prognoses between different types of brain tumors, we aim to highlight study results that focus specifically on meningioma patient cohorts to ensure that our conclusions are generalizable to this patient population.

MAJOR RESEARCH FINDINGS
Extended Hospital Length of Stay

Hospital LOS is a well-described outcome among patients with meningioma, with an extensive body of literature characterizing predictors of prolonged LOS. Studies examining extended LOS among patients with meningioma can be best understood as pertaining to 1 of 3 categories: (1) tumor-specific and surgery-specific factors, (2) patient age and frailty, and (3) socioeconomic disparities.

Tumor-specific and Surgery-specific Factors

There are a number of operative and tumor-specific factors that have been demonstrated to influence hospital LOS among patients with meningioma. A study by Sharma and colleagues found that patients with posterior cranial fossa tumors had a significantly higher risk of prolonged hospital LOS compared with patients with anterior fossa tumor in multivariate analysis (relative risk = 1.20, $P < .0001$).[5] Recent study by Seaman

Department of Neurosurgery, Johns Hopkins University School of Medicine, 1800 Orleans Street, Baltimore, MD 21231, USA
* Corresponding author.
E-mail address: dmukher1@jhmi.edu

Neurosurg Clin N Am 34 (2023) 493–504
https://doi.org/10.1016/j.nec.2023.02.016

Table 1
Key studies examining high-value care outcomes in patients with meningioma

Extended LOS	Nonroutine Discharge Disposition	High Hospital Costs	Unplanned Readmission
Bateman et al,[19] 2005 PMID: 16284557	Bateman et al,[19] 2005 PMID: 16284557	Grossman et al.,[21] 2011 PMID: 21492731	McKee et al.,[35] 2018 PMID: 30010072
Grossman et al.,[21] 2011 PMID: 21492731	Curry et al.,[50] 2005 PMID: 16028755	Nosova et al.,[15] 2013 PMID: 23273964	Lin et al.,[81] 2020 PMID: 32779026
Dickinson et al,[30] 2013 PMID: 23607067	Ambekar et al,[51] 2013 PMID: 23852621	Mukherjee et al,[43] 2013 PMID: 23084348	Theriault et al,[36] 2020 PMID: 33002880
Nosova et al,[15] 2013 PMID: 23273964	Muhlestein et al,[62] 2016 PMID: 29868316	Abou-Al-Shaar et al,[67] 2018 PMID: 30064026	Hauser et al,[80] 2020 PMID: 32654076
Mukherjee et al,[43] 2013 PMID: 23084348	Brandel et al,[61] 2018 PMID: 29606044	McKee et al,[35] 2018 PMID: 30010072	Cole et al,[37] 2022 PMID: 35216859
Bir et al,[7] 2016 PMID: 26805681	Slot et al,[52] 2018 PMID: 29430269	Reese et al,[68] 2019 PMID: 30872202	Howard et al,[91] 2022 PMID: 35445630
Sarkiss et al,[17] 2016 PMID: 27297242	Sharma et al,[5] 2019 PMID: 31323403	Spinazzi et al,[16] 2019 PMID: 30309806	Jimenez et al,[13] 2022 PMID: 34896348
Lagman et al,[14] 2018 PMID: 30456031	Jimenez et al,[60] 2020 PMID: 32652275	Cannizzaro et al,[72] 2020 PMID: 32962243	
McKee et al,[35] 2018 PMID: 30010072	Theriault et al,[36] 2020 PMID: 33002880	Jimenez et al,[49] 2021 PMID: 33567369	
Steinberger et al,[26] 2018 PMID: 28919230	Jimenez et al,[49] 2021 PMID: 33567369	Randhawa et al,[28] 2021 PMID: 34062298	
Sharma et al,[5] 2019 PMID: 31323403	Muhlestein et al,[63] 2021 PMID: 33483747	Jackson et al,[42] 2022 PMID: 34982878	
Spinazzi et al,[16] 2019 PMID: 30309806	Cole et al,[37] 2022 PMID: 35216859		
Theriault et al,[36] 2020 PMID: 33002880	Jimenez et al,[13] 2022 PMID: 34896348		
Li et al,[8] 2020 PMID: 32682250			
Seaman et al,[6] 2020 PMID: 35769807			
Dicpinigaitis et al,[38] 2021 PMID: 34495456			
Jimenez et al,[49] 2021 PMID: 33567369			
Neef et al,[11] 2021 PMID: 34298814			
Rafiq et al,[27] 2021 PMID: 34245986			
Randhawa8 et al,[28] 2021 PMID: 34062298			
Cole et al,[37] 2022 PMID: 35216859			
Jackson et al,[42] 2022 PMID: 34982878			
Jimenez et al,[13] 2022 PMID: 34896348			
Varela et al,[18] 2022 PMID: 35442224			

and colleagues, studying different minimally invasive approaches for anterior skull base meningiomas, found that patients undergoing supraorbital approaches had significantly shorter LOS (3.4 days) compared with those undergoing endoscopic endonasal approaches (EEA; 6.1 days, $P < .001$), possibly related to the need for prolonged lumbar drainage in the EEA cohort.[6] A study by Bir and colleagues highlighted the utility of neuronavigation in reducing average LOS in patients with meningioma ($P = .008$), which could potentially be explained by higher intraoperative surgical precision and thus less inadvertent trauma and resulting postoperative complications.[7] A 2020 study by Li and colleagues suggests that patients who receive lower volumes of intraoperative colloid infusion have shorter postoperative LOS (linear regression coefficient [coef] = 0.006, $P < .001$).[8] Although research has yet to demonstrate definitive causal associations between a positive fluid balance and adverse postoperative outcomes in patients with meningioma, potential mechanisms of harm via excess fluid administration include hemodilution and possible coagulopathies, elevated venous pressure resulting in decreased vascular perfusion pressure gradients, and interstitial edema.[9,10]

Research by Neef and colleagues found that red blood cell transfusion was associated with significant longer LOS ($P < .0001$) among patients undergoing primary meningioma resection.[11] Studies by Jimenez and colleagues reinforced the well-known associations between nonelective admission and prolonged LOS (>4 days) among patients with skull-base (odds ratio [OR] = 19.74, $P < .0001$) and patients with nonskull base meningioma (OR = 6.25, $P < .0001$), and they also demonstrated increased surgical duration was independently associated with prolonged LOS (OR = 1.36, $P < .001$), validating earlier findings by Lagman and colleagues.[12–14] Jimenez and colleagues also demonstrated that patients with nonskull base meningioma with larger tumor volumes (OR = 1.01, $P = .0022$) and patients with skull base meningioma with lower American Society of Anesthesiologists physical status scores (OR = 1.22, $P = .0025$) were significantly more likely to have prolonged LOS.[12,13] Regarding the influence of postoperative hospital course on LOS, results by Nosova and colleagues demonstrated that urinary tract infections (UTIs) among patients with meningioma added 2.3 days to total LOS, whereas data by Spinazzi and colleagues suggest that occurrence of venous thromboembolic events (VTEs) also resulted in significantly longer hospitalizations (18.8 vs 6.6 days; $P < .001$).[15,16]

Interestingly, studies by Sarkiss and colleagues and Varela and colleagues have demonstrated the day of the week that a patient undergoes surgery is significantly associated with prolonged LOS, with the underlying mechanism likely due to earlier access to services such as physical therapy and social work in addition to overall more efficient care coordination if the surgery is done toward the beginning of the week.[17,18] Specifically, Sarkiss and colleagues' results found a statistically significant decreased LOS (<3 days) in patients with meningioma who underwent surgery from Monday to Wednesday compared with those who received surgery from Thursday to Friday ($P = .045$) while Varela and colleagues similarly found the day of surgery to be independently associated with extended LOS (OR = 1.91, $P = .03$).[17,18]

Patient Age and Frailty

Regarding predictive factors for extended LOS, many studies within the neurosurgical literature have focused on the effects of advanced age among patients with meningioma undergoing tumor resection.[19–26] Results from early investigations such as those by Bateman and colleagues and Patil and colleagues suggested that older patient age was significantly associated with increased hospital LOS, and a recent meta-analysis of 13 retrospective studies by Rafiq and colleagues demonstrating significantly higher LOS in older (10.8 days) patients compared with younger patients (6.8 days, $P < .0001$) has validated the robustness of this association.[19,20,27] Increased LOS among older patients with meningioma is likely driven by an increased number of comorbidities such as diabetes mellitus and lower functional reserves among this population when undergoing surgery, with the notion of "functional reserves" being closely related to the concept of "frailty."[27,28] Frailty can be conceptualized as an age-related decrease in the physiologic capacity of multiple organ systems that causes an increased susceptibility to stressors in an individual.[29] Studies by Dickinson and colleagues and Kolakshyapati and colleagues highlighting the use of patient weight and body mass index (BMI) to prognosticate outcomes in patients with meningioma, and these studies can be seen as early efforts to develop a frailty phenotype.[30,31] Many different tools exist to quantify frailty, with popular frailty metrics including the Charlson Comorbidity Index (CCI), the 11-factor modified frailty index (mFI-11), and the 5-factor modified frailty index (mFI-5).[32–34] McKee and colleagues found that increasing CCI score (0 vs ≥ 4, OR = 2.51, $P = .0042$) was significantly and independently associated with prolonged LOS ($\geq$10 days).[35] Theriault and colleagues found that each point increase in mFI-11 score was associated with an increase of LOS by 1.7 days on average in multivariate analysis (P = .046) when controlling for age, BMI, sex, and tumor size.[36] These findings were validated in a recent article by Cole and colleagues, which found an mFI-5 score of 3 or greater as being significantly and independently associated with extended LOS of 7 days or greater.[37]

Given the assumption that frailty is an age-related decline of physiologic reserves, more recent investigations have begun to directly compare the predictive abilities of age and frailty.[38–40] Among patients with meningioma specifically, one comparative analysis between age and frailty was conducted by Dicpinigaitis and colleagues using data from the National (Nationwide) Inpatient Sample.[41] The study found that increasing mFI-11 score (OR = 1.20, P < .001) but not age (OR = 1.01, P = .85) was significantly and independently associated with extended LOS greater than 7 days in multivariate analysis. Further, the authors noted that mFI-11 demonstrated superior discrimination (area under the receiver operating characteristic curve [AUC] = 0.61, 95% confidence interval [CI] = 0.59 to 0.63) for predicting extended LOS compared with age (AUC = 0.56, CI = 0.54 to 0.58). These recent research findings highlight the possibility that advanced age may only be predictive for high-value postoperative outcomes when accompanied by the decreased physiologic reserves and medical comorbidities that are better quantified by frailty indices. Further research will be needed to better delineate the role of both age and frailty in predicting postoperative outcomes in patients with meningioma, as well as to determine whether frailty measures attempting to capture "physiologic age" should supplant simpler measures of chronologic age in this population.[41]

Health-care disparities in hospital length of stay
Much research has been dedicated toward better understanding the cause and effects of health-care disparities in the surgical treatment of patients with meningioma. Pivotal work by Jackson and colleagues found that African-American patients were significantly more likely to have longer postoperative LOS (P = .0053), and they also noted that African-American patients were more likely to present through the emergency department than an outpatient clinic (P < .0001), were more likely to have lower Karnofsky Performance scores (KPS; P = .023), and more frequently had

peritumoral edema (P = .0017) compared with White patients.[42] In addition to validating results from earlier studies, Jackson and colleagues' results highlight the importance of later, more advanced disease presentation as a major contributor to increased morbidity and poorer high-value health-care outcomes among minority patients seeking neurosurgical care.[35,42,43] Ongoing efforts to increase access to health care and remove barriers to accessing subspeciality care will remain a vitally important research topic moving forward.[42,44–46]

Nonroutine discharge disposition
Studies describing predictors of discharge disposition among patients with meningioma can be understood as either focusing on patient-related or procedure-related factors. Patient-specific factors, such as functional status and medical comorbidities, can ideally be optimized through strategies such as prehabilitation.[47–49] However, procedure-related factors, such as having surgery at a low-volume hospital, could be addressed via centralization of meningioma surgery at specialty care centers.[50]

Patient-specific Factors
Regarding patient-specific factors that predict nonroutine discharge disposition, Bateman and colleagues first established an association between patient age of 70 years or older and discharge to a location other than home (53.2% vs 16.6%, P < .001).[19] The association between older patient age and nonroutine discharge was further validated in studies by Ambekar and colleagues (age $\geq$80 years, OR = 7.5, P < .001), Slot and colleagues (age $\geq$65 years, 48% vs 20%, P = .004), and Jimenez and colleagues (OR = 1.06, P = .0020).[12,51,52] Similar to the significantly higher rates of prolonged LOS among older patients with meningioma, the higher rates of nonroutine discharge seen among this patient population are likely driven by an increased number of medical comorbidities, lower functional reserves, and increased frailty.[27,28,36,37] Specifically, Theriault and colleagues found that higher mFI-11 scores were significantly and independently associated with increased likelihood of discharge to a higher level of posthospitalization care (P = .001), whereas Cole and colleagues demonstrated that an mFI-5 score of 3 or greater was significantly associated with discharge to a location other than home (OR = 9.34, P < .001).[36,37] Jimenez and colleagues also noted that greater mFI-5 scores were significantly and independently associated with nonroutine discharge (OR = 1.48, P = .039) among patients

with nonskull base meningioma.[13] Importantly, unlike research focusing on quantifying predictors of prolonged LOS among patients with meningioma, there has not yet been a direct comparison of the prognostic abilities of both age and frailty for quantifying nonroutine discharge among patients with meningioma. Studies aiming to determine whether nonroutine discharge risk is better predicted by chronologic age or by frailty metrics would be an important goal for future research efforts.

Aside from patient age and frailty, trends in racial and economic disparities have been noted in research examining patient-specific predictors of nonroutine discharge disposition among patients with meningioma. Ambekar and colleagues found that African-American patients (OR = 1.23, $P < .001$) and patients with Medicare insurance coverage (OR = 4.1, $P < .001$) were significantly more likely to experience nonroutine discharge relative to counterparts.[51] Interestingly, significant associations between patient sex and nonroutine discharge disposition have also been found among patients with meningioma. Results by Ambekar and colleagues established a significant association between female sex and lower odds of nonroutine discharge disposition (OR = 0.83, $P < .001$), findings which were later validated by Jimenez and colleagues with their results demonstrating a significant association between male sex and higher odds of nonroutine discharge (OR = 2.46, $P = .0090$) in a cohort of patients with nonskull base meningiomas.[13,51] Although these results may point toward important sex-based differences in outcomes among patients with meningioma, further research will be needed to better characterize potential mechanisms driving these findings, especially considering the direction and magnitude of associations between patient sex and discharge disposition vary widely in the surgical literature.[53–55]

Marital status is another important patient-specific factor that likely has implications for discharge disposition among patients with meningioma. Unmarried patients with nonskull base meningiomas were found to experience significantly higher odds of nonroutine discharge (OR = 2.17, $P = .024$) in multivariate analysis. Although this association may be driven by the lack of caregiver support at home, as postulated by prior authors, further research specifically in patients with meningioma will be necessary to confirm this hypothesis.[13,56,57]

Tumor size and location have also been shown to be key prognostic variables for discharge disposition in patients with meningioma. Among patients with skull base meningioma, Jimenez and colleagues found tumor volume to be significantly

and independently associated with nonroutine discharge (OR = 1.02, $P = .0052$), whereas Sharma and colleagues noted that skull base patients with posterior fossa tumors were significantly less likely to be discharged home compared with patients with tumors in the anterior fossa (OR = 0.54, $P < .001$).[5,12] Among patients with nonskull base meningioma, Jimenez and colleagues found that patients with parasagittal/parafalcine or intraventricular meningiomas were significantly more likely to experience nonroutine discharge compared with patients with convexity meningiomas.[13] The authors attribute this finding as likely being due to higher complication rates resulting from the proximity of these tumors to important draining veins, thus portending more challenging surgical resections.[13,58,59] Earlier study by Jimenez and colleagues also found that higher mFI-5 score (OR = 2.06; $P = .0088$), Simpson grade IV resection (OR = 4.22; $P = .0062$), and occurrence of any postoperative complication (OR = 2.89; $P = .031$) were independent predictors of nonroutine discharge disposition among a cohort of 154 patients with parasagittal/parafalcine meningioma.[60] Brandel and colleagues found that a longer interval between preoperative endovascular embolization to tumor resection was significantly associated with nonroutine discharge (OR 1.33, $P = .004$).[61] The authors postulate that patients who are selected for preoperative embolization represent a subset of high-risk meningiomas that will likely require additional clinical needs and more extensive postoperative care, which would explain higher rates of discharge to specialized care facilities rather than home.[61]

Within the high-value outcomes literature, studies have begun to integrate a number of different patient-specific factors using machine learning approaches to produce predictions about a specific meningioma patient's probability of experiencing nonroutine discharge disposition after surgery. A 2016 article by Muhlestein and colleagues created an ensemble learning algorithm using 76 unique data points (ie, age, race, sex, BMI) from 611 operations.[62] The authors found that the AUC of their ensemble model (0.78) was significantly higher than that of a comparable logistic regression model (0.71, $P = .01$), and they noted that the variables in their ensemble model, which most strongly influenced predictive performance included tumor size, presentation at the emergency department, body mass index, convexity location, and preoperative motor deficit.[62] Further work by Muhlestein and colleagues utilized a natural language processing (NLP) algorithm trained on multi-institutional meningioma patient data, preoperative notes, and radiology reports to predict nonhome discharge disposition. The authors noted good discrimination (AUC>0.7) on both internal and holdout validation datasets, and they also found that preoperative notes were the most influential factor within the model's final prediction.[63]

Procedure-related Factors

Regarding procedure-related factors that impact discharge disposition among patients with meningioma, a study by Curry and colleagues in 2005 found that adverse discharge was significantly less likely at high-volume hospitals in multivariate analysis (OR = 0.71, $P < .001$) and that odds of adverse discharge among patients being treated by higher caseload providers was significantly lower than counterparts (OR = 0.71, $P < .001$).[50] Similarly, Ambekar and colleagues also found that patients with meningioma treated at high case-volume centers (OR = 0.8, $P < .001$) and by high case-volume physicians (OR = 0.63, $P < .001$) had significantly lower rates of hospital discharge to facilities other than home.[51] The investigators also noted that teaching hospitals had significantly lower rates of adverse discharge compared with nonteaching hospitals (OR = 0.8, $P < .001$), that patients admitted over the weekend were significantly more likely to be discharged to a facility other than home (OR = 1.8, $P < .001$), and that patients undergoing surgery on their first day of admission had a significantly lower rate of adverse discharge outcome (OR = 0.4, $P < .001$) compared with patients undergoing later surgeries.

High hospital costs

Drivers of hospital costs and charges can be understood as factors that increase a patient's utilization of health-care services, and these factors can be separated into preoperative, intraoperative, and postoperative factors. Importantly, there is a distinction between *charges*, which are the amounts a health-care provider sets for services before any discounts, and *costs*, which depends on who is being charged for health-care services. To providers such as surgeons, cost is the expense incurred to deliver health-care services to patients, whereas to patients, cost is the amount paid out-of-pocket for health-care services. To payers such as insurance companies, cost is the amount they pay to providers for services rendered.[64,65] Given the often close connection between charges and costs, these 2 metrics will be analyzed as one outcome for the purposes of this review.[66]

Preoperative factors that influence hospital cost/charges are those that serve as a proxy for a patient's functional status or disease severity,

and thus whether they will require more extensive health-care resources and longer LOS to allow for safe resection of their meningiomas.[15,16,67,68] Structural and procedure-related factors such as hospital volume and surgeon experience also play key roles in preoperative risk stratification given that they influence patient risk for postoperative complications and secondary health-care services, resulting in increased hospital costs.[69-71]

Regarding preoperative factors that influence hospital charges, results by Grossman and colleagues highlight frailty as measured by the CCI as an independent predictor of increased hospital charges (coef = 1,964, $P = .002$), whereas Mukherjee and colleagues demonstrated African-American patients were significantly more likely to have higher hospital charges compared with Caucasian counterparts (OR = 1.85, $P < .0001$).[21,43] Jackson and colleagues' findings that African-American patients presented with lower KPS ($P = .023$), more frequently had peritumoral edema ($P = .0017$), and had significantly higher hospitalization costs ($P = .046$) compared with White patients validated earlier research findings regarding the effects of preoperative functional status and racial disparities on hospital charges, underscoring the mechanism of later disease presentation due to limited health-care access as a potential explanation for these data.[12,35,42,43,72] Abou-Al-Shaar and colleagues found maximum meningioma size to be significantly and independently associated with hospital cost ($\beta = 0.1$, $P = .01$), findings which were validated by Jimenez and colleagues in a cohort of patients with skull base meningioma.[12,67] Findings regarding the effect of BMI on hospital charges have generally found a positive association between greater BMI and higher hospital charges. McKee and colleagues found obesity (OR = 2.31, $P < .0001$) to be significantly associated with higher hospital charges in patients with meningioma generally, whereas Jimenez and colleagues found higher BMI (OR = 1.07, $P = .0026$) to be associated with higher hospital charges among patients with skull base meningioma specifically.[12,35]

Additional preoperative factors that have been shown to influence hospital charges among patients with meningioma include female sex (OR = 0.80, $P < .0001$), lower income (OR = 0.51, $P < .0001$), Medicaid insurance (OR = 0.61, $P < .0001$), Medicare insurance (OR = 0.71, $P < .0001$), rural patient residence (OR = 0.66, $P < .001$), teaching hospital location (OR = 0.73, $P = .023$), and greater surgeon years of experience (OR = 0.96, $P = .027$), all of which are significantly associated with lower odds of excess hospital charges.[12,35] Additional predictors of high charges include tobacco use (OR = 1.75, $P < .0001$), diabetes mellitus (OR = 1.27, $P = .020$), and having surgery at a high volume center (OR = 3.95, $P < .0001$).[28,35]

There has been limited research into intraoperative factors predicting increased hospital cost aside from longer surgery duration, which was established as an independent predictor of higher cost among patients with skull base meningioma (OR = 1.50, $P < .0001$), presumably due to increased utilization of OR staff and resources in longer surgeries.[12] Quantifying the impact of both well-known intraoperative variables, such as resident participation in surgery, as well as newer technologies currently being implemented into OR workflows, such as intraoperative tumor diagnosis via Raman spectroscopy, on hospital charges would be productive avenues for future efforts in high-value meningioma research.[73–75]

Although the effect of complicated postoperative courses incurring higher hospital costs among patients is well established within the neurosurgical oncology literature generally, there is a relative dearth quantifying these associations in patients with meningioma specifically.[76–78] Among the few studies examining the financial impact of postoperative complications following meningioma resection, the associations between postoperative UTIs (increase in hospital charges of US$18,473 in women and US$19,963 among men) and VTEs (US$195,837 in patients with VTEs vs US$74,434 for non-VTE patients; $P < .001$) on increased hospital charges has been quantified by Nosova and colleagues and Spinazzi and colleagues, respectively.[15,16] A recent study by Jin and colleagues highlighted postneurosurgical status epilepticus (PNSE) as an important postoperative complication associated with considerable mortality and cost. Given that patients undergoing meningioma resection have greater odds of developing an early PNSE compared with patients undergoing resection of metastatic tumors (adjusted odds ratio [aOR] = 2.701, $P = .003$), future research should aim to quantify the implications of PNSE on high-value health-care outcomes in patients with meningioma.[79]

Unplanned readmission

The final high-value care metric to be highlighted within meningioma patient outcomes research is hospital readmission. Although the exact timeframe of readmission can vary between studies (ie, 30-day or 90-day readmission), predictors for readmission in this patient population can be conceptualized broadly as factors that either (1) prevent patients from getting their required care

outside of the hospital or (2) directly contribute to the deterioration of their health and functional status, putting patients at the risk of emergent medical/surgical intervention.

One important risk factor that may prevent patients from receiving needed medical care outside of the hospital is their insurance status. Work by Hauser and colleagues found that, compared with patients with meningioma with private insurance, those who were insured through Medicaid (OR = 1.40, $P = .035$) or Medicare (OR = 1.47, $P = .002$) had significantly higher odds of 90-day readmission on multivariable analysis.[80] These findings supported earlier results by McKee and colleagues, which also found higher odds of 30-day readmission among patients with meningioma with Medicare compared with those with private insurance (OR = 1.30, $P = .012$).[35] Lin and colleagues also found that Medicare (OR = 1.53, $P < .0001$) and Medicaid (OR = 1.47, $P < .0001$) insurance status were associated with significantly higher odds of 90-day readmission compared with private insurance.[81] Jimenez and colleagues later validated these findings in patients with non-skull base meningioma specifically, with their findings demonstrating a significant and independent association between Medicare, Medicaid, or uninsured coverage and 90-day readmission (OR = 2.46, $P = .010$).[13] Regarding how insurance status affects patients' readmission risk, earlier literature has examined how public insurance coverage, specifically Medicaid coverage, can minimize close neurosurgical postoperative follow-up, thus leaving initially mild postoperative issues unresolved until emergency department presentation and admission for intervention is required.[80,82,83] As discussed by Hauser and colleagues, one potential solution to this issue is attempting to engage Medicaid and Medicare patients in primary care soon after a hospital discharge to hopefully reduce readmission rates among this population.[80,84,85]

In addition to insurance status, patient race/ethnicity and income serve as additional proxies for socioeconomic disparities that increase patients' readmission risk by preventing close postoperative follow-up and access to necessary subspeciality care.[45,86–88] Specifically, McKee and colleagues found that Black patients with meningioma (OR = 1.38, $P < .001$) and those of Hispanic ethnicity (OR = 1.41, $P = .0043$) were significantly and independently more likely to experience a 30-day hospital readmission relative to Caucasian counterparts, whereas Lin and colleagues demonstrated that patients with meningioma in the 51st to 75th percentile of income were significantly less likely to experience a 90-day readmission compared with patients in the 0 to 25th percentile when adjusting for key demographic and clinical characteristics (OR = 0.87, P = .02).[35,81] Jimenez and colleagues also noted that marital status was significantly and independently associated with increased odds of a 90-day readmission (OR = 2.49, P = .0081), likely explained by earlier findings that married patients and individuals with larger social networks have decreased rates of readmission due to a greater sense of interconnectedness and purpose at home.[13,89,90]

The role of patient sex in influencing readmission risk after meningioma surgery has been highlighted in studies by McKee and colleagues and Lin and colleagues, who found complementary results of significantly lower odds of a 30-day readmission among female patients with meningioma (OR = 0.71, P < .0001) and significantly higher odds of a 90-day readmission among male patients (OR = 1.28, P < .0001), respectively.[35,81] However, a recent study by Howard and colleagues failed to find significant differences in a 30-day (P = .49) or 90-day (P = .49) readmission based on patient sex when matching for key clinical characteristics in a cohort of 349 patients with meningioma.[91] Further research will be needed to determine whether these sex-based differences are mostly due to disparities in care access, lack of support outside of the hospital, or whether there are meaningful sex-based differences in baseline health states between these 2 groups that puts men at higher risk for postoperative deterioration compared with women.[92]

Finally, indicators of patient health and functional status play a key role in quantifying potential readmission risk. Patient age of 65 years or older (OR = 1.32, P = .0090) and CCI score of 4 or greater (OR = 1.52, P = .016) were both established as risk-factors for a 30-day hospital readmission by McKee and colleagues.[35] Theriault and colleagues and Cole and colleagues later validated both the mFI-11 (P = .025) and the mFI-5 (OR = 2.31, P < .01) as independent predictors of readmission among patients with meningioma, respectively.[36,37] Further, Lin and colleagues established that greater illness severity (quantified by the All Patient Refined-Diagnosis Related Groups, OR = 1.15, P = .010), nonroutine discharge (OR = 1.53, P < .0001), and prolonged LOS (OR = 1.31, P < .0001) were all significant predictors of a 90-day readmission, highlighting the role of short-term high-value care metrics in prognosticating a patient's risk of subsequent readmission.[81]

Future directions for high-value care research

There are several open avenues for investigation in meningioma high-value outcomes research. One approach, which has arisen in the neurosurgical literature, is optimizing postoperative pathways by attempting to minimize intensive care unit LOS in appropriate patients, thus more efficiently utilizing health-care resources.[93–96] Given that many meningiomas are resected electively, preoperative risk stratification may be a feasible strategy within this patient population; future research efforts should aim to quantify the influence of this high-value approach to care in patients with meningioma, especially considering the efficacy and cost-effectiveness seen in early results by Osorio and colleagues and Young and colleagues.[95,96] Another approach that warrants further investigation is the use of predictive modeling to provide risk-stratification and prognostication at the level of the individual patient. Open-access calculators show promise in allowing clinicians to provide patients with personalized counseling regarding their predictive postoperative courses. Following rigorous external validation, such tools could be used in clinical workflows to further optimize high-value care outcomes.[12,13,63] An additional underutilized analytics technique within neurosurgery that should be used in future high-value meningioma research is Bayesian inference, which aims to directly quantify statistical uncertainty and provides rigorous estimates of effect sizes in a way that is not possible with traditional frequentist inference.[97] Key results by Angevine and colleagues in spinal surgery have highlighted the novel and complementary statistical information that Bayesian techniques can add to traditional inference methods, and utilization of this approach toward optimizing high-value care outcomes in patients with meningioma should be explored.[98]

SUMMARY

High-value care outcomes research in meningioma surgery focuses on optimizing the following outcomes: hospital LOS, discharge disposition, hospital costs/charges, and hospital readmission. Each of the 4 domains has unique risk-factors and drivers of adverse outcomes, and the body of literature exploring each outcome can be categorized in unique ways. However, common themes that emerge for all 4 outcomes include preoperative risk-stratification and medical optimization of high-risk patients, with frailty metrics playing a key role in all outcomes. Further, while the current body of literature on outcomes can be understood by analyzing each outcome separately, outcomes clearly influence each other and working toward optimizing one domain (such as decreasing LOS) will likely lead to improvements in other high-value care domains (such as lower hospital charges). Additional research utilizing meningioma-specific patient data aimed at personalizing risk-stratification via predictive analytics and novel methods of statistical analysis will be an important goal for future research efforts.

CLINICS CARE POINTS

- High-value care outcomes research involves optimization of 4 key metrics: hospital LOS, discharge disposition, charges, and readmission.
- Frailty is a measure that has wide-applicability in optimizing high-value care outcomes among patients with meningioma.
- More meningioma-specific, high-value research is warranted, given the unique baseline health characteristics and prognosis of this population among all patients with brain tumors.

FINANCIAL DISCLOSURE

The authors received no financial support for the research, authorship, and/or publication of this article.

CONFLICT OF INTEREST

On behalf of all authors, the corresponding author states that there is no conflict of interest.

REFERENCES

1. Porter ME. What is Value in Health Care? N Engl J Med 2010;363(26):2477–81.
2. Tsevat J, Moriates C. Value-Based Health Care Meets Cost-Effectiveness Analysis. Ann Intern Med 2018;169(5):329–32.
3. Ostrom QT, Gittleman H, Fulop J, et al. CBTRUS statistical Report: primary brain and central nervous system tumors diagnosed in the United States in 2008-2012. Neuro Oncol 2015;17:iv1–62.
4. Cohen SA. A review of demographic and infrastructural factors and potential solutions to the physician and nursing shortage predicted to impact the growing us elderly population. J Public Heal Manag Pract 2009;15(4):352–62.
5. Sharma M, Ugiliweneza B, Boakye M, et al. Feasibility of Bundled Payments in Anterior, Middle, and Posterior Cranial Fossa Skull Base Meningioma Surgery: MarketScan Analysis of Health Care Utilization and Outcomes. World Neurosurg 2019;131: e116–27.
6. Seaman SC, Ali MS, Marincovich A, et al. Minimally Invasive Approaches to Anterior Skull Base Meningiomas. J Neurol Surg B Skull Base 2022;83(3): 254–64.
7. Bir SC, Konar SK, Maiti TK, et al. Utility of Neuronavigation in Intracranial Meningioma Resection: A Single-Center Retrospective Study. World Neurosurg 2016;90:546–55.e1.
8. Li Y-T, Wang M, Gu Z-Y, et al. Effect of intraoperative fluid administration on postoperative complications and length of stay following meningioma resection: A retrospective analysis. J Clin Anesth 2020;67: 109985.
9. Ince C. Hemodynamic coherence and the rationale for monitoring the microcirculation. Crit Care 2015; 19(Suppl 3):S8.
10. Silversides JA, Perner A, Malbrain MLNG. Liberal versus restrictive fluid therapy in critically ill patients. Intensive Care Med 2019;45(10):1440–2.
11. Neef V, Konig S, Monden D, et al. Clinical Outcome and Risk Factors of Red Blood Cell Transfusion in Patients Undergoing Elective Primary Meningioma Resection. Cancers 2021;13(14).
12. Jimenez AE, Khalafallah AM, Lam S, et al. Predicting High-Value Care Outcomes After Surgery for Skull Base Meningiomas. World Neurosurg 2021;149: e427–36.
13. Jimenez AE, Chakravarti S, Liu S, et al. Predicting High-Value Care Outcomes Following Surgery for Non-Skull Base Meningiomas. World Neurosurg 2022;159:e130–8.
14. Lagman C, Sheppard JP, Beckett JS, et al. Red Blood Cell Transfusions Following Resection of Skull Base Meningiomas: Risk Factors and Clinical Outcomes. J Neurol Surg B Skull Base 2018;79(6): 599–605.
15. Nosova K, Nuno M, Mukherjee D, et al. Urinary tract infections in meningioma patients: Analysis of risk factors and outcomes. J Hosp Infect 2013;83(2): 132–9.
16. Spinazzi EF, Shastri D, Raikundalia M, et al. Impact of venous thromboembolism during admission for meningioma surgery on hospital charges and postoperative complications. J Clin Neurosci 2019;59: 218–23.
17. Sarkiss CA, Papin JA, Yao A, et al. Day of Surgery Impacts Outcome: Rehabilitation Utilization on Hospital Length of Stay in Patients Undergoing Elective Meningioma Resection. World Neurosurg 2016;93: 127–32.
18. Varela S, Garcia J, Kazim SF, et al. Letter: Association of Late Week Nonhome Discharge With Increased Length of Stay in Intracranial Meningioma Resection Patients. Neurosurgery 2022;90(6): e186–8.
19. Bateman BT, Pile-Spellman J, Gutin PH, et al. Meningioma resection in the elderly: nationwide inpatient

sample, 1998-2002. Neurosurgery 2005;57(5): 866–72.

20. Patil CG, Veeravagu A, Lad SP, et al. Craniotomy for resection of meningioma in the elderly: A multicentre, prospective analysis from the national surgical quality improvement program. J Neurol Neurosurg Psychiatry 2010;81(5):502–5.

21. Grossman R, Mukherjee D, Chang DC, et al. Preoperative Charlson comorbidity score predicts postoperative outcomes among older intracranial meningioma patients. World Neurosurg 2011;75(2): 279–85.

22. Poon MT-C, Fung LH-K, Pu JK-S, et al. Outcome comparison between younger and older patients undergoing intracranial meningioma resections. J Neuro Oncol 2013;114(2):219–27.

23. Connolly ID, Cole T, Veeravagu A, et al. Craniotomy for Resection of Meningioma: An Age-Stratified Analysis of the MarketScan Longitudinal Database. World Neurosurg 2015;84(6):1864–70.

24. Yamamoto J, Takahashi M, Idei M, et al. Clinical features and surgical management of intracranial meningiomas in the elderly. Oncol Lett 2017;14(1): 909–17.

25. Eksi MS, Canbolat C, Akbas A, et al. Elderly Patients with Intracranial Meningioma: Surgical Considerations in 228 Patients with a Comprehensive Analysis of the Literature. World Neurosurg 2019;132: e350–65.

26. Steinberger J, Bronheim RS, Vempati P, et al. Morbidity and Mortality of Meningioma Resection Increases in Octogenarians. World Neurosurg 2018; 109:e16–23.

27. Rafiq R, Katiyar V, Garg K, et al. Comparison of outcomes of surgery for intracranial meningioma in elderly and young patients – A systematic review and meta-analysis. Clin Neurol Neurosurg 2021; 207:106772.

28. Randhawa KS, Choi CB, Shah AD, et al. Impact of Diabetes Mellitus on Adverse Outcomes After Meningioma Surgery. World Neurosurg 2021;152:e429–35.

29. Dent E, Martin FC, Bergman H, et al. Management of frailty: opportunities, challenges, and future directions. Lancet 2019;394(10206):1376–86.

30. Dickinson H, Carico C, Nuno M, et al. The effect of weight in the outcomes of meningioma patients. Surg Neurol Int 2013;4:45.

31. Kolakshyapati M, Ikawa F, Abiko M, et al. Multivariate risk factor analysis and literature review of postoperative deterioration in Karnofsky Performance Scale score in elderly patients with skull base meningioma. Neurosurg Focus 2018;44(4):E14.

32. Khalafallah AM, Huq S, Jimenez AE, et al. The 5-factor modified frailty index: an effective predictor of mortality in brain tumor patients. J Neurosurg 2020;1–9.

33. Huq S, Khalafallah AM, Jimenez AE, et al. Predicting Postoperative Outcomes in Brain Tumor Patients With a 5-Factor Modified Frailty Index. Neurosurgery 2020;8(1):147–54.

34. Pazniokas J, Gandhi C, Theriault B, et al. The immense heterogeneity of frailty in neurosurgery: a systematic literature review. Neurosurg Rev 2021; 44(1):189–201.

35. McKee SP, Yang A, Gray M, et al. Intracranial Meningioma Surgery: Value-Based Care Determinants in New York State, 1995–2015. World Neurosurg 2018; 118:e731–44.

36. Theriault BC, Pazniokas J, Adkoli AS, et al. Frailty predicts worse outcomes after intracranial meningioma surgery irrespective of existing prognostic factors. Neurosurg Focus 2020;49(4):E16.

37. Cole KL, Kazim SF, Thommen R, et al. Association of baseline frailty status and age with outcomes in patients undergoing intracranial meningioma surgery: Results of a nationwide analysis of 5818 patients from the National Surgical Quality Improvement Program (NSQIP) 2015-2019. Eur J Surg Oncol 2022; 48(7):1671–7.

38. Dicpinigaitis AJ, Kalakoti P, Schmidt M, et al. Associations of Baseline Frailty Status and Age with Outcomes in Patients Undergoing Vestibular Schwannoma Resection. JAMA Otolaryngol - Head Neck Surg. 2021;147(7):608–14.

39. Dicpinigaitis AJ, Hanft S, Cooper JB, et al. Comparative associations of baseline frailty status and age with postoperative mortality and duration of hospital stay following metastatic brain tumor resection. Clin Exp Metastasis 2022;39(2):303–10.

40. Thommen R, Kazim SF, Cole KL, et al. Worse Pituitary Adenoma Surgical Outcomes Predicted by Increasing Frailty, Not Age. World Neurosurg 2022; 161:e347–54.

41. Dicpinigaitis AJ, Kazim SF, Schmidt MH, et al. Association of baseline frailty status and age with postoperative morbidity and mortality following intracranial meningioma resection. J Neuro Oncol 2021;155(1): 45–52.

42. Jackson HN, Hadley CC, Khan AB, et al. Racial and Socioeconomic Disparities in Patients With Meningioma: A Retrospective Cohort Study. Neurosurgery 2022;90(1):114–23.

43. Mukherjee D, Patil CG, Todnem N, et al. Racial disparities in medicaid patients after brain tumor surgery. J Clin Neurosci 2013;20(1):57–61.

44. Mukherjee D, Zaidi HA, Kosztowski T, et al. Disparities in access to neuro-oncologic care in the United States. Arch Surg 2010;145(3):247–53.

45. Curry WT, Carter BS, Barker FG. Racial, ethnic, and socioeconomic disparities in patient outcomes after craniotomy for tumor in adult patients in the United States, 1988-2004. Neurosurgery 2010;66(3): 427–37.

46. Bhambhvani HP, Rodrigues AJ, Medress ZA, et al. Racial and socioeconomic correlates of treatment

and survival among patients with meningioma: a population-based study. J Neuro Oncol 2020; 147(2):495–501.

47. Rathi P, Coleman S, Durbin-Johnson B, et al. Effect of day of the week of primary total hip arthroplasty on length of stay at a university-based teaching medical center. Am J Orthop 2014;43(12):E299–303.

48. Nielsen PR, Andreasen J, Asmussen M, et al. Costs and Quality of Life for Prehabilitation and Early Rehabilitation After Surgery of the Lumbar Spine. BMC Health Serv Res 2008;8:209.

49. Jimenez AE, Shah PP, Khalafallah AM, et al. Patient-Specific Factors Drive Intensive Care Unit and Total Hospital Length of Stay in Operative Patients with Brain Tumor. World Neurosurg 2021;153:e338–48.

50. Curry WT, McDermott MW, Carter BS, et al. Craniotomy for meningioma in the United States between 1988 and 2000: Decreasing rate of mortality and the effect of provider caseload. J Neurosurg 2005; 102(6):977–86.

51. Ambekar S, Sharma M, Madhugiri VS, et al. Trends in intracranial meningioma surgery and outcome: A Nationwide Inpatient Sample database analysis from 2001 to 2010. J Neuro Oncol 2013;114(3): 299–307.

52. Slot KM, Peters JVM, Vandertop WP, et al. Meningioma surgery in younger and older adults: patient profile and surgical outcomes. Eur Geriatr Med 2018;9(1):95–101.

53. Nuno M, Mukherjee D, Elramsisy A, et al. Racial and gender disparities and the role of primary tumor type on inpatient outcomes following craniotomy for brain metastases. Ann Surg Oncol 2012;19(8): 2657–63.

54. Benton JA, Ramos RDLG, Gelfand Y, et al. Prolonged length of stay and discharge disposition to rehabilitation facilities following single-level posterior lumbar interbody fusion for acquired spondylolisthesis. Surg Neurol Int 2020;11:411.

55. Elsamadicy AA, Freedman IG, Koo AB, et al. Influence of gender on discharge disposition after spinal fusion for adult spine deformity correction. Clin Neurol Neurosurg 2020;194:105875.

56. Konda SR, Gonzalez LJ, Johnson JR, et al. Marriage Status Predicts Hospital Outcomes Following Orthopedic Trauma. Geriatr Orthop Surg Rehabil 2020;11. 215145931989864.

57. Huq S, Khalafallah AM, Patel P, et al. Predictive Model and Online Calculator for Discharge Disposition in Brain Tumor Patients. World Neurosurg 2021; 146:e786–98.

58. Sughrue ME, Rutkowski MJ, Shangari G, et al. Results with judicious modern neurosurgical management of parasagittal and falcine meningiomas: Clinical article. J Neurosurg 2011;114(3):731–7.

59. Chen H, Lai R, Tang X, et al. Lateral Intraventricular Anaplastic Meningioma: A Series of 5 Patients at a Single Institution and Literature Review. World Neurosurg 2019;131:e1–11.

60. Jimenez A, Khalafallah A, Huq S, et al. Predictors of Nonroutine Discharge Disposition Among Parasagittal/Parafalcine Meningioma Patients. World Neurosurg 2020;142:e344–9.

61. Brandel MG, Rennert RC, Wali AR, et al. Impact of preoperative endovascular embolization on immediate meningioma resection outcomes. Neurosurg Focus 2018;44(4):1–7.

62. Muhlestein WE, Akagi DS, Kallos JA, et al. Using a Guided Machine Learning Ensemble Model to Predict Discharge Disposition following Meningioma Resection. J Neurol Surgery, Part B Skull Base 2018;79(2):123–30.

63. Muhlestein WE, Monsour MA, Friedman GN, et al. Predicting Discharge Disposition following Meningioma Resection Using a Multi-Institutional Natural Language Processing Model. Neurosurgery 2021; 88(4):838–45.

64. Moriates C, Arora V, Shah N. Understanding value-based healthcare. McGraw-Hill; 2015.

65. Arora V, Moriates C, Shah N. The Challenge of Understanding Health Care Costs and Charges. AMA J ethics 2015;17(11):1046–52.

66. Muhlestein WE, Akagi DS, McManus AR, et al. Machine learning ensemble models predict total charges and drivers of cost for transsphenoidal surgery for pituitary tumor. J Neurosurg 2019;131(2): 507–16.

67. Abou-Al-Shaar H, Azab MA, Karsy M, et al. Assessment of Costs in Open Microsurgery and Stereotactic Radiosurgery for Intracranial Meningiomas. World Neurosurg 2018;119:e357–65.

68. Reese JC, Twitchell S, Wilde H, et al. Analysis of Treatment Cost Variation Among Multiple Neurosurgical Procedures Using the Value-Driven Outcomes Database. World Neurosurg 2019;126:e914–20.

69. Zacharia BE, Deibert C, Gupta G, et al. Incidence, cost, and mortality associated with hospital-acquired conditions after resection of cranial neoplasms. Neurosurgery 2014;74(6):638–47.

70. Trinh VT, Davies JM, Berger MS. Surgery for primary supratentorial brain tumors in the United States, 2000-2009: effect of provider and hospital caseload on complication rates. J Neurosurg 2015;122(2):280–96.

71. Ramakrishna R, Hsu W-C, Mao J, et al. Surgeon Annual and Cumulative Volumes Predict Early Postoperative Outcomes After Brain Tumor Resection. World Neurosurg 2018;114:e254–66.

72. Cannizzaro D, Tropeano MP, Zaed I, et al. Intracranial Meningiomas in the Elderly: Clinical, Surgical and Economic Evaluation. A Multicentric Experience. Cancers 2020;12(9).

73. Nguyen AV, Coggins WS, Jain RR, et al. Effect of an additional neurosurgical resident on procedure length, operating room time, estimated blood loss,

and post-operative length-of-stay. Br J Neurosurg 2020;34(6):611–5.

74. Hollon TC, Pandian B, Adapa AR, et al. Near real-time intraoperative brain tumor diagnosis using stimulated Raman histology and deep neural networks. Nat Med 2020;26(1):52–8.

75. Djirackor L, Halldorsson S, Niehusmann P, et al. Intraoperative DNA methylation classification of brain tumors impacts neurosurgical strategy. Neuro-oncology Adv. 2021;3(1):vdab149.

76. De la Garza-Ramos R, Kerezoudis P, Tamargo RJ, et al. Surgical complications following malignant brain tumor surgery: An analysis of 2002-2011 data. Clin Neurol Neurosurg 2016;140:6–10.

77. Guan J, Karsy M, Bisson EF, et al. Patient-level factors influencing hospital costs and short-term patient-reported outcomes after transsphenoidal resection of sellar tumors. Neurosurgery 2018; 83(4):726–31.

78. Patel S, Chiu RG, Rosinski CL, et al. Risk Factors for Hyponatremia and Perioperative Complications With Malignant Intracranial Tumor Resection in Adults: An Analysis of the Nationwide Inpatient Sample from 2012 to 2015. World Neurosurg 2020;144:e876–82.

79. Jin MC, Parker JJ, Zhang M, et al. Status epilepticus after intracranial neurosurgery: incidence and risk stratification by perioperative clinical features. J Neurosurg 2021;1–13.

80. Hauser BM, Gupta S, Xu E, et al. Impact of insurance on hospital course and readmission after resection of benign meningioma. J Neuro Oncol 2020;149(1):131–40.

81. Lin M, Min E, Orloff EA, et al. Predictors of readmission after craniotomy for meningioma resection: a nationwide readmission database analysis. Acta Neurochir 2020;162(11):2637–46.

82. El-Sayed AM, Ziewacz JE, Davis MC, et al. Insurance status and inequalities in outcomes after neurosurgery. World Neurosurg 2011;76(5):459–66.

83. Kim H, McConnell KJ, Sun BC. Comparing Emergency Department Use Among Medicaid and Commercial Patients Using All-Payer All-Claims Data. Popul Health Manag 2017;20(4):271–7.

84. Gao W, Keleti D, Donia TP, et al. Postdischarge engagement decreased hospital readmissions in Medicaid populations. Am J Manag Care 2018; 24(7):e200–6.

85. Wiest D, Yang Q, Wilson C, et al. Outcomes of a City-wide Campaign to Reduce Medicaid Hospital Readmissions With Connection to Primary Care Within 7 Days of Hospital Discharge. JAMA Netw Open 2019;2(1):e187369.

86. Meuter RFI, Gallois C, Segalowitz NS, et al. Overcoming language barriers in healthcare: A protocol for investigating safe and effective communication when patients or clinicians use a second language. BMC Health Serv Res 2015;15:371.

87. Nayeri A, Brinson PR, Weaver KD, et al. Factors Associated with Low Socioeconomic Status Predict Poor Postoperative Follow-up after Meningioma Resection. J Neurol Surgery, Part B Skull Base 2016;77(3):226–30.

88. Timmins CL. The impact of language barriers on the health care of Latinos in the United States: a review of the literature and guidelines for practice. J Midwifery Wom Health 2002;47(2):80–96.

89. Rodriguez-Artalejo F, Guallar-Castillon P, Herrera MC, et al. Social Network as a Predictor of Hospital Readmission and Mortality Among Older Patients With Heart Failure. J Card Fail 2006;12(8):621–7.

90. Pedersen MK, Mark E, Uhrenfeldt L. Hospital readmission: Older married male patients' experiences of life conditions and critical incidents affecting the course of care, a qualitative study. Scand J Caring Sci 2018;32(4):1379–89.

91. Howard SD, Kvint S, Borja AJ, et al. Matched analysis of patient gender and meningioma resection outcomes. Br J Neurosurg 2022;1–7.

92. Aghi MK, Eskandar EN, Carter BS, et al. Increased prevalence of obesity and obesity-related postoperative complications in male patients with meningiomas. Neurosurgery 2007;61(4):751–4.

93. Florman JE, Cushing D, Keller LA, et al. A protocol for postoperative admission of elective craniotomy patients to a non-ICU or step-down setting. J Neurosurg 2017;127(6):1392–7.

94. de Almeida CC, Boone MD, Laviv Y, et al. The Utility of Routine Intensive Care Admission for Patients Undergoing Intracranial Neurosurgical Procedures: A Systematic Review. Neurocrit Care 2018;28(1):35–42.

95. Osorio JA, Safaee MM, Viner J, et al. Cost-effectiveness development for the postoperative care of craniotomy patients: A safe transitions pathway in neurological surgery. Neurosurg Focus 2018;44(5):1–5.

96. Young JS, Chan AK, Viner JA, et al. A Safe Transitions Pathway for post-craniotomy neurological surgery patients: high-value care that bypasses the intensive care unit. J Neurosurg 2020;134(5):1386–91.

97. Fornacon-Wood I, Mistry H, Johnson-Hart C, et al. Understanding the Differences Between Bayesian and Frequentist Statistics. Int J Radiat Oncol Biol Phys 2022;112(5):1076–82.

98. Angevine PD, Bray D, Cloney M, et al. Uncertainty in the relationship between sagittal alignment and patient-reported outcomes. Neurosurgery 2020; 86(4):485–91.

Printed and bound by CPI Group (UK) Ltd, Croydon, CR0 4YY

08/05/2025

01864715-0017